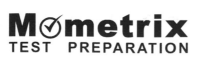

FREE Study Skills Videos/DVD Offer

Dear Customer,

Thank you for your purchase from Mometrix! We consider it an honor and a privilege that you have purchased our product and we want to ensure your satisfaction.

As part of our ongoing effort to meet the needs of test takers, we have developed a set of Study Skills Videos that we would like to give you for <u>FREE</u>. These videos cover our *best practices* for getting ready for your exam, from how to use our study materials to how to best prepare for the day of the test.

All that we ask is that you email us with feedback that would describe your experience so far with our product. Good, bad, or indifferent, we want to know what you think!

To get your FREE Study Skills Videos, you can use the **QR code** below, or send us an **email** at <u>studyvideos@mometrix.com</u> with *FREE VIDEOS* in the subject line and the following information in the body of the email:

- The name of the product you purchased.
- Your product rating on a scale of 1-5, with 5 being the highest rating.
- Your feedback. It can be long, short, or anything in between. We just want to know your impressions and experience so far with our product. (Good feedback might include how our study material met your needs and ways we might be able to make it even better. You could highlight features that you found helpful or features that you think we should add.)

If you have any questions or concerns, please don't hesitate to contact me directly.

Thanks again!

Sincerely,

Jay Willis
Vice President
<u>jay.willis@mometrix.com</u>
1-800-673-8175

Mometrix
TEST PREPARATION

Mometrix
TEST PREPARATION

PTCB
Exam Study Guide 2022-2023

3 Full-Length Practice Tests

Pharmacy Technician Certification Secrets Review Book

4th Edition

Written and edited by Mometrix Test Prep

Printed in the United States of America

This paper meets the requirements of ANSI/NISO Z39.48-1992 (Permanence of Paper).

Mometrix offers volume discount pricing to institutions. For more information or a price quote, please contact our sales department at sales@mometrix.com or 888-248-1219.

Mometrix Media LLC is not affiliated with or endorsed by any official testing organization. All organizational and test names are trademarks of their respective owners.

Paperback
ISBN 13: 978-1-5167-2058-3
ISBN 10: 1-5167-2058-X

DEAR FUTURE EXAM SUCCESS STORY

First of all, **THANK YOU** for purchasing Mometrix study materials!

Second, congratulations! You are one of the few determined test-takers who are committed to doing whatever it takes to excel on your exam. **You have come to the right place.** We developed these study materials with one goal in mind: to deliver you the information you need in a format that's concise and easy to use.

In addition to optimizing your guide for the content of the test, we've outlined our recommended steps for breaking down the preparation process into small, attainable goals so you can make sure you stay on track.

We've also analyzed the entire test-taking process, identifying the most common pitfalls and showing how you can overcome them and be ready for any curveball the test throws you.

Standardized testing is one of the biggest obstacles on your road to success, which only increases the importance of doing well in the high-pressure, high-stakes environment of test day. Your results on this test could have a significant impact on your future, and this guide provides the information and practical advice to help you achieve your full potential on test day.

Your success is our success

We would love to hear from you! If you would like to share the story of your exam success or if you have any questions or comments in regard to our products, please contact us at **800-673-8175** or **support@mometrix.com**.

Thanks again for your business and we wish you continued success!

Sincerely,
The Mometrix Test Preparation Team

> **Need more help? Check out our flashcards at:**
> **http://mometrixflashcards.com/PTCB**

TABLE OF CONTENTS

Introduction

Thank you for purchasing this resource! You have made the choice to prepare yourself for a test that could have a huge impact on your future, and this guide is designed to help you be fully ready for test day. Obviously, it's important to have a solid understanding of the test material, but you also need to be prepared for the unique environment and stressors of the test, so that you can perform to the best of your abilities.

For this purpose, the first section that appears in this guide is the **Secret Keys**. We've devoted countless hours to meticulously researching what works and what doesn't, and we've boiled down our findings to the five most impactful steps you can take to improve your performance on the test. We start at the beginning with study planning and move through the preparation process, all the way to the testing strategies that will help you get the most out of what you know when you're finally sitting in front of the test.

We recommend that you start preparing for your test as far in advance as possible. However, if you've bought this guide as a last-minute study resource and only have a few days before your test, we recommend that you skip over the first two Secret Keys since they address a long-term study plan.

If you struggle with **test anxiety**, we strongly encourage you to check out our recommendations for how you can overcome it. Test anxiety is a formidable foe, but it can be beaten, and we want to make sure you have the tools you need to defeat it.

Secret Key #1 – Plan Big, Study Small

There's a lot riding on your performance. If you want to ace this test, you're going to need to keep your skills sharp and the material fresh in your mind. You need a plan that lets you review everything you need to know while still fitting in your schedule. We'll break this strategy down into three categories.

Information Organization

Start with the information you already have: the official test outline. From this, you can make a complete list of all the concepts you need to cover before the test. Organize these concepts into groups that can be studied together, and create a list of any related vocabulary you need to learn so you can brush up on any difficult terms. You'll want to keep this vocabulary list handy once you actually start studying since you may need to add to it along the way.

Time Management

Once you have your set of study concepts, decide how to spread them out over the time you have left before the test. Break your study plan into small, clear goals so you have a manageable task for each day and know exactly what you're doing. Then just focus on one small step at a time. When you manage your time this way, you don't need to spend hours at a time studying. Studying a small block of content for a short period each day helps you retain information better and avoid stressing over how much you have left to do. You can relax knowing that you have a plan to cover everything in time. In order for this strategy to be effective though, you have to start studying early and stick to your schedule. Avoid the exhaustion and futility that comes from last-minute cramming!

Study Environment

The environment you study in has a big impact on your learning. Studying in a coffee shop, while probably more enjoyable, is not likely to be as fruitful as studying in a quiet room. It's important to keep distractions to a minimum. You're only planning to study for a short block of time, so make the most of it. Don't pause to check your phone or get up to find a snack. It's also important to **avoid multitasking**. Research has consistently shown that multitasking will make your studying dramatically less effective. Your study area should also be comfortable and well-lit so you don't have the distraction of straining your eyes or sitting on an uncomfortable chair.

 The time of day you study is also important. You want to be rested and alert. Don't wait until just before bedtime. Study when you'll be most likely to comprehend and remember. Even better, if you know what time of day your test will be, set that time aside for study. That way your brain will be used to working on that subject at that specific time and you'll have a better chance of recalling information.

Finally, it can be helpful to team up with others who are studying for the same test. Your actual studying should be done in as isolated an environment as possible, but the work of organizing the information and setting up the study plan can be divided up. In between study sessions, you can discuss with your teammates the concepts that you're all studying and quiz each other on the details. Just be sure that your teammates are as serious about the test as you are. If you find that your study time is being replaced with social time, you might need to find a new team.

Secret Key #2 – Make Your Studying Count

You're devoting a lot of time and effort to preparing for this test, so you want to be absolutely certain it will pay off. This means doing more than just reading the content and hoping you can remember it on test day. It's important to make every minute of study count. There are two main areas you can focus on to make your studying count.

Retention

It doesn't matter how much time you study if you can't remember the material. You need to make sure you are retaining the concepts. To check your retention of the information you're learning, try recalling it at later times with minimal prompting. Try carrying around flashcards and glance at one or two from time to time or ask a friend who's also studying for the test to quiz you.

To enhance your retention, look for ways to put the information into practice so that you can apply it rather than simply recalling it. If you're using the information in practical ways, it will be much easier to remember. Similarly, it helps to solidify a concept in your mind if you're not only reading it to yourself but also explaining it to someone else. Ask a friend to let you teach them about a concept you're a little shaky on (or speak aloud to an imaginary audience if necessary). As you try to summarize, define, give examples, and answer your friend's questions, you'll understand the concepts better and they will stay with you longer. Finally, step back for a big picture view and ask yourself how each piece of information fits with the whole subject. When you link the different concepts together and see them working together as a whole, it's easier to remember the individual components.

Finally, practice showing your work on any multi-step problems, even if you're just studying. Writing out each step you take to solve a problem will help solidify the process in your mind, and you'll be more likely to remember it during the test.

Modality

Modality simply refers to the means or method by which you study. Choosing a study modality that fits your own individual learning style is crucial. No two people learn best in exactly the same way, so it's important to know your strengths and use them to your advantage.

For example, if you learn best by visualization, focus on visualizing a concept in your mind and draw an image or a diagram. Try color-coding your notes, illustrating them, or creating symbols that will trigger your mind to recall a learned concept. If you learn best by hearing or discussing information, find a study partner who learns the same way or read aloud to yourself. Think about how to put the information in your own words. Imagine that you are giving a lecture on the topic and record yourself so you can listen to it later.

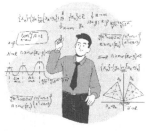

For any learning style, flashcards can be helpful. Organize the information so you can take advantage of spare moments to review. Underline key words or phrases. Use different colors for different categories. Mnemonic devices (such as creating a short list in which every item starts with the same letter) can also help with retention. Find what works best for you and use it to store the information in your mind most effectively and easily.

3

Secret Key #3 – Practice the Right Way

Your success on test day depends not only on how many hours you put into preparing, but also on whether you prepared the right way. It's good to check along the way to see if your studying is paying off. One of the most effective ways to do this is by taking practice tests to evaluate your progress. Practice tests are useful because they show exactly where you need to improve. Every time you take a practice test, pay special attention to these three groups of questions:

- The questions you got wrong
- The questions you had to guess on, even if you guessed right
- The questions you found difficult or slow to work through

This will show you exactly what your weak areas are, and where you need to devote more study time. Ask yourself why each of these questions gave you trouble. Was it because you didn't understand the material? Was it because you didn't remember the vocabulary? Do you need more repetitions on this type of question to build speed and confidence? Dig into those questions and figure out how you can strengthen your weak areas as you go back to review the material.

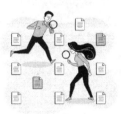 Additionally, many practice tests have a section explaining the answer choices. It can be tempting to read the explanation and think that you now have a good understanding of the concept. However, an explanation likely only covers part of the question's broader context. Even if the explanation makes perfect sense, **go back and investigate** every concept related to the question until you're positive you have a thorough understanding.

As you go along, keep in mind that the practice test is just that: practice. Memorizing these questions and answers will not be very helpful on the actual test because it is unlikely to have any of the same exact questions. If you only know the right answers to the sample questions, you won't be prepared for the real thing. **Study the concepts** until you understand them fully, and then you'll be able to answer any question that shows up on the test.

It's important to wait on the practice tests until you're ready. If you take a test on your first day of study, you may be overwhelmed by the amount of material covered and how much you need to learn. Work up to it gradually.

On test day, you'll need to be prepared for answering questions, managing your time, and using the test-taking strategies you've learned. It's a lot to balance, like a mental marathon that will have a big impact on your future. Like training for a marathon, you'll need to start slowly and work your way up. When test day arrives, you'll be ready.

Start with the strategies you've read in the first two Secret Keys—plan your course and study in the way that works best for you. If you have time, consider using multiple study resources to get different approaches to the same concepts. It can be helpful to see difficult concepts from more than one angle. Then find a good source for practice tests. Many times, the test website will suggest potential study resources or provide sample tests.

Practice Test Strategy

If you're able to find at least three practice tests, we recommend this strategy:

UNTIMED AND OPEN-BOOK PRACTICE

Take the first test with no time constraints and with your notes and study guide handy. Take your time and focus on applying the strategies you've learned.

TIMED AND OPEN-BOOK PRACTICE

Take the second practice test open-book as well, but set a timer and practice pacing yourself to finish in time.

TIMED AND CLOSED-BOOK PRACTICE

Take any other practice tests as if it were test day. Set a timer and put away your study materials. Sit at a table or desk in a quiet room, imagine yourself at the testing center, and answer questions as quickly and accurately as possible.

Keep repeating timed and closed-book tests on a regular basis until you run out of practice tests or it's time for the actual test. Your mind will be ready for the schedule and stress of test day, and you'll be able to focus on recalling the material you've learned.

Secret Key #4 – Pace Yourself

Once you're fully prepared for the material on the test, your biggest challenge on test day will be managing your time. Just knowing that the clock is ticking can make you panic even if you have plenty of time left. Work on pacing yourself so you can build confidence against the time constraints of the exam. Pacing is a difficult skill to master, especially in a high-pressure environment, so **practice is vital**.

Set time expectations for your pace based on how much time is available. For example, if a section has 60 questions and the time limit is 30 minutes, you know you have to average 30 seconds or less per question in order to answer them all. Although 30 seconds is the hard limit, set 25 seconds per question as your goal, so you reserve extra time to spend on harder questions. When you budget extra time for the harder questions, you no longer have any reason to stress when those questions take longer to answer.

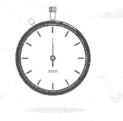

Don't let this time expectation distract you from working through the test at a calm, steady pace, but keep it in mind so you don't spend too much time on any one question. Recognize that taking extra time on one question you don't understand may keep you from answering two that you do understand later in the test. If your time limit for a question is up and you're still not sure of the answer, mark it and move on, and come back to it later if the time and the test format allow. If the testing format doesn't allow you to return to earlier questions, just make an educated guess; then put it out of your mind and move on.

On the easier questions, be careful not to rush. It may seem wise to hurry through them so you have more time for the challenging ones, but it's not worth missing one if you know the concept and just didn't take the time to read the question fully. Work efficiently but make sure you understand the question and have looked at all of the answer choices, since more than one may seem right at first.

Even if you're paying attention to the time, you may find yourself a little behind at some point. You should speed up to get back on track, but do so wisely. Don't panic; just take a few seconds less on each question until you're caught up. Don't guess without thinking, but do look through the answer choices and eliminate any you know are wrong. If you can get down to two choices, it is often worthwhile to guess from those. Once you've chosen an answer, move on and don't dwell on any that you skipped or had to hurry through. If a question was taking too long, chances are it was one of the harder ones, so you weren't as likely to get it right anyway.

On the other hand, if you find yourself getting ahead of schedule, it may be beneficial to slow down a little. The more quickly you work, the more likely you are to make a careless mistake that will affect your score. You've budgeted time for each question, so don't be afraid to spend that time. Practice an efficient but careful pace to get the most out of the time you have.

Secret Key #5 – Have a Plan for Guessing

When you're taking the test, you may find yourself stuck on a question. Some of the answer choices seem better than others, but you don't see the one answer choice that is obviously correct. What do you do?

The scenario described above is very common, yet most test takers have not effectively prepared for it. Developing and practicing a plan for guessing may be one of the single most effective uses of your time as you get ready for the exam.

In developing your plan for guessing, there are three questions to address:

- When should you start the guessing process?
- How should you narrow down the choices?
- Which answer should you choose?

When to Start the Guessing Process

Unless your plan for guessing is to select C every time (which, despite its merits, is not what we recommend), you need to leave yourself enough time to apply your answer elimination strategies. Since you have a limited amount of time for each question, that means that if you're going to give yourself the best shot at guessing correctly, you have to decide quickly whether or not you will guess.

Of course, the best-case scenario is that you don't have to guess at all, so first, see if you can answer the question based on your knowledge of the subject and basic reasoning skills. Focus on the key words in the question and try to jog your memory of related topics. Give yourself a chance to bring the knowledge to mind, but once you realize that you don't have (or you can't access) the knowledge you need to answer the question, it's time to start the guessing process.

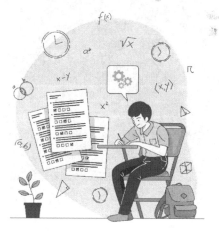

It's almost always better to start the guessing process too early than too late. It only takes a few seconds to remember something and answer the question from knowledge. Carefully eliminating wrong answer choices takes longer. Plus, going through the process of eliminating answer choices can actually help jog your memory.

Summary: Start the guessing process as soon as you decide that you can't answer the question based on your knowledge.

How to Narrow Down the Choices

The next chapter in this book (**Test-Taking Strategies**) includes a wide range of strategies for how to approach questions and how to look for answer choices to eliminate. You will definitely want to read those carefully, practice them, and figure out which ones work best for you. Here though, we're going to address a mindset rather than a particular strategy.

Your odds of guessing an answer correctly depend on how many options you are choosing from.

Number of options left	5	4	3	2	1
Odds of guessing correctly	20%	25%	33%	50%	100%

You can see from this chart just how valuable it is to be able to eliminate incorrect answers and make an educated guess, but there are two things that many test takers do that cause them to miss out on the benefits of guessing:

- Accidentally eliminating the correct answer
- Selecting an answer based on an impression

We'll look at the first one here, and the second one in the next section.

To avoid accidentally eliminating the correct answer, we recommend a thought exercise called **the $5 challenge**. In this challenge, you only eliminate an answer choice from contention if you are willing to bet $5 on it being wrong. Why $5? Five dollars is a small but not insignificant amount of money. It's an amount you could afford to lose but wouldn't want to throw away. And while losing

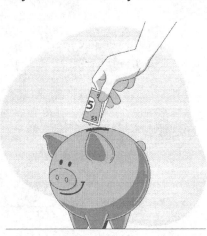

$5 once might not hurt too much, doing it twenty times will set you back $100. In the same way, each small decision you make—eliminating a choice here, guessing on a question there—won't by itself impact your score very much, but when you put them all together, they can make a big difference. By holding each answer choice elimination decision to a higher standard, you can reduce the risk of accidentally eliminating the correct answer.

The $5 challenge can also be applied in a positive sense: If you are willing to bet $5 that an answer choice *is* correct, go ahead and mark it as correct.

Summary: Only eliminate an answer choice if you are willing to bet $5 that it is wrong.

8

Which Answer to Choose

You're taking the test. You've run into a hard question and decided you'll have to guess. You've eliminated all the answer choices you're willing to bet $5 on. Now you have to pick an answer. Why do we even need to talk about this? Why can't you just pick whichever one you feel like when the time comes?

The answer to these questions is that if you don't come into the test with a plan, you'll rely on your impression to select an answer choice, and if you do that, you risk falling into a trap. The test writers know that everyone who takes their test will be guessing on some of the questions, so they intentionally write wrong answer choices to seem plausible. You still have to pick an answer though, and if the wrong answer choices are designed to look right, how can you ever be sure that you're not falling for their trap? The best solution we've found to this dilemma is to take the decision out of your hands entirely. Here is the process we recommend:

Once you've eliminated any choices that you are confident (willing to bet $5) are wrong, select the first remaining choice as your answer.

Whether you choose to select the first remaining choice, the second, or the last, the important thing is that you use some preselected standard. Using this approach guarantees that you will not be enticed into selecting an answer choice that looks right, because you are not basing your decision on how the answer choices look.

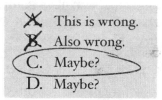

This is not meant to make you question your knowledge. Instead, it is to help you recognize the difference between your knowledge and your impressions. There's a huge difference between thinking an answer is right because of what you know, and thinking an answer is right because it looks or sounds like it should be right.

Summary: To ensure that your selection is appropriately random, make a predetermined selection from among all answer choices you have not eliminated.

Test-Taking Strategies

This section contains a list of test-taking strategies that you may find helpful as you work through the test. By taking what you know and applying logical thought, you can maximize your chances of answering any question correctly!

It is very important to realize that every question is different and every person is different: no single strategy will work on every question, and no single strategy will work for every person. That's why we've included all of them here, so you can try them out and determine which ones work best for different types of questions and which ones work best for you.

Question Strategies

⊘ READ CAREFULLY

Read the question and the answer choices carefully. Don't miss the question because you misread the terms. You have plenty of time to read each question thoroughly and make sure you understand what is being asked. Yet a happy medium must be attained, so don't waste too much time. You must read carefully and efficiently.

⊘ CONTEXTUAL CLUES

Look for contextual clues. If the question includes a word you are not familiar with, look at the immediate context for some indication of what the word might mean. Contextual clues can often give you all the information you need to decipher the meaning of an unfamiliar word. Even if you can't determine the meaning, you may be able to narrow down the possibilities enough to make a solid guess at the answer to the question.

⊘ PREFIXES

If you're having trouble with a word in the question or answer choices, try dissecting it. Take advantage of every clue that the word might include. Prefixes can be a huge help. Usually, they allow you to determine a basic meaning. *Pre-* means before, *post-* means after, *pro-* is positive, *de-* is negative. From prefixes, you can get an idea of the general meaning of the word and try to put it into context.

⊘ HEDGE WORDS

Watch out for critical hedge words, such as *likely, may, can, sometimes, often, almost, mostly, usually, generally, rarely,* and *sometimes*. Question writers insert these hedge phrases to cover every possibility. Often an answer choice will be wrong simply because it leaves no room for exception. Be on guard for answer choices that have definitive words such as *exactly* and *always*.

⊘ SWITCHBACK WORDS

Stay alert for *switchbacks*. These are the words and phrases frequently used to alert you to shifts in thought. The most common switchback words are *but, although,* and *however*. Others include *nevertheless, on the other hand, even though, while, in spite of, despite,* and *regardless of*. Switchback words are important to catch because they can change the direction of the question or an answer choice.

⊘ FACE VALUE

When in doubt, use common sense. Accept the situation in the problem at face value. Don't read too much into it. These problems will not require you to make wild assumptions. If you have to go beyond creativity and warp time or space in order to have an answer choice fit the question, then you should move on and consider the other answer choices. These are normal problems rooted in reality. The applicable relationship or explanation may not be readily apparent, but it is there for you to figure out. Use your common sense to interpret anything that isn't clear.

Answer Choice Strategies

⊘ ANSWER SELECTION

The most thorough way to pick an answer choice is to identify and eliminate wrong answers until only one is left, then confirm it is the correct answer. Sometimes an answer choice may immediately seem right, but be careful. The test writers will usually put more than one reasonable answer choice on each question, so take a second to read all of them and make sure that the other choices are not equally obvious. As long as you have time left, it is better to read every answer choice than to pick the first one that looks right without checking the others.

⊘ ANSWER CHOICE FAMILIES

An answer choice family consists of two (in rare cases, three) answer choices that are very similar in construction and cannot all be true at the same time. If you see two answer choices that are direct opposites or parallels, one of them is usually the correct answer. For instance, if one answer choice says that quantity x increases and another either says that quantity x decreases (opposite) or says that quantity y increases (parallel), then those answer choices would fall into the same family. An answer choice that doesn't match the construction of the answer choice family is more likely to be incorrect. Most questions will not have answer choice families, but when they do appear, you should be prepared to recognize them.

⊘ ELIMINATE ANSWERS

Eliminate answer choices as soon as you realize they are wrong, but make sure you consider all possibilities. If you are eliminating answer choices and realize that the last one you are left with is also wrong, don't panic. Start over and consider each choice again. There may be something you missed the first time that you will realize on the second pass.

⊘ AVOID FACT TRAPS

Don't be distracted by an answer choice that is factually true but doesn't answer the question. You are looking for the choice that answers the question. Stay focused on what the question is asking for so you don't accidentally pick an answer that is true but incorrect. Always go back to the question and make sure the answer choice you've selected actually answers the question and is not merely a true statement.

⊘ EXTREME STATEMENTS

In general, you should avoid answers that put forth extreme actions as standard practice or proclaim controversial ideas as established fact. An answer choice that states the "process should be used in certain situations, if..." is much more likely to be correct than one that states the "process should be discontinued completely." The first is a calm rational statement and doesn't even make a definitive, uncompromising stance, using a hedge word *if* to provide wiggle room, whereas the second choice is far more extreme.

⊘ BENCHMARK

As you read through the answer choices and you come across one that seems to answer the question well, mentally select that answer choice. This is not your final answer, but it's the one that will help you evaluate the other answer choices. The one that you selected is your benchmark or standard for judging each of the other answer choices. Every other answer choice must be compared to your benchmark. That choice is correct until proven otherwise by another answer choice beating it. If you find a better answer, then that one becomes your new benchmark. Once you've decided that no other choice answers the question as well as your benchmark, you have your final answer.

⊘ PREDICT THE ANSWER

Before you even start looking at the answer choices, it is often best to try to predict the answer. When you come up with the answer on your own, it is easier to avoid distractions and traps because you will know exactly what to look for. The right answer choice is unlikely to be word-for-word what you came up with, but it should be a close match. Even if you are confident that you have the right answer, you should still take the time to read each option before moving on.

General Strategies

⊘ TOUGH QUESTIONS

If you are stumped on a problem or it appears too hard or too difficult, don't waste time. Move on! Remember though, if you can quickly check for obviously incorrect answer choices, your chances of guessing correctly are greatly improved. Before you completely give up, at least try to knock out a couple of possible answers. Eliminate what you can and then guess at the remaining answer choices before moving on.

⊘ CHECK YOUR WORK

Since you will probably not know every term listed and the answer to every question, it is important that you get credit for the ones that you do know. Don't miss any questions through careless mistakes. If at all possible, try to take a second to look back over your answer selection and make sure you've selected the correct answer choice and haven't made a costly careless mistake (such as marking an answer choice that you didn't mean to mark). This quick double check should more than pay for itself in caught mistakes for the time it costs.

⊘ PACE YOURSELF

It's easy to be overwhelmed when you're looking at a page full of questions; your mind is confused and full of random thoughts, and the clock is ticking down faster than you would like. Calm down and maintain the pace that you have set for yourself. Especially as you get down to the last few minutes of the test, don't let the small numbers on the clock make you panic. As long as you are on track by monitoring your pace, you are guaranteed to have time for each question.

⊘ DON'T RUSH

It is very easy to make errors when you are in a hurry. Maintaining a fast pace in answering questions is pointless if it makes you miss questions that you would have gotten right otherwise. Test writers like to include distracting information and wrong answers that seem right. Taking a little extra time to avoid careless mistakes can make all the difference in your test score. Find a pace that allows you to be confident in the answers that you select.

12

⊘ KEEP MOVING

Panicking will not help you pass the test, so do your best to stay calm and keep moving. Taking deep breaths and going through the answer elimination steps you practiced can help to break through a stress barrier and keep your pace.

Final Notes

The combination of a solid foundation of content knowledge and the confidence that comes from practicing your plan for applying that knowledge is the key to maximizing your performance on test day. As your foundation of content knowledge is built up and strengthened, you'll find that the strategies included in this chapter become more and more effective in helping you quickly sift through the distractions and traps of the test to isolate the correct answer.

Now that you're preparing to move forward into the test content chapters of this book, be sure to keep your goal in mind. As you read, think about how you will be able to apply this information on the test. If you've already seen sample questions for the test and you have an idea of the question format and style, try to come up with questions of your own that you can answer based on what you're reading. This will give you valuable practice applying your knowledge in the same ways you can expect to on test day.

Good luck and good studying!

Four-Week PTCB Study Plan

On the next few pages, we've provided an optional study plan to help you use this study guide to its fullest potential over the course of four weeks. If you have eight weeks available and want to spread it out more, spend two weeks on each section of the plan.

Below is a quick summary of the subjects covered in each week of the plan.

- Week 1: Abbreviations and Terminology & Medications
- Week 2: Federal Requirements, Patient Safety and Quality Assurance, Order Entry and Processing
- Week 3: State Requirements and Practice Standards, Inventory Management, Administrative and Management, Health and Wellness, Billing and Reimbursement
- Week 4: Practice Tests

Please note that not all subjects will take the same amount of time to work through.

Three full-length practice tests are included in this study guide. We recommend saving the third test and any additional tests for after you've completed the study plan. Take these practice tests without any reference materials a day or two before the real thing as practice runs to get you in the mode of answering questions at a good pace.

Week 1: Abbreviations and Terminology & Medications

INSTRUCTIONAL CONTENT

First, read carefully through the Abbreviations and Terminology & Medications chapters in this book, checking off your progress as you go:

- ❏ Medical Root Words
- ❏ Medical Suffixes
- ❏ Medical Prefixes
- ❏ Medical Terms
- ❏ Abbreviations Used in the Pharmacy
- ❏ Generic Names, Brand Names, and Classifications of Medications
- ❏ Therapeutic Equivalence
- ❏ Common and Life-Threatening Drug Interactions and Contraindications
- ❏ Dosage Forms and Routes of Administration
- ❏ Common and Severe Medication Side Effects, Adverse Effects, and Allergies
- ❏ Indications of Medications and Dietary Supplements
- ❏ Drug Stability
- ❏ Narrow-Therapeutic-Index-Medications
- ❏ Incompatibilities Related to Nonsterile Compounding and Reconstitution
- ❏ Proper Storage of Medications

As you read, do the following:

- Highlight any sections, terms, or concepts you think are important
- Draw an asterisk (*) next to any areas you are struggling with
- Watch the review videos to gain more understanding of a particular topic
- Take notes in your notebook or in the margins of this book

After you've read through everything, go back and review any sections that you highlighted or that you drew an asterisk next to, referencing your notes along the way.

Week 2: Federal Requirements, Patient Safety and Quality Assurance, Order Entry and Processing

INSTRUCTIONAL CONTENT

First, read carefully through the Federal Requirements, Patient Safety and Quality Assurance, and Order Entry and Processing chapters in this book, checking off your progress as you go:

- ❏ Handling and Disposal of Pharmaceutical Substances and Waste
- ❏ Controlled Substance Prescriptions and DEA Controlled Substance Schedules
- ❏ Substances
- ❏ Restricted Drug Programs and Related Medication Processing
- ❏ FDA Requirements
- ❏ High Alert/High Risk and LASA Medications
- ❏ Error-Prevention Strategies
- ❏ Issues That Require Pharmacist Intervention
- ❏ Event Reporting Procedures
- ❏ Types of Prescription Errors
- ❏ Hygiene and Cleaning Standards
- ❏ Procedures to Compound Nonsterile Products
- ❏ Formulas and Calculations
- ❏ Equipment/Supplies Required for Drug Administration
- ❏ Lot Numbers, Expiration Dates, and NDC Numbers
- ❏ Procedures for Identifying and Returning Medications and Supplies

As you read, do the following:

- Highlight any sections, terms, or concepts you think are important
- Draw an asterisk (*) next to any areas you are struggling with
- Watch the review videos to gain more understanding of a particular topic
- Take notes in your notebook or in the margins of this book

After you've read through everything, go back and review any sections that you highlighted or that you drew an asterisk next to, referencing your notes along the way.

16

Week 3: State Requirements and Practice Standards, Inventory Management, Administrative and Management, Health and Wellness, Billing and Reimbursement

INSTRUCTIONAL CONTENT

First, read carefully through the State Requirements and Practice Standards, Inventory Management, Administrative and Management, Health and Wellness, and Billing and Reimbursement chapters in this book, checking off your progress as you go:

- ❏ Licensure, Registration, and/or Certification of Pharmacy Technicians
- ❏ Roles and Responsibilities of Pharmacy Employees
- ❏ Facilities, Equipment, and Supply
- ❏ Procedures to Address Improperly Stored Inventory
- ❏ Automated Equipment Inventory Management
- ❏ Formulary or Approved/Preferred Product List
- ❏ Suitable Alternatives for Ordering
- ❏ Medication Quality Control System Requirements
- ❏ Inventory Control Practices and Record Keeping
- ❏ Procedures to Perform Physical Inventory
- ❏ Administrative and Management
- ❏ Factors That Can Influence Effects of Medications
- ❏ Devices Commonly Dispense by Pharmacies
- ❏ Compliance and the Medication Adherence Ratio
- ❏ Characteristics of Reimbursement Policies and Plans
- ❏ Strategies to Resolve Third-Party Rejected Claims
- ❏ Reimbursement Models
- ❏ Procedures to Coordinate Benefits
- ❏ Level-of-Service Billing

As you read, do the following:

- Highlight any sections, terms, or concepts you think are important
- Draw an asterisk (*) next to any areas you are struggling with
- Watch the review videos to gain more understanding of a particular topic
- Take notes in your notebook or in the margins of this book

After you've read through everything, go back and review any sections that you highlighted or that you drew an asterisk next to, referencing your notes along the way.

Week 4: Practice Tests

Your success on test day depends not only on how many hours you put into preparing, but also on whether you prepared the right way. It's good to check along the way to see if your studying is paying off. One of the most effective ways to do this is by taking practice tests to evaluate your progress. Practice tests are useful because they show exactly where you need to improve. Every time you take a practice test, pay special attention to these three groups of questions:

- The questions you got wrong
- The questions you had to guess on, even if you guessed right
- The questions you found difficult or slow to work through

This will show you exactly what your weak areas are, and where you need to devote more study time. Ask yourself why each of these questions gave you trouble. Was it because you didn't understand the material? Was it because you didn't remember the vocabulary? Do you need more repetitions on this type of question to build speed and confidence? Dig into those questions and figure out how you can strengthen your weak areas as you go back to review the material.

PRACTICE TEST #1

Now that you've read over the instructional content, it's time to take a practice test. Complete Practice Test #1. Take this test with **no time constraints**, and feel free to reference the applicable sections of this guide as you go. Once you've finished, check your answers against the provided answer key. For any questions you answered incorrectly, review the answer rationale, and then **go back and review** the applicable sections of the book. The goal in this stage is to understand why you answered the question incorrectly, and make sure that the next time you see a similar question, you will get it right.

PRACTICE TEST #2

Next, complete Practice Test #2. This time, give yourself **1 hour and 50 minutes** to complete all of the questions. You should again feel free to reference the guide and your notes, but be mindful of the clock. If you run out of time before you finish all of the questions, mark where you were when time expired, but go ahead and finish taking the practice test. Once you've finished, check your answers against the provided answer key, and as before, review the answer rationale for any that you answered incorrectly and then go back and review the associated instructional content. Your goal is still to increase understanding of the content but also to get used to the time constraints you will face on the test.

As you go along, keep in mind that the practice test is just that: practice. Memorizing these questions and answers will not be very helpful on the actual test because it is unlikely to have any of the same exact questions. If you only know the right answers to the sample questions, you won't be prepared for the real thing. **Study the concepts** until you understand them fully, and then you'll be able to answer any question that shows up on the test.

Abbreviations and Terminology

MEDICAL ROOT WORDS

A root word is part of a word that tells us the primary meaning of the word. In medical terminology, the root of the word is usually in Latin. Knowing the meanings of the Latin root words helps us understand what the word means even if we have never seen it before.

Root Word	Meaning
Acous, audi	Hearing
Adip	Fat
Alges	Pain
Andr	Male
Aneur	Widening
Angi	Vessel
Aort	Aorta
Arthr	Joint
Cardi	Heart
Carp	Wrist
Cere	Cerebrum (part of brain)
Crani	Skull
Cutane, derm	Skin
Dactyl	Finger, toe
Encephal	Brain
Esthes	Sensation
Gastr	Stomach
Gynec	Women
Hem, hemat	Blood
Hepat	Liver
Hyster	Uterus
Ichthy	Dry, scaly
Kerat	Hard
Lapar	Abdomen
Lord	Curve
Mamm, mast	Breast

Root Word	Meaning
My	Muscle
Myel	Spinal cord
Necr	Death
Nephr	Kidney
Neur	Nerve
Ocul, ophthalm, optic	Eye
Pector	Chest
Ped, pod	Foot
Phalang	Bones of the fingers and toes
Phas	Speech
Pneum	Lung, air
Psycho	Mind
Pulmon	Lung
Onych	Nail
Oste	Bone
Prurit, psor	Itching
Rhin	Nose
Scoli	Bent
Somat	Body
Sten	Narrow
Stern	Sternum, breastbone
Tars	Ankle
Thromb	Clot
Ven	Vein

MEDICAL SUFFIXES

Many medical words are Latin in origin, so knowing parts of the Latin words can help us define medical terms. A suffix is the ending of a word. Knowing the suffix of a word can help us understand what the word means, even if we haven't seen that word before.

Suffix	Meaning
-ac, -al, -ar, -ary	Pertaining to
-algia, -dynia	Pain
-asthenia	Weakness
-cele	Hernia, bulging
-cyesis	Pregnancy
-ectasis	Dilation
-ectomy	Surgical removal
-edema	Swelling
-emesis	Vomiting
-emia	Blood condition
-esthenia	Lack of sensation
-genic	Producing, forming
-gram	Record
-iatry	Treatment
-icle	Small
-itis	Inflammation
-lepsy	Seizure
-lith	Stone
-lysis	Breaking down
-malacia	Softening
-megaly	Enlargement

Suffix	Meaning
-oma	Tumor
-opia, -opsia	Vision
-orexia	Appetite
-paresis	Partial paralysis
-pathy	Disease
-pepsia	Digestion
-phagia	Swallowing
-phasia	Speech
-philic	Attraction
-plegia	Paralysis, stroke
-pnea	Breathing
-rrhage	To burst
-rrhea	Discharge
-sclerosis	To harden
-spasm	Involuntary contraction
-stasis	Stop, control
-stomy	Artificial opening
-trophy	Growth, nourishment
-uria	Urination

Review Video: Drug Suffixes
Visit mometrix.com/academy and enter code: 882876

MEDICAL PREFIXES

A prefix is the beginning of a word.

Prefix	Meaning		Prefix	Meaning
A-, An-	Without		Inter-	Between
Ambi-	Both		Intra-	Within
Ante-	Before		Iso-	Equal
Anti-	Against		Leuk-	White
Auto-	Self		Lip-	Fat
Bi-	Two, both		Macro-	Large
Brady-	Slow		Mal-	Poor
Circum-	Around		Medi-, meso-, mid-	Middle
Cirrh-	Yellow		Meta-	Beyond, after
Con-	With		Micro-	Small
Contra-	Against		Mono-	One
Dia-	Completely		Multi-	Many
Dipl-	Double		Neo-	New
Dis-	Separate, apart		Pachy-	Heavy, thick
Dys-	Painful, difficult		Pan-	All
Ec-	Away, out of		Para-	Near, abnormal
Ecto-	Outside		Peri-	Around
En-	In		Poly-	Many
Endo-	Within		Post-, retro-	After
Epi-	Above		Pre-, pro-	Before
Eso-	Inward		Pseudo-	FALSE
Eu-	Normal, good		Super-, supra-	Above
Exo-	Outside		Sym-, syn-	With
Hemi-	Half		Tachy-	Fast
Heter-	Different		Trans-	Across
Hyper-	Above, over		Tri-	Three
Hypo-	Below, under		Uni-	One
Im-	Not, without		Xero-	Dry
Immune-	Immunity			
Infra-	Below, under			

MEDICAL TERMS

Medical Terms Associated WITH Medical Conditions

Definitions of common medical conditions include:

- **Myocardial infarction**: Heart attack (hint: "myo" means muscle, "cardi" means heart, and "infarction" means tissue death). When a blood clot obstructs blood flow to the heart, the heart muscles cannot get enough oxygen and the tissue eventually dies.
- **Pulmonary embolism**: Blood clot in the lung (hint: "pulm" means lung, and an embolism is a blood clot).
- **Benign prostatic hyperplasia**: Enlarged prostate (hint: "hyper" means greater than normal).
- **Thrombus**: A blood clot that develops in a blood vessel (hint: "thromb" means clot).
- **Embolism**: A thrombus that breaks off and gets stuck in another blood vessel.
- **Hypertension**: High blood pressure (hint: "hyper" means greater than normal).
- **Hypotension**: Low blood pressure (hint: "hypo" means less than normal).

21

- **Hyperglycemia**: High blood glucose (hint: "glyc" means sugar or glucose, and "emia" refers to a condition of the blood). This is the main clinical feature of diabetes mellitus.
- **Neuropathy**: A disease of the nerves, usually resulting in nerve pain or unusual sensations (hint: "neur" refers to nerves, and "pathy" means disease).

MEDICAL TERMS USED TO DESCRIBE ADVERSE EFFECTS OF MEDICATIONS

Key terms describing adverse effects of medications include the following:

- **Hypoglycemia**: Low blood glucose (hint: "hypo" means less than normal). This is a common adverse effect of antidiabetic medications.
- **Hyperkalemia**: High blood potassium levels (hint: "hyper" means above, and the chemical abbreviation for potassium is "K").
- **Hypokalemia**: Low blood potassium levels. This is a common adverse effect of diuretics or water tablets.
- **Orthostatic hypotension**: Low blood pressure upon standing, which often leads to dizziness and blurred vision.
- **Fatigue**: Tiredness, drowsiness, or sleepiness.
- **Malaise**: A general feeling of discomfort or illness.
- **Dyspepsia**: Heartburn, indigestion, bloating, or abdominal pain (hint: "dys" means painful, and "pepsia" means digestion).
- **Pruritus**: Itching.
- **Diaphoresis**: Sweating.
- **Alopecia**: Hair loss.
- **Myalgia**: Muscle pain (hint: "my" refers to muscles, and "algia" means pain).
- **Edema**: Swelling
- **Xerostomia**: Dry mouth (hint: "xero" means dry, and "stomy" refers to an opening such as the mouth).
- **Anuria**: Lack of urination (hint: "an" means without, and "urea" means urination). Oliguria may also be used to refer to reduced urination.

ABBREVIATIONS USED IN THE PHARMACY

Common medical abbreviations:

Abbreviation	Meaning
ACE	Angiotensin-converting enzyme
ADH	Antidiuretic hormone
ADR	Adverse drug reaction
AF, AFib	Atrial fibrillation (a type of heart arrhythmia)
BMI	Body mass index
BP	Blood pressure
BPH	Benign prostatic hyperplasia
CNS	Central nervous system
CVS	Cardiovascular system
DEA	Drug Enforcement Administration
DMARD	Disease-modifying antirheumatic drug
DVT	Deep vein thrombosis
ECG/EKG	Electrocardiogram
ED	Erectile dysfunction
FDA	Food and Drug Administration

GFR	Glomerular filtration rate (measure of kidney function)
HBP	High blood pressure
HIV	Human immunodeficiency virus
HRT	Hormone replacement therapy
HSV	Herpes simplex virus
HTN	Hypertension
Ig	Immunoglobulin
INR	International normalized ratio (a test used to dose warfarin)
IR	Immediate release
LMWH	Low-molecular-weight heparin
MDI	Metered-dose inhaler
MI	Myocardial infarction (heart attack)
MR	Modified release (formulation)
MRI	Magnetic resonance imaging
MRSA	Methicillin-resistant Staphylococcus aureus
N/V/D	Nausea, vomiting, and diarrhea
NSAID	Nonsteroidal anti-inflammatory drug
NSTEMI	Non-ST elevation myocardial infarction (ST refers to the ST segment)
OTC	Over-the-counter
PCA	Patient-controlled analgesia
PE	Pulmonary embolism
PPI	Proton pump inhibitor (acid suppressor)
PRN	As needed
SR	Sustained release (long acting)
SSRI	Selective serotonin reuptake inhibitor (antidepressant)
STEMI	ST elevation myocardial infarction
TB	Tuberculosis
TCA	Tricyclic antidepressant
TIA	Transient ischemic attack (ministroke)
VTE	Venous thromboembolism
XR	Extended release (long acting)

Medications

Transform passive reading into active learning! After immersing yourself in this chapter, put your comprehension to the test by taking a quiz. The insights you gained will stay with you longer this way. Scan the QR code to go directly to the chapter quiz interface for this study guide. If you're using a computer, simply visit the bonus page at **mometrix.com/bonus948/ptcb** and click the Chapter Quizzes link.

Generic Names, Brand Names, and Classifications of Medications

BRAND NAME AND GENERIC NAME

The brand name for a drug is its advertised name assigned by the original inventor. The generic name is its chemical, scientific, or nonproprietary name. The generic name is always listed on the label of the container, but a brand name is not required for generic versions. For example, when you go to the store to purchase household cleaner, you will have the choice of purchasing Clorox (brand name) or the store brand of bleach cleaner (generic name).

The same system applies to pharmacy. If you browse the OTC section of your local pharmacy for the nasal spray Flonase (brand name), you will also have the option to purchase a generic version labeled fluticasone. Both product labels are required to contain the generic name of fluticasone.

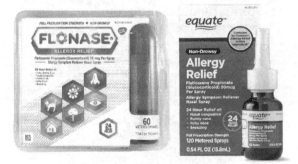

Inventors/manufacturers of a new drug will file for a patent, which gives them exclusive rights to produce that drug for the next 20 years. During this period, the drug will only be available as a brand-name product. Once the patent expires, other companies will be allowed to produce generic versions of the drug once they obtain Food and Drug Administration (FDA) approval and prove that the ingredients and formulation are equivalent to the branded product.

ANTIHYPERTENSIVE DRUGS

Beta-blockers and alpha-blockers block the fight-or-flight response in our bodies that triggers increased heart rate, increased force of contraction of the heart, and increased blood pressure. By blocking this response, beta blockers lower heart rate and blood pressure to treat hypertension.

Calcium channel blockers prevent calcium from entering the cells of the heart and blood vessel walls. Because calcium is needed for muscle contraction, calcium channel blockers reduce the force of contraction of the heart and the muscles surrounding blood vessels, resulting in lower blood pressure.

ACE inhibitors block angiotensin-converting enzyme, which is responsible for producing a substance called angiotensin II. Angiotensin II narrows blood vessels and helps the body retain water, which leads to a rise in blood pressure.

Diuretics decrease the volume of blood by promoting water loss in the urine. This volume loss results in lower blood pressure.

Hypertension means high blood pressure, so antihypertensive medications help lower blood pressure. High blood pressure is one of the most common conditions treated with medication. There are many classes of cardiovascular drugs that are prescribed in the treatment of high blood pressure. The most common classes of medications are beta-blockers (they end in the suffix "-olol"), calcium channel blockers (most end in "-pine"), angiotensin-converting enzyme (ACE) inhibitors (end with the suffix "-pril"), alpha-blockers (end in "-zosin"), and diuretics (there are various naming systems, but some end in "-thiazide").

Classification	Generic Name	Brand Name
Beta-blocker	Atenolol	Tenormin
Beta-blocker	Metoprolol	Lopressor, Toprol
Beta-blocker	Nadolol	Corgard
Beta-blocker	Propranolol	Inderal
Calcium channel blocker	Amlodipine	Norvasc
Calcium channel blocker	Diltiazem	Cardizem, Cartia, Tiazac
Calcium channel blocker	Nifedipine	Procardia
Calcium channel blocker	Verapamil	Calan
ACE inhibitor	Benazepril	Lotensin
ACE inhibitor	Captopril	APO-Captopril
ACE inhibitor	Enalapril	Vasotec
ACE inhibitor	Lisinopril	Zestril
ACE inhibitor	Ramipril	Altace
Alpha-blocker	Prazosin	Minipress
Alpha-blocker	Doxazosin	Cardura
Diuretic	Hydrochlorothiazide	APO-Hydro
Diuretic	Furosemide	Lasix
Diuretic	Spironolactone	Aldactone

DRUGS USED TO TREAT HEART FAILURE

Heart failure occurs when a patient's heart is not functioning efficiently, often as a result of a heart attack or cardiovascular disease. These patients get chest pain (angina) when they exert themselves and overwork their heart. They will be prescribed an antianginal agent, also referred to as nitrates, to use to prevent or treat angina pains. Heart failure patients are usually prescribed antihypertensive medications and diuretics as well to lower blood pressure and reduce the rate and force of the contraction of the heart. Some patients may have an irregularity in their heartbeat, which is treated with antiarrhythmic medications.

Vasodilators and antianginal agents cause vasodilation (widening) of blood vessels, which lowers blood pressure. Antihypertensive medications and diuretics also reduce blood pressure. Lower blood pressures reduce the strain on an overworked heart to reduce angina pains.

Antiarrhythmic drugs help restore a normal heart rhythm and improve the efficiency of the heart.

Drug Classification	Generic Name	Brand Name
Vasodilator	Hydralazine	Apresoline
Antianginal	Nitroglycerin	Nitrostat, Nitrolingual, Rectiv
Antianginal	Isosorbide mononitrate	(None currently on the market)
Antiarrhythmic	Amiodarone	Nexterone
Antiarrhythmic	Digoxin	Lanoxin

ANTIARRHYTHMIC DRUGS

An arrhythmia is an irregularity in the rate or rhythm at which the heart beats. The most common types of arrhythmias are ventricular tachycardia and atrial fibrillation.

Some classes of medications that are used to treat hypertension are also used to treat arrhythmias, including beta-blockers (end in "-olol") and calcium channel blockers. These medications slow the heart rate and are used to treat tachycardias. Tachycardia is a type of heart arrhythmia in which the heart beats too fast. Several other classes of antiarrhythmic drugs also exist. The common antiarrhythmic drugs are used to treat tachycardias and/or atrial fibrillation. You may notice that many of the brand names for antiarrhythmic drugs contain the root words "pace" or "rhythm," which is helpful for indicating that they are used to control the pace or rhythm of the heart.

Generic Name	Brand Name
Metoprolol	Lopressor, Toprol
Atenolol	Tenormin
Sotalol	Betapace
Verapamil	Calan SR, Verelan
Amiodarone	Pacerone, Nexterone
Propafenone	Rythmol
Disopyramide	Norpace
Flecainide	Tambocor
Digoxin	Lanoxin

HYPERCHOLESTEROLEMIA AND ANTIHYPERLIPIDEMIC MEDICATIONS

Hypercholesterolemia is defined as high cholesterol levels. Cholesterol is a lipid molecule that is transported in the blood and is linked to cardiovascular disease. Most antihyperlipidemic medications inhibit the enzyme HMG-CoA reductase, which is involved in the production of cholesterol in the body. HMG-CoA reductase inhibitors are commonly referred to as **statins** because they end in the suffix "-statin." Some antihyperlipidemic medications, such as ezetimibe, work by inhibiting the absorption of cholesterol in the gastrointestinal tract. Cholestyramine and colestipol act by binding to and removing bile salts in the gastrointestinal tract. Because cholesterol is used by the body to make bile salts, removing bile salts helps use up excess cholesterol to make more bile salts. Cholesterol or bile salt binding antihyperlipidemic medications are usually well tolerated, but some patients experience abdominal cramping, constipation, nausea, or vomiting.

Generic Name	Brand Name
Ezetimibe	Zetia
Pravastatin	(None currently on the market)
Simvastatin	Zocor
Atorvastatin	Lipitor

Generic Name	Brand Name
Rosuvastatin	Crestor
Cholestyramine	Questran
Colestipol	Colestid

BLOOD THINNERS

Thrombolytics dissolve blood clots that have already formed, whereas antiplatelets and anticoagulants are blood thinners that prevent blood clot formation. Antiplatelets prevent the platelets in the blood from sticking together and forming a clot. Anticoagulants prevent the formation of fibrin, a protein that holds blood clots together.

Thrombolytics, also called clot busters, are used in emergency situations to break up clots associated with a stroke, pulmonary embolism, or heart attack.

Antiplatelets and anticoagulants are given to at-risk patients to prevent clot formation. Patients who are hospitalized or immobile after surgery are usually prescribed an anticoagulant to prevent clots from forming in their legs. Patients who have heart arrhythmias, such as atrial fibrillation, are also at higher risk of clot formation and may be prescribed an anticoagulant. Other risk factors that may justify the use of a blood thinner include cardiovascular disease or history of stroke, heart attack, or pulmonary embolism.

Commonly prescribed **blood thinners** include the following:

Drug Classification	Generic Name	Brand Name
Anticoagulant	Warfarin	Coumadin
Anticoagulant	Heparin	(None currently on the market)
Anticoagulant	Enoxaparin	Lovenox
Anticoagulant	Rivaroxaban	Xarelto
Anticoagulant	Apixaban	Eliquis
Anticoagulant	Dabigatran	Pradaxa
Antiplatelet	Aspirin	Bayer
Antiplatelet	Clopidogrel	Plavix
Antiplatelet	Prasugrel	Effient
Antiplatelet	Ticagrelor	Brilinta
Antiplatelet	Dipyridamole	Persantine
Thrombolytic	Alteplase	Activase, Cathflo

> **Review Video: Heparin - An Injectable Anti-Coagulant**
> Visit mometrix.com/academy and enter code: 127426
>
> **Review Video: Warfarin - Uses and Side Effects**
> Visit mometrix.com/academy and enter code: 844117
>
> **Review Video: Antiplatelets and Thrombolytics**
> Visit mometrix.com/academy and enter code: 711284

RESPIRATORY AGENTS

Respiratory medications include tablets, capsules, inhalers, and nebulizer solutions. Commonly treated respiratory conditions include asthma, emphysema, chronic obstructive pulmonary disease (COPD), bronchitis, flu, cold, and allergies.

- **Antihistamines** reduce inflammation by inhibiting histamine, a chemical messenger in the body that promotes inflammation. Antihistamines are used to treat allergies such as hay fever, flu symptoms, and cold symptoms.
- **Decongestants** constrict the blood vessels in the nose to reduce mucus buildup and congestion. Decongestants are used to treat head and sinus congestions associated with colds and flus.
- **Antitussives** prevent coughing and are used to treat cold and flu symptoms. The mechanism of action varies depending upon the specific medication. Some medications soothe the lining of the throat, whereas others act on cough reflex centers in the brain.
- **Expectorants** help thin the mucus that builds up during a cold or respiratory illness. They help patients with productive coughs bring up excess mucus and relieve chest congestion.
- **Bronchodilators** dilate or open the airways to make it easier for patients to breathe. They are used to treat respiratory diseases, such as asthma and chronic obstructive pulmonary disease (COPD), but they can also be used short term during a respiratory illness to help relieve shortness of breath.
- **Corticosteroids** are anti-inflammatory medications that are used to treat a wide range of diseases, including respiratory illnesses.

RESPIRATORY MEDICATIONS

Medications that can be purchased over the counter (OTC) without a prescription are italicized in the table below. Pseudoephedrine is a special case because, although it can be purchased without a prescription, it is kept behind the pharmacy counter and the customer must show identification and sign for it in order to purchase it.

Drug Classification	Generic Name	Brand Name
Antihistamine	Loratadine	Claritin, Alavert
Antihistamine	Cetirizine	Zyrtec
Antihistamine	Fexofenadine	Allegra
Antihistamine	Chlorpheniramine	Chlor-Trimeton
Antihistamine	Diphenhydramine	Benadryl
Antihistamine	Promethazine	Phenergan
Decongestant	Pseudoephedrine	Sudafed
Decongestant	Phenylephrine	Sudafed-PE
Antitussive	Dextromethorphan	Delsym
Antitussive	Codeine (used in combination cough syrups)	Phenergan with codeine
Expectorant	Guaifenesin	Robitussin, Mucinex
Bronchodilator	Albuterol	Ventolin, Airomir
Bronchodilator	Levalbuterol	Xopenex
Bronchodilator	Ipratropium	Atrovent
Bronchodilator	Formoterol	Perforomist
Bronchodilator	Salmeterol	Serevent
Corticosteroid	Budesonide	Pulmicort
Corticosteroid	Beclomethasone	Qvar

Drug Classification	Generic Name	Brand Name
Corticosteroid	Mometasone	Asmanex
Corticosteroid	Fluticasone	Flovent
Corticosteroid	Triamcinolone	Hexatrione, Kenalog
Antiasthmatic drug (leukotriene receptor antagonist)	Montelukast	Singulair

ANALGESICS

Analgesics are medications that are used to reduce pain. They can be given in the form of a tablet/capsule, oral liquid, or parenteral injection. Most nonsteroidal anti-inflammatory drugs (NSAIDs) as well as aspirin and acetaminophen are available over the counter (OTC). Opioids are stronger, have more side effects, and have a higher potential for abuse, so they are prescription only. Most opioids are classified as controlled substances.

Commonly used **analgesics**:

Drug Classification	Generic Name	Brand Name	Legal Classification
Salicylate	Aspirin	Bayer	OTC
NSAID	Ibuprofen	Motrin, Advil	OTC
NSAID	Naproxen	Aleve	OTC
NSAID	Celecoxib	Celebrex	R only, noncontrolled
Non-aspirin, non-NSAID	Acetaminophen	Tylenol	OTC
Opiate	Tramadol	Ultram	Sch IV
Opiate	Acetaminophen with codeine Promethazine with codeine	Tylenol with Codeine (None currently on the market)	Sch II if >90 mg per dosage unit Sch III if <90 mg per dosage unit Sch V if ≤200 mg per 100 mL or 100 g
Opiate	Hydrocodone	Hysingla, Zoyhydro	Sch II
Opiate	Hydromorphone	Dilaudid	Sch II
Opiate	Morphine	MS Contin, Duramorph, Infumorph, Mitigo	Sch II
Opiate	Oxycodone	Oxycontin, Oxaydo, Roxicodone, Roxybond	Sch II
Opiate	Meperidine	Demerol	Sch II

ANTIBIOTICS

Antibiotics are used to treat bacterial or microbial infections. Broad-spectrum antibiotics are less specific and kill a wide range of bacteria, but they have more side effects. Narrow-spectrum antibiotics are more specific and are used to treat infections when the bacterial cause is known.

Commonly prescribed **antibiotics**:

Class	Drug Examples	Class Details
Penicillins	Amoxicillin, penicillin, ampicillin	Broad-spectrum antibiotics used to treat respiratory infections.
Cephalosporins	Cefaclor (Cefaclor), cefixime (Suprax)	Broad-spectrum antibiotics.
Tetracyclines	Tetracycline, doxycycline (Vibramycin, Monodoxyne), minocycline (Minocin, Solodyn)	Broad-spectrum, but many bacteria are resistant. Used to treat acne.
Macrolides	Erythromycin (Erythrocin), clarithromycin (Biaxin)	Similar spectrum to penicillins, so they are used as an alternative in penicillin allergy. Used to treat respiratory infections, acne, and chlamydia.
Quinolones	Ciprofloxacin (Cipro), levofloxacin (Levaquin)	Narrower spectrum, commonly used to treat pneumonia.
Sulfonamides (sulfa drugs)	Sulfamethoxazole-trimethoprim (Bactrim)	Used to treat urinary tract infections.
Glycopeptides	Vancomycin	Narrow spectrum, used to treat MRSA (IV only). Oral vancomycin is used to treat colitis and *Clostridium difficile*.

ANTIVIRAL MEDICATIONS

Antiviral medications are used to treat viral infections. Viruses are different in structure and behavior than bacteria and require different types of medications to eradicate them. In general, drug names that end in "-vir" are antiviral drugs. Some viral infections are short term (e.g., influenza), whereas others are chronic and require life-long treatment (e.g., human immunodeficiency virus [HIV]). In addition to therapeutic medications, there are several vaccinations that are used to prevent viral infections before the patient becomes infected (e.g., flu vaccine, hepatitis B vaccine).

Commonly prescribed **antiviral medications**:

Generic Name	Brand Name	Indication
Acyclovir	(None currently on the market)	Herpes infections
Valacyclovir	Valtrex	Herpes infections
Oseltamivir	Tamiflu	Influenza viruses
Zanamivir	Relenza	Influenza viruses
Emtricitabine and tenofovir disoproxil fumarate	Truvada	HIV prevention in at-risk patients
Dolutegravir, abacavir, and lamivudine	Triumeq	HIV
Dolutegravir	Tivicay	HIV
Tenofovir alafenamide and emtricitabine	Descovy	HIV
Elvitegravir, cobicistat, emtricitabine, and tenofovir alafenamide	Genvoya	HIV

Generic Name	Brand Name	Indication
Darunavir and ritonavir	Prezista	HIV
Ledipasvir and sofosbuvir	Harvoni	Hepatitis C
Sofosbuvir and velpatasvir	Epclusa	Hepatitis C

ANTIFUNGAL MEDICATIONS

Fungi differ from bacteria and viruses in their structure and behavior, so a different set of medications are required to treat a fungal infection. Antifungal medications can easily be identified because they either end in the suffix "-conazole" or "-fungin." However, there are always exceptions to the rule and there are a few antifungal medications that do not follow this naming rule. Common types of fungal infections include oral thrush, vaginal candidiasis (yeast infection), athlete's foot, jock itch, and fungal skin infections. Most of these conditions are minor and can be treated with OTC medications. The OTC medications are italicized in the table below. Occasionally, fungal infections can get into the body and cause more serious widespread infections, meningitis, or pneumonia.

Generic Name	Brand Name
Caspofungin	Cancidas
Micafungin	Mycamine
Clotrimazole	*Gyne-Lotrimin* (cream is OTC; tablets are R-only)
Fluconazole	Diflucan
Itraconazole	Sporanox
Miconazole	*Cavilon*, Desenex
Terbinafine	*Lamisil* (cream is OTC; tablets are R-only)
Amphotericin B	(None currently on the market)
Nystatin	Nyamyc, Nystop
Griseofulvin	(None currently on the market)

CANCER DRUGS

Drugs used to treat cancer are also called antineoplastic agents or anticancer agents.

- **Antimetabolites** inhibit cancer cell growth by interfering with their metabolism (cellular processes).
- Examples: methotrexate (Rasuvo, Otrexup, Trexall), fluorouracil, mercaptopurine (Purixan), capecitabine (Xeloda), azathioprine (Imuran)
- **Alkylating agents and antitumor antibiotics** interfere with and cause damage to DNA. This prevents cancer cells from replicating or growing.
- Examples: cyclophosphamide (Procytox), temozolomide (Temodar), carmustine, daunorubicin, bleomycin
- **Hormonal anticancer therapies** are used to treat cancers that require certain hormones to grow (e.g., breast cancer, prostate cancer). By blocking the necessary hormone, these therapies inhibit the growth of cancer cells. These therapies are more selective and have fewer classic antineoplastic agent side effects.
- Examples: tamoxifen (Soltamox), letrozole (Femara), anastrozole (Arimidex), bicalutamide (Casodex), leuprolide (Lupron, Eligard)
- **Radioactive isotopes** act in a similar way to radiation therapy. The radiation enters cancer cells and causes damage, preventing the cells from growing and dividing. Example: cesium-137

THYROID DISORDERS AND MEDICATIONS

Hypothyroidism is defined as thyroid hormone levels that are too low, and **hyperthyroidism** is defined as thyroid hormone levels that are too high. Recall that the prefix "hypo-" means less than normal or low and "hyper-" means greater than normal or high. The thyroid gland sits low in the front of the neck and is responsible for secreting thyroid hormone. This gland is part of the body's endocrine system, which is responsible for secreting hormones that regulate body processes. Hypothyroidism is more common than hyperthyroidism in the United States and is easily treatable with hormone replacement therapy. Symptoms of hypothyroidism include fatigue, weakness, joint pain, sensitivity to cold, weight gain, hair thinning, depression, impaired memory, slow heart rate, and irregular menstrual periods. Symptoms of hyperthyroidism are essentially the opposite: restlessness, tremors, intolerance to heat, weight loss, increased appetite, sweating, anxiety, rapid heart rate, and agitation.

Indication	Generic Name	Brand Name
Hypothyroidism	Levothyroxine	Synthroid, Levoxyl
Hypothyroidism	Liothyronine	Cytomel
Hyperthyroidism	Propylthiouracil	Halycil

ORAL ANTIHYPERGLYCEMIC DRUGS

Diabetes is caused by either a lack of insulin or reduced sensitivity to insulin. Insulin is a hormone that shuttles glucose from the blood into the tissues. The mechanism of action for common oral antihyperglycemic drugs are as follows:

- **Biguanides** decrease glucose production in the liver, decrease absorption of glucose in the intestines, and improve glucose uptake into tissues.
- **Alpha-glucosidase inhibitors** delay the digestion of carbohydrates in the intestines, thereby slowing the release of glucose into the blood.
- **Sulfonylureas** stimulate the release of insulin from the pancreas.
- **Thiazolidinediones** decrease glucose production in the liver and enhance the sensitivity of tissues to insulin, allowing them to take up more glucose from the blood.
- **DPP-4 inhibitors** promote insulin production by increasing the levels of a hormone called glucagon-like peptide-1 (GLP-1).
- **SGLT-2 inhibitors** inhibit a sodium-glucose transporter in the kidney, which promotes the excretion of glucose in the urine.

Commonly used **oral antihyperglycemic drugs** include the following:

Drug Class	Generic Name	Brand Name
Biguanide	Metformin	Glucophage
Alpha-glucosidase inhibitor	Acarbose	(None currently on the market)
Sulfonylurea	Glipizide	Glucotrol
Sulfonylurea	Glyburide	Glynase
Sulfonylurea	Glimepiride	Amaryl
Thiazolidinedione	Pioglitazone	Actos
Thiazolidinedione	Rosiglitazone	(None currently on the market)
DPP inhibitor	Saxagliptin	Onglyza
DPP-4 inhibitor	Sitagliptin	Januvia
DPP-4 inhibitor	Linagliptin	Tradjenta
SGLT-2 inhibitor	Canagliflozin	Invokana

| SGLT-2 inhibitor | Dapagliflozin | Farxiga |
| SGLT-2 inhibitor | Empagliflozin | Jardiance |

DIABETES MELLITUS

Diabetes mellitus is a chronic disease in which patients have too much glucose in their blood. It is related to dysfunction of insulin, a hormone that shuttles glucose from the blood into the tissues. In diabetics, either too little insulin is being produced or the tissues are not sensitive or responsive enough to insulin. Because insulin is not shuttling glucose from the blood into the tissues, glucose builds up in the blood.

- **Type 1 diabetes** is a genetic disorder that is diagnosed at a young age. Immune cells in the body attack and destroy the beta cells in the pancreas that produce insulin. Therefore, type 1 diabetics must replace the missing insulin using insulin injections.
- **Type 2 diabetes** is characterized by decreased sensitivity to insulin. Although there may also be reduced insulin production, the tissues are not responding to the insulin that is present. Type 2 diabetes is usually diagnosed later in life. Although there are genetic risk factors, lifestyle factors such as obesity increase the risk of getting the disease. Type 2 diabetes can be treated by diet and lifestyle modifications, oral or injectable antihyperglycemic medications, and insulin.

> **Review Video: Diabetes Mellitus: Diet, Exercise, & Medication**
> Visit mometrix.com/academy and enter code: 774388
>
> **Review Video: Diabetes Mellitus**
> Visit mometrix.com/academy and enter code: 501396
>
> **Review Video: Diabetes Mellitus: Complications**
> Visit mometrix.com/academy and enter code: 996788

MEDICATIONS TREATING DIABETES

Insulin injections replace insulin that is missing or lacking in the body. They are usually used to treat type 1 diabetes, but they may also be used in type 2 diabetes. Common side effects of using insulin are hypoglycemia, weight gain, and injection site reactions.

Incretin mimetics are a newer class of injectable antihyperglycemic drugs. They increase the activity of the hormone GLP-1, which increases insulin production, decreases glucagon (stored glucose) release, slows glucose digestion, and reduces appetite. Because they do not replace insulin, they are only used in type 2 diabetes. Incretin mimetics are becoming increasing popular because they have a low risk of causing hypoglycemia and they help patients lose weight.

Amylin mimetics decrease the production of glucagon (stored glucose), slow gastric emptying (this slows glucose digestion), enhances satiety (the feeling of fullness after a meal), and cause weight loss. They are not very popular because they can cause severe hypoglycemia. However, they can be used in combination with insulin in type 1 or type 2 diabetics who have failed other regimens.

Drug Class	Generic Name	Brand Name
Incretin mimetic	Liraglutide	Victoza
Incretin mimetic	Exenatide	Byetta, Bydureon BCise
Amylin mimetic	Pramlintide	SymlinPen

HYPOGLYCEMIA

Diabetes mellitus is defined by hyperglycemia (high blood glucose). Treatments for diabetes aim to lower blood glucose. Therefore, many antihyperglycemic medications can cause hypoglycemia (low blood glucose). Some classes of antihyperglycemic medications have a higher risk of causing hypoglycemia (e.g., sulfonylureas, insulin, amylin mimetics) than others.

Hypoglycemia is a potentially serious side effect of antihyperglycemic medications. If too high of a dose is administered or if a patient does not eat enough carbohydrates, the patient's blood glucose levels can become too low. Symptoms of hypoglycemia include tremors, dizziness, sweating, hunger, irritability, slurred speech, anxiety, and headache.

If hypoglycemia is suspected, the patient should be given a sugary snack or drink, glucose tablets, or a glucagon injection (if the patient is unconscious) as soon as possible. If left untreated, hypoglycemia can cause the patient to pass out, have a seizure, or even die.

Glucose tablets	Glucolift, Dex4, Relion
Glucose oral gel	Dex4, Glutose, Transcend
Glucagon injection	GlucaGen

INSULIN REGIMENS

Basal bolus regimen (first-line, preferred regimen)

The basal bolus regimen involves injecting a long-acting insulin once or twice daily in addition to injecting a dose of rapid-acting insulin before every meal.

Insulin Type/Generic Name	Brand Name	Duration
Rapid-Acting Insulins		
Insulin glulisine	Apidra	1–3 hours
Insulin aspart	NovoLog	3–5 hours
Insulin lispro	Humalog, Admelog	3–4 hours
Long-Acting Insulins		
Insulin glargine	Lantus	24 hours
Insulin detemir	Levemir	18–24 hours

Twice-daily mixed insulin regimen

The mixed insulin regimen involves the patient injecting a mixture of intermediate- and short-acting insulin twice daily. This regimen does not provide as steady of an insulin level compared to the basal bolus regimen, and it increases the patient's risk for a hypoglycemic event.

Insulin Type/Generic Name	Brand Name	Duration
Short-Acting Insulins		
Insulin regular	Novolin R, Humulin R	4–6 hours
Intermediate-Acting Insulins		
Insulin NPH	Novolin N, Humulin N	10–18 hours
Premixed Formulations		
70% Insulin NPH + 30% insulin regular	Novolin 70/30 Humulin 70/30	
50% Insulin NPH + 30% insulin regular	Humulin 50/50	

ACNE AND ACNE TREATMENTS

Acne occurs when oil glands in the skin become blocked, infected, and inflamed. Acne is common in teenagers because puberty causes overproduction of skin oils. Acne treatments include antibiotics to treat the infection, exfoliants that remove excess dead skin and oils to prevent blockage of glands, and retinoids that decrease oil production.

Some topical treatments are available as OTC medications. The oral retinoid isotretinoin is reserved for severe cases of acne that have not responded to topical therapies or oral antibiotics. Isotretinoin can cause serious birth defects if taken during pregnancy, so it is part of an iPledge risk evaluation and mitigation strategy (REMS) program that places restrictions on its use.

Commonly prescribed acne medications are below. Those available OTC are italicized.

Drug Classification	Generic Name	Brand Name
Topical antibiotic	Clindamycin	Cleocin T
Topical antibiotic	Erythromycin	Erygel
Topical antibiotic	*Benzoyl peroxide*	*PanOxyl*
Topical antibiotic	Dapsone	Aczone
Topical antibiotic/exfoliant	Azelaic acid	Finacea
Topical exfoliant	*Salicylic acid*	*Stridex, Noxzema, Neutrogena, Clearasil*
Oral antibiotic	Tetracycline	(None currently on the market)
Oral antibiotic	Erythromycin	Erythrocin, E.E.S.
Oral antibiotic	Doxycycline	Vibramycin
Oral antibiotic	Minocycline	Minocin
Topical retinoid	Tretinoin	Retin-A
Topical retinoid	Adapalene	Differin
Topical retinoid	Tazarotene	Tazorac
Oral retinoid	Isotretinoin	Accutane, Amnesteem, Claravis

HEARTBURN AND GASTROESOPHAGEAL REFLUX DISEASE

Heartburn is a burning sensation in the chest caused by acid from the stomach entering the esophagus. Gastroesophageal reflux disease (GERD) is the medical term for heartburn. Gastric acid in the stomach moves upward into the esophagus, causing discomfort and a burning sensation. Treatments for heartburn, or GERD, include medications that reduce the amount of acid in the stomach. Antacids act quickly by combining with existing stomach acid and neutralizing it. Acid reducers, such as proton pump inhibitors (PPIs) or histamine-$_2$ antagonists (H$_2$ blockers) prevent the production of stomach acid. Therefore, they take longer to start working than antacids. Many of these medications are available as OTC formulas (they are italicized in the table).

Drug Classification	Generic Name	Brand Name
Antacid	*Calcium carbonate*	*Tums, Rolaids*
Antacid	*Magnesium hydroxide*	*Milk of Magnesia, Maalox*
PPI	*Lansoprazole*	*Prevacid*
PPI	Dexlansoprazole	Dexilant
PPI	*Omeprazole*	*Prilosec*
PPI	*Esomeprazole*	*Nexium*
PPI	Rabeprazole	Aciphex
PPI	Pantoprazole	Protonix
H$_2$ blocker	*Famotidine*	*Pepcid*

CONSTIPATION

Constipation is defined as hard stools or difficulty with bowel movements. Common causes include dehydration (reduced fluid intake), lack of fiber in the diet, lack of exercise, and medications. Opioid pain medications are a common cause of constipation.

Drug Classification	Generic Name	Brand Name
Bulk-forming laxative	Psyllium	Metamucil
Bulk-forming laxative	Methylcellulose	Citrucel
Stool softener	Docusate	Colace
Osmotic laxative	Magnesium salts (magnesium hydroxide, magnesium citrate, magnesium sulfate), Epsom salts	Milk of Magnesia
Osmotic laxative	Sodium phosphate	Fleet Enema
Osmotic laxative	Polyethylene glycol	MiraLAX
Stimulant laxative	Senna	Senokot, Ex-Lax
Stimulant laxative	Bisacodyl	Dulcolax
Stimulant laxative	Glycerin	Avedana Glycerin, Fleet Liquid Glycerin Supp

TYPES OF LAXATIVES

The mechanisms of action for various laxatives are as follows:

- **Bulk-forming laxatives** absorb water into the stool to increase its bulkiness so that it moves along the colon easier. They usually start working within 2–3 days.
- **Stool softeners** are emollients (oils) that soften and lubricate the stool, making it easier to pass. Their onset of action is 2–3 days.
- **Osmotic laxatives** pull water into the colon to hydrate the stool. They start working in 1–3 days.
- **Stimulant laxatives** stimulate bowel movements by causing local irritation to the lining of the bowel. Stimulants work more quickly than other laxatives. Glycerin works within 30 minutes, whereas senna and bisacodyl work within 6–12 hours.

DIARRHEA

Diarrhea is defined as loose, runny, or frequent bowel movements. Diarrhea can be caused by overeating in general and by certain foods, illnesses, and medications. Foods that commonly cause diarrhea include spicy foods and meals high in carbohydrates. Cold and flu viruses can cause diarrhea as well as bacterial infections, such as food poisoning and traveler's diarrhea. Medications that commonly cause diarrhea include antibiotics, magnesium-containing antacids, and antineoplastic agents (chemotherapy). Patients with diarrhea can lose a lot of water in their stool, so it is important to drink water or electrolyte drinks to stay hydrated.

There are two OTC medications available to treat diarrhea. **Loperamide (Imodium)** is an opioid agonist that slows the movement of food along the digestive tract. **Bismuth subsalicylate (Pepto-Bismol)** works as an antacid as well as reduces the frequency of bowel movements.

The prescription-only medication **diphenoxylate 2.5 mg/atropine 0.025 mg (Lomotil)** can be prescribed to treat cases of diarrhea that are not resolved by OTC Imodium. The diphenoxylate ingredient in Lomotil is an opioid agonist that helps slow down the digestive system. Because it contains an opioid ingredient, Lomotil is a schedule V controlled substance.

NAUSEA AND VOMITING

Nausea and vomiting can be caused by gastrointestinal issues, such as infection or obstruction. Certain medical disorders can also cause nausea and vomiting including headaches or migraines, pregnancy, recent surgery, motion sickness, ear infections, vertigo (dizziness), and drug or alcohol withdrawal. Many medications include nausea and vomiting as a common side effect: antibiotics, antivirals, cancer treatments (chemotherapy), opioid pain medications, NSAIDs (e.g., naproxen, ibuprofen), antidepressants, digoxin, theophylline, iron supplements. Patients who have been vomiting should try to remain hydrated by drinking water or electrolyte drinks. Untreated vomiting can lead to dehydration, electrolyte imbalances, and postsurgical complications in patients who have recently had surgery.

Medications that are used to treat nausea and vomiting are called antiemetics. Some antiemetics are available as OTC medicines (they are italicized in the table), whereas others require a prescription.

Generic Name	Brand Name
Ondansetron	Zofran
Granisetron	Sancuso, Sustol
Promethazine	Phenergan
Prochlorperazine	Compro
Aprepitant	Emend
Dexamethasone	Dexabliss, DoubleDex
Dimenhydrinate	*Driminate*
Diphenhydramine	*Benadryl*
Meclizine	*Bonine, Travel-Ease*

ANEMIA

Anemia occurs when there are not enough healthy red blood cells to carry oxygen around the body. Symptoms include fatigue (tiredness), shortness of breath, headache, rapid heart rate, pale skin, dizziness, difficulty concentrating, and leg cramps. Potential dietary causes include inadequate intake of iron, folic acid, or vitamin B_{12}. In addition, some medications interfere with iron absorption, including tetracyclines, antacids, and acid reducers. Reduced absorption also occurs in patients with alcoholism, Crohn's disease, ulcerative colitis, or a history of gastric bypass or bowel resection. Disease states such as cancer, rheumatoid arthritis, and kidney disease also increase anemia risk. Infants, elderly, pregnant, lactating, and menstruating patients are at higher risk. Blood loss from trauma, surgery, gastrointestinal ulcers, or heavy menstruation can also lead to anemia.

Treatment of anemia depends upon the cause but may include iron, folic acid, or vitamin B_{12} supplements. Patients with kidney disease may require injections of erythropoietin, a hormone produced in the kidney that stimulates red blood cell production. Italicized drugs are available over the counter.

Generic Name	Brand Name
Ferrous sulfate	*Fer-in-Sol, Ferosol*
Ferrous gluconate	*Ferate*
Ferrous fumarate	*Ferretts, Fumerin*
Folic acid	*FA-8*
Vitamin B_{12} (cyanocobalamin)	Dodex
Polysaccharide iron complex (IV only)	*Myferon, Ferrex*
Epoetin alfa (IV only)	Procrit, Epogen
Darbepoetin alfa	Aranesp

RHEUMATOID ARTHRITIS

Rheumatoid arthritis is an autoimmune disease that causes the body's own immune system to attack the joints. It affects about 1% of the population and is far more common in women than men. There is a strong genetic component to the disease, but it is also known to have environmental triggers, such as infection. Disease progression varies greatly among individuals, but symptoms usually begin in the patient's late 20s or early 30s. Diagnosis is based on the patient's symptoms as well as a lab test for rheumatoid factor.

Symptoms of rheumatoid arthritis include fatigue, joint pain, joint swelling, and morning stiffness. Although these symptoms seem very nonspecific, the chronic morning joint stiffness is a key symptom in diagnosis. Rheumatoid arthritis is a progressive disease, and without effective treatment, permanent joint damage can occur. The joints that are usually affected include the fingers, wrists, ankles, elbows, shoulders, hips, knees, and jaw.

TREATMENTS

Disease-modifying antirheumatic drugs (DMARDs) halt disease progression and prevent joint damage. The downsides are that they become less effective over time and they are associated with significant side effects, such as increased infection risk, liver damage, and infertility.

Biologic drugs are newer, more expensive treatments that target specific molecules to prevent disease progression. Most biologics are subcutaneous injections that can be administered at home by patients after an initial training session. However, some biologics (e.g., Remicade) can only be administered intravenously at an infusion center. Like DMARDs, many biologics are associated with an increased risk of infection.

Nonsteroidal anti-inflammatory drugs (NSAIDs) are used to control joint pain and inflammation. Most rheumatoid arthritis patients take an NSAID long term and should be aware that long-term NSAID use can cause stomach ulcers. Taking NSAIDs with food or in combination with an acid reducer can help prevent this.

Medications for rheumatoid arthritis:

Drug Classification	Generic Name	Brand Name
Biologic	Adalimumab	Humira
Biologic	Etanercept	Enbrel
Biologic	Infliximab	Remicade
Biologic	Abatacept	Orencia
Biologic	Tocilizumab	Actemra
DMARD	Leflunomide	Arava
DMARD	Methotrexate	Otrexup, Rasuvo, Trexall
DMARD	Hydroxychloroquine	Plaquenil
DMARD	Sulfasalazine	Azulfidine
DMARD	Azathioprine	Imuran
DMARD	Tofacitinib	Xeljanz
NSAID	Diclofenac	Cambia, Lofena, Zipsor
NSAID	Ibuprofen	Motrin
NSAID	Naproxen	Naprosyn, Aleve
NSAID	Meloxicam	Anjeso
NSAID	Celecoxib	Celebrex

OSTEOPOROSIS

Osteoporosis is defined as low bone mineral density that results in deterioration of bone tissue, bone fragility, and increased risk of bone fracture. Symptoms include bone pain, bone fractures, and loss of height. Risk factors for osteoporosis include being elderly, cigarette smoking, ethnicity (Caucasians and Asians are at higher risk), alcoholism, sex (females are at higher risk), family history, low calcium and/or vitamin D intake, and sedentary lifestyle. Certain medical conditions can also reduce bone density and lead to osteoporosis: acquired immunodeficiency syndrome, anorexia, hyperthyroidism, hyperparathyroidism, inflammatory bowel disease, type 1 diabetes mellitus, rheumatoid arthritis, chronic kidney disease, and COPD. In addition, some classes of medications can increase the risk of developing osteoporosis: anticonvulsants, glucocorticoids (steroids), long-term heparin therapy, high doses of thyroid hormone, hormonal antineoplastic agents, antivirals, antidepressants, and acid reducers.

Medications commonly used to treat **osteoporosis**:

Drug Classification	Generic Name	Brand Name
Bisphosphonate	Ibandronate	(None currently on the market)
Bisphosphonate	Risedronate	Actonel
Bisphosphonate	Alendronate	Fosamax
Calcium supplement	Calcium citrate	Citracal
Calcium supplement	Calcium carbonate	Tums
Estrogen receptor modulator	Raloxifene	Evista

Review Video: Osteoporosis
Visit mometrix.com/academy and enter code: 421205

GOUT

Gout is a disease caused by the buildup of uric acid in the joints. This leads to joint pain, inflammation, and swelling. Patients may also experience fever, chills, and general body aches. Gout occurs in about 1% of the population and is far more common in men. Gout usually attacks one joint at a time, and symptoms last for 1–2 weeks if left untreated. Commonly affected joints include the ankle, heel, knee, wrist, fingers, and elbow.

Uric acid is a product of the metabolism of ribose, a sugar that is found in RNA. Patients with gout should avoid foods that are high in ribose, including red meats, seafood, sugary drinks, processed foods, and alcohol.

Drug treatment of gout includes anti-inflammatory drugs to reduce joint pain and swelling, uricosuric agents that promote the excretion of excess uric acid in the urine, and xanthine oxidase inhibitors that stop the production of uric acid.

Drug Classification	Generic Name	Brand Name
Uricosuric drug	Probenecid	(None currently on the market)
Xanthine oxidase inhibitor	Allopurinol	Zyloprim, Aloprim
Xanthine oxidase inhibitor	Febuxostat	Uloric
Anti-inflammatory	Colchicine	Colcrys
Anti-inflammatory (NSAID)	Indomethacin	Indocin

PARKINSON'S DISEASE

Parkinson's disease (PD) is a chronic, progressive neuromuscular disorder in which the brain has difficulty communicating with the muscles. In PD, there is a progressive degeneration of cells in the brain that produce dopamine, a neurotransmitter that is involved in muscle movements. Therefore, drug treatments aim to replace or enhance the activity of dopamine.

The cause of PD is not fully known, although it is known to have genetic links as well as environmental risk factors, such as infection, trauma, and medication use. Antipsychotic medications usually act on dopamine and aim to block the effects of dopamine. Therefore, antipsychotic medications cause Parkinson-like side effects, which are usually reversible with discontinued use.

Symptoms of PD include tremors, muscle rigidity (stiffness), akinesia (an inability to initiate movement), bradykinesia (slowed movements), postural instability, abnormal gait (walk), difficulty standing, drooling, decreased blinking, dysphagia (difficulty swallowing), dysphasia (difficulty speaking), constipation, and urinary incontinence.

MEDICATIONS TREATING PD

One of the causes of PD is a reduction in the levels of dopamine in the brain. Dopamine is a neurotransmitter that is involved in muscle movement. Most drug treatments for PD aim to replace or enhance the effects of dopamine. Mechanisms of actions are as follows:

- **Dopaminergic drugs** mimic dopamine in the body by binding to and stimulating dopamine receptors.
- **MAO-B inhibitors** block an enzyme called monoamine oxidase type B that breaks down dopamine in the body. Preventing the breakdown of dopamine leads to an increase in dopamine levels.
- **Anticholinergic drugs** block the effects of acetylcholine, another neurotransmitter that is involved in muscle movements.

Drug Classification	Generic Name	Brand Name
Dopaminergic	Carbidopa-levodopa	Sinemet
Dopaminergic	Bromocriptine	Parlodel
Dopaminergic	Pramipexole	Mirapex ER
Dopaminergic	Rotigotine	Neupro (patch available)
MAO-B inhibitor	Selegiline	Eldepryl, Zelapar
MAO-B inhibitor	Rasagiline	Azilect
MAO-B inhibitor	Amantadine	Gocovri, Osmolex
Anticholinergic	Benztropine	Cogentin

ALZHEIMER'S DISEASE

Cholinesterase inhibitors are the recommended first line treatment of mild Alzheimer's disease (AD). One of the key neurological changes in AD is significantly reduced levels of the neurotransmitter acetylcholine. Cholinesterase inhibitors increase acetylcholine levels by blocking the enzyme acetylcholinesterase, which is responsible for breaking down acetylcholine. These drugs are usually started at a low dose and gradually titrated up to minimize side effects.

***N*-Methyl-D-aspartate (NMDA) receptor antagonists (blockers)** are used to treat moderate to severe cases of AD. *N*-Methyl-D-aspartate (NMDA) receptors release glutamate and are overactive in AD. The buildup of glutamate is one of the causes of neurological dysfunction and cell death in AD. NMDA receptor antagonists block the actions of NMDA receptors and reduce glutamate levels.

Drug Classification	Generic Name	Brand Name
Cholinesterase inhibitor	Donepezil	Aricept
Cholinesterase inhibitor	Rivastigmine	Exelon (patch is available)
Cholinesterase inhibitor	Galantamine	Razadyne
NMDA receptor antagonist	Memantine	Namenda

ATTENTION-DEFICIT/HYPERACTIVITY DISORDER

Attention-deficit/hyperactivity disorder (ADHD) is defined by a persistent pattern of inattention, hyperactivity, and/or impulsiveness that interferes with daily activities.

Stimulants are the first-line treatment for ADHD. Stimulants increase levels of dopamine in the brain, which is a neurotransmitter that is associated with attention, motivation, and pleasure. All of the stimulants used to treat ADHD are schedule II controlled substances with a high potential for abuse. Therefore, prescriptions cannot be received by telephone or fax and refills are not allowed. Stimulants can also be used to treat narcolepsy (daytime drowsiness) and are used by military pilots to maintain wakefulness.

Nonstimulants are used as a second-line treatment if stimulants have failed. These medications are prescription only but are not controlled substances.

Therapeutic Category	Generic Name	Brand Name
Stimulant	Methylphenidate	Ritalin, Methylin, Metadate, Concerta, Daytrana
Stimulant	Dexmethylphenidate	Focalin
Stimulant	Dextroamphetamine	Dexedrine
Stimulant	Lisdexamfetamine	Vyvanse
Stimulant	Dextroamphetamine-amphetamine	Adderall
Nonstimulant	Atomoxetine	Strattera
Nonstimulant	Guanfacine	Intuniv

MEDICATIONS TO PREVENT MIGRAINES

Patients who experience recurring migraines may be prescribed a preventative therapy to reduce the frequency of attacks and improve their responsiveness to on-demand treatments. Although the exact cause of migraine disorders is not known, there are genetic risk factors as well as known environmental triggers. Environmental triggers vary among individuals, but they often include weather or air pressure changes, bright lights, chemical fumes, hormonal changes during the menstrual cycle, and certain foods (e.g., red wine, beer, cheeses, etc.). Trigger avoidance is an important part of migraine prevention.

Medications that are normally used to treat hypertension or heart failure, such as beta-blockers and calcium channel blockers, have proven to be effective in preventing migraines. Drugs that act on the central nervous system (CNS), including antidepressants and anticonvulsant drugs, also play a role in migraine prevention.

Medications that are commonly prescribed to prevent migraines:

Drug Classification	Generic Name	Brand Name
Beta-blocker	Propranolol	Inderal
Beta-blocker	Metoprolol	Toprol, Lopressor
Beta-blocker	Atenolol	Tenormin
Antidepressant	Amitriptyline	Elavil
Antidepressant	Fluoxetine	Prozac
Calcium channel blocker	Diltiazem	Cartia, Cardizem
Calcium channel blocker	Verapamil	Calan SR
Anticonvulsant	Valproate	Depakene
Anticonvulsant	Gabapentin	Neurontin
Anticonvulsant	Topiramate	Topamax

DRUGS USED DURING MIGRAINE ATTACKS

Migraines are a severe form of headache associated with pain in the front and sides of the head (usually only one side of the head is affected), nausea, vomiting, and sensitivity to light and sound. Some patients also experience aural, visual, or sensory symptoms. There may also be prodromal symptoms that occur before the migraine begins, such as mood changes, fatigue, or neck pain.

- **Nonsteroidal anti-inflammatory drugs (NSAIDs)** help reduce some of the pain associated with headaches, although their ability to relieve migraine symptoms is limited.
- **Selective serotonin receptor agonists (triptans)** are taken on an as-needed basis at the first sign of a migraine. They start acting relatively quickly, within 10–60 minutes depending upon the drug. The potential adverse effects are relatively minor: dizziness, flushing, neck pain or stiffness, and fatigue. Triptans are available in a variety of dosage forms in order to get past the nausea and vomiting that many patients experience during a migraine, including orally disintegrating tablets, nasal sprays, transdermal patches, and infusions.

Therapeutic Classification	Generic Name	Brand Name
Triptan	Sumatriptan	Imitrex
Triptan	Eletriptan	Relpax
Triptan	Rizatriptan	Maxalt
Triptan	Zolmitriptan	Zomig
Triptan	Naratriptan	(None currently on the market)
NSAID	Ibuprofen	Motrin, Advil
NSAID	Naproxen	Naprosyn, Aleve

MEDICATIONS TO TREAT SEIZURE DISORDERS

Drugs used to treat epilepsy are referred to as antiepileptics or anticonvulsants. Epilepsy is notoriously difficult to treat, and not all patients respond to drug treatments. Antiepileptic medications are a diverse group of medications with many different mechanisms of action. Benzodiazepines (normally used to treat anxiety) may also be used to treat some seizure types. Each type of seizure disorder has a preferred drug regimen that involves the specific antiepileptic drugs that work best for that condition. Most patients will start out on the recommended first-line monotherapy (one-drug treatment), and a second adjunctive therapy will be added if the patient is not responding.

Medications commonly used to treat seizure disorders (epilepsy):

Generic Name	Brand Name
Phenytoin	Dilantin, Phenytek
Carbamazepine	Tegretol
Oxcarbazepine	Trileptal
Tiagabine	Gabitril
Ethosuximide	Zarontin
Phenobarbital	Sezaby
Primidone	Mysoline
Perampanel	Fycompa
Felbamate	Felbatol
Valproic acid/ Divalproex sodium	Depakote
Clobazam	Onfi
Eslicarbazepine	Aptiom
Ezogabine	(None currently on the market)
Vigabatrin	Sabril
Zonisamide	Zonegran
Lacosamide	Vimpat
Lamotrigine	Lamictal
Topiramate	Topamax
Levetiracetam	Keppra
Gabapentin	Neurontin
Pregabalin	Lyrica

GLAUCOMA DRUGS

Glaucoma is an eye condition characterized by increased pressure in the eye. Glaucoma is treated using eye drops that act locally and have minimal adverse effects.

Initial treatment is with either a **prostaglandin** drug (they end in "-prost") or a **beta-blocker** (they end in "-olol"). Prostaglandins stimulate drainage of fluid from the eye, and beta-blockers prevent the production of fluid. Prostaglandins are more popular because they are administered once daily at bedtime, whereas most beta-blockers are administered twice daily. Treatment is started with a single drug; additional drugs are added if required.

Second-line add-on treatments include **carbonic anhydrase inhibitors** (they end in "-zolamide") and **alpha-agonists** (they end in "-onidine"), which decrease the production of fluid in the eye. Most of these eye drops must be applied three times a day.

Drug Classification	Generic Name	Brand Name
Beta-blocker	Betaxolol	Betoptic
Beta-blocker	Timolol	Timoptic
Beta-blocker	Levobunolol	(None currently on the market)
Prostaglandin	Bimatoprost	Lumigan
Prostaglandin	Latanoprost	Xalatan
Prostaglandin	Travoprost	Travatan
Carbonic anhydrase inhibitor	Dorzolamide	(None currently on the market)
Carbonic anhydrase inhibitor	Brinzolamide	Azopt
Alpha-agonist	Brimonidine	Alphagan

OPHTHALMIC DROPS

Antibiotic eye drops are used to treat bacterial **eye infections**, such as conjunctivitis. Ciprofloxacin and gentamicin are available in eye drop form and are commonly prescribed to treat conjunctivitis.

Patients who experience **seasonal allergies** often use an antihistamine eye drop such as olopatadine to treat their symptoms.

Some anti-inflammatory medications are available in eye drop form to treat **eye inflammation**. Inflammation can occur in the eye due to infection or recent eye surgery. Corticosteroids, such as budesonide and prednisolone, and NSAIDs, such as flurbiprofen and ketorolac, are available in eye drop form for treating inflammation.

Dry eye is another condition for which patients seek treatment using eye drops. Most of these treatments contain harmless lubricants or saline, and most are available as OTC medications.

Drug Classification	Generic Name	Brand Name
Antibiotic	Ciprofloxacin	Ciloxan
Antibiotic	Gentamicin	Gentak
Antihistamine	Olopatadine	Pataday
Antihistamine	Azelastine	(None currently on the market)
Anti-inflammatory	Prednisolone	Pred Forte
Anti-inflammatory	Flurbiprofen	(None currently on the market)
Anti-inflammatory	Ketorolac	Acular
Eye lubricant	Propylene glycol	Systane

OTIC DROPS

Antibiotic ear drops are used to treat bacterial **ear infections**, such as swimmer's ear or otitis media. Common antibiotics used in the ear include ciprofloxacin, neomycin, and polymyxin b. If necessary, ophthalmic drops can also be administered into the ear.

Anti-inflammatory corticosteroid drugs are also available in otic form to treat **ear inflammation**. Because ear inflammation is usually associated with an infection, anti-inflammatory drugs are usually an ingredient in combination ear drops that also contain an antibiotic. Common drugs used to treat ear inflammation include dexamethasone and hydrocortisone.

Earwax buildup is another common condition for which patients seek treatment using ear drops. Most of these treatments contain a weak acid (e.g., acetic acid) or an oily substance that helps soften earwax and make it easier to remove. Many earwax softening treatments are available as OTC formulas.

Drug Classification	Generic Name	Brand Name
Antibiotic/anti-inflammatory	Ciprofloxacin, dexamethasone	Ciprodex
Antibiotic/anti-inflammatory	Neomycin, polymyxin b, hydrocortisone	(None currently on the market)
Ear wax softener	Acetic acid (vinegar)	Acetasol HC
Ear wax softener	Carbamide peroxide	Clinere

DRUGS USED TO TREAT BIPOLAR DISORDER

Bipolar disorder is a mood disorder characterized by alternating highs (mania) and lows (depression). Many **mood stabilizer drugs** were originally developed to treat epilepsy but were found to be effective in treating bipolar disorder as well. Most mood stabilizers have a narrow therapeutic index (a narrow safe dosage range), so extra monitoring and blood tests are often involved. Many of the drugs in this class also have the potential to cause serious side effects, such as increased risk of infection, electrolyte imbalances, birth defects, liver damage, and kidney damage. Mood stabilizers also interact with many other medications, so refer any computer alerts to a pharmacist.

Antipsychotic drugs have a long list of commonly experienced side effects. These include drowsiness, weight gain, orthostatic hypotension (dizziness upon standing), dry mouth, constipation, and urinary retention. Because they block dopamine, they also cause Parkinson-like side effects including involuntary muscle spasms (dystonia), restlessness, bradykinesia (slow movements), and tremors.

Examples of different classes of drugs used to treat **bipolar disorder**:

Drug Classification	Generic Name	Brand Name
Antipsychotic	Aripiprazole	Abilify
Antipsychotic	Risperidone	Risperdal
Antipsychotic	Quetiapine	Seroquel
Antipsychotic	Olanzapine	Zyprexa
Mood stabilizer	Lithium	Lithobid
Mood stabilizer	Lamotrigine	Lamictal
Mood stabilizer	Valproate	Epilim, Depakote
Mood stabilizer	Carbamazepine	Tegretol

SCHIZOPHRENIA TREATMENT AND ANTIPSYCHOTIC DRUGS

Schizophrenia is a psychological disorder associated with delusions, hallucinations, disorganized speech, personality and mood disorders, and behavioral symptoms. Overactivity of dopamine plays a major role in the disorder, so most **antipsychotic drug treatments** target and block dopamine. Because Parkinson's disease is characterized by a lack of dopamine, antipsychotic medications can cause Parkinson-like side effects, such as tremors, involuntary muscle spasms (dystonia), restlessness, and bradykinesia (slow movements). Older, conventional antipsychotics tend to have more Parkinson-like side effects. Newer, atypical antipsychotics have fewer Parkinson-like side effects and usually cause more significant weight gain, elevations in cholesterol levels, and hyperglycemia. Clozapine requires extra lab tests and monitoring as part of a REMS program because it causes a rare but serious side effect that reduces the body's ability to fight infection.

The generic and brand names of commonly prescribed antipsychotic drugs:

Generic Name	Brand Name
Aripiprazole	Abilify
Risperidone	Risperdal
Ziprasidone	Geodon
Quetiapine	Seroquel
Olanzapine	Zyprexa
Haloperidol	Haldol
Clozapine	Clozaril

Fluphenazine	(None currently on the market)
Lurasidone	Latuda
Asenapine	Saphris

ANTIDEPRESSANTS

Depression is characterized by low mood, fatigue, body aches, sleep disturbances, appetite changes, anxiety, and suicidal thoughts. Treatment usually involves a selective serotonin reuptake inhibitor (SSRI), serotonin-norepinephrine reuptake inhibitor (SNRI), or TCA, although antipsychotics and other classes of antidepressants can be used in resistant depression.

- **Tricyclic antidepressants (TCAs)** increase the concentration of serotonin and norepinephrine in the brain. They cause significant sedation, increased heart rate, hypotension, increased risk of arrhythmia, weight gain, sexual dysfunction, dry mouth, and urinary retention.
- **Selective serotonin reuptake inhibitors (SSRIs)** increase the concentration of serotonin in the brain. They are the most popular class of antidepressant because they are safer than other medications. Adverse effects are limited to headache, fatigue, insomnia, nausea, and sexual dysfunction.
- **Serotonin-norepinephrine reuptake inhibitors (SNRIs)** increase the concentration of serotonin and norepinephrine in the brain. Possible adverse effects are similar to those of SSRIs.

The generic and brand names of commonly prescribed antidepressants:

Drug Classification	Generic Name	Brand Name
TCA	Amitriptyline	Elavil
TCA	Nortriptyline	Pamelor
TCA	Doxepin	Silenor
TCA	Clomipramine	Anafranil
SSRI	Citalopram	Celexa
SSRI	Escitalopram	Lexapro
SSRI	Fluoxetine	Prozac
SSRI	Paroxetine	Paxil
SSRI	Sertraline	Zoloft
SNRI	Venlafaxine	Effexor
SNRI	Desvenlafaxine	Pristiq
SNRI	Duloxetine	Cymbalta

BENZODIAZEPINES AND HYPNOTICS

Benzodiazepines are a class of medication that enhances the action of gamma-aminobutyric acid, a neurotransmitter that relaxes the neurons. Benzodiazepines are used to treat a variety of conditions including anxiety, epilepsy, alcohol withdrawal, insomnia, obsessive-compulsive disorder, and post-traumatic stress. Due to their relaxing and euphoric effects, benzodiazepines have a high potential for abuse and are classified as schedule IV controlled substances. Long-term use is not recommended because tolerance develops quickly. Patients are encouraged to use these medications on an as-needed basis. Other adverse effects include significant sedation, dizziness, confusion, and blurred vision. Elderly patients should be particularly cautious because these adverse effects increase the risk of falls. Patients should also be advised not to take benzodiazepines with alcohol or opiate pain medications.

The **hypnotic Z-drugs** are benzodiazepine-like medications used to treat insomnia. They have similar side effects and are also schedule IV controlled substances. They include zolpidem, zopiclone, eszopiclone, and zaleplon.

The generic and brand names for commonly prescribed **benzodiazepines and hypnotics**:

Generic Name	Brand Name	Indications (Uses)
Alprazolam	Xanax	Anxiety, insomnia
Chlordiazepoxide	Librium	Alcohol withdrawal
Clonazepam	Klonopin	Anxiety
Diazepam	Valium	Anxiety
Lorazepam	Ativan	Anxiety
Temazepam	Restoril	Anxiety, insomnia
Triazolam	Halcion	Insomnia
Zolpidem	Ambien	Insomnia
Zaleplon	(None currently on the market)	Insomnia
Eszopiclone	Lunesta	Insomnia

HORMONE REPLACEMENT THERAPIES

After menopause, women experience a decline in estrogen levels. This causes menopausal symptoms such as hot flashes, vaginal dryness, and osteoporosis. Some women are placed on **estrogen hormone replacement therapy** to combat menopausal symptoms and reduce the risk of osteoporosis. However, estrogen replacement can cause adverse effects such as breast tenderness, acne, blood clots, and increased risk of breast cancer.

Men may require **testosterone hormone replacement therapy**. Symptoms of testosterone deficiency include decreased sexual desire and decreased energy. Testosterone replacement therapy may be prescribed to combat these symptoms. Side effects of testosterone replacement therapy include raised cholesterol levels, fluid retention, and liver failure. Testosterone also helps the body build muscle, so it is often abused by body builders. Therefore, testosterone products are schedule III controlled substances.

The generic and brand names for commonly prescribed hormone replacement therapies:

Generic Name	Brand Name
Testosterone	Androgel
Estradiol vaginal cream	Estrace
Estradiol pessary	Vagifem
Estradiol vaginal ring	Estring, Femring
Estradiol tablets	Estrace, Femtrace
Estradiol patch	Vivelle-Dot, Climara
Conjugated estrogens tablets and cream	Premarin
Estradiol/levonorgestrel patch	Climara Pro
Estradiol/norethindrone patch	CombiPatch
Estradiol/norethindrone tablets	Activella
Conjugated estrogen/medroxyprogesterone tablets	Prempro

COMBINED HORMONAL CONTRACEPTIVES

Combined oral contraceptives (COCs) contain an estrogen and a progesterone. COCs are available as daily tablets, once-weekly patches, and once-monthly vaginal rings. There are hundreds of oral COCs available on the market that contain different strengths and different forms of hormones in order to help women regulate their menstrual cycle.

Common adverse effects of COCs include breast tenderness, nausea, vomiting, headache, high blood pressure, weight gain, and breakthrough vaginal bleeding. The estrogens in COCs increase the risk of developing breast cancer and blood clots.

The different combined oral contraceptive (COC) products:

Dosage Form	Generic Name	Brand Names
Oral tablet	Ethinyl estradiol/ norethindrone	Loestrin, Necon, Nortrel, Ortho Novum
Oral tablet	Ethinyl estradiol/ levonorgestrel	Aviane, Levora, Trivora, Seasonique, Jolessa
Oral tablet	Ethinyl estradiol/ drospirenone	Yasmin, Ocella, Yaz
Oral tablet	Ethinyl estradiol/ norgestrel	Cryselle, Elinest, Low Ogestrel
Oral tablet	Ethinyl estradiol/ desogestrel	Apri, Cyred, Mircette, Pimtrea
Oral tablet	Ethinyl estradiol/ norgestimate	Estarylla, Mili, TriLinya
Patch	Ethinyl estradiol/ norelgestromin	Xulane, Zafemy
Vaginal ring	Ethinyl estradiol/ etonogestrel	NuvaRing

PROGESTERONE-ONLY CONTRACEPTIVES

Progesterone-only contraceptives (POCs) are safer than birth controls that contain estrogen because there is a lower risk of blood clot and breast cancer development. Additionally, POCs are safe to use in women who are breastfeeding, whereas estrogen-containing products are not. Common side effects of POCs include weight gain, irregular menstrual periods, acne, breast tenderness, fatigue, and depression.

Oral tablets should be taken daily at the same time each day for 21 days, followed by a 7-day tablet-free period during menstruation. With POCs, it is important that patients are compliant because missing a dose by 3 hours or more constitutes a missed dose. If a dose is missed, another form of contraceptive must be used for at least 2 days.

For patients who do not want to take a tablet every day, there are several more convenient formulations available. Long-acting **medroxyprogesterone injections** only need to be administered every 3 months. **Subdermal implants** are placed under the skin for up to 3 years, and **intrauterine devices** are effective for up to 5 years.

Dosage Form	Generic Name	Brand Name
Oral tablet	Norethindrone	Aygestin, Camila
Long-acting injection	Medroxyprogesterone	Depo-Provera
Implant/Subdermal injection	Etonogestrel	Nexplanon
Intrauterine device (IUD)	Levonorgestrel	Mirena

MEDICATIONS FOR URINARY SYSTEM DISORDERS

Classes medications that target the urinary system include:

- **Alpha-blockers**, such as tamsulosin and finasteride, improve urine flow in patients with benign prostatic hyperplasia or prostate enlargement. They relax the muscles of the prostate and bladder to alleviate the symptoms of urinary retention associated with prostate cancer. Common side effects include headache, hypotension, and erectile dysfunction.
- **Alpha-reductase inhibitors** block the conversion of testosterone into a molecule that contributes to prostate enlargement. These are used to treat urinary retention caused by prostate issues in patients where alpha-blockers have failed.
- **Anticholinergic drugs**, such as solifenacin and tolterodine, relax the bladder to treat symptoms of overactive bladder and urinary urgency.
- **Phosphodiesterase (PDE) inhibitors** (end in "-afil") are used to treat erectile dysfunction by increasing blood flow to the penis. Common side effects include headache and nausea. PDE inhibitors should not be used in combination with nitrate drugs that are used to treat chest pain.

The different classes of medications used to treat urinary system disorders, including prostate enlargement, overactive bladder, and erectile dysfunction:

Drug Classification	Generic Name	Brand Name
Alpha-blocker	Tamsulosin	Flomax
Alpha-blocker	Doxazosin	Cardura
Alpha-blocker	Terazosin	APO-Terazosin
Alpha-blocker	Alfuzosin	Uroxatral
Alpha-reductase inhibitor	Dutasteride	Avodart
Alpha-reductase inhibitor	Finasteride	Proscar
Anticholinergic	Solifenacin	Vesicare
Anticholinergic	Tolterodine	Detrol
Anticholinergic	Oxybutynin	Ditropan
PDE inhibitor	Sildenafil	Viagra
PDE inhibitor	Tadalafil	Cialis

CHILDHOOD VACCINATIONS

Childhood vaccination recommendations per CDC guidelines are as follows:

- The annual **influenza vaccine** (Afluria, Flulaval, Fluzone, Fluarix) is recommended for all children over 6 months old.
- The **DTaP vaccine** (Daptacel, Infanrix, Kinrix, Pediarix, Pentacel, Quadracel, Vaxelis) protects against diphtheria, tetanus, and pertussis (whooping cough). Infants receive initial doses starting at 6 weeks, or children 7 years and older receive the **Tdap vaccine** (Adacel or Boostrix) as a catch up vaccine. Children age 11 also receive the Tdap vaccine routinely.
- **Hepatitis B vaccination** (Engerix-B, Recombivax HB) and **hepatitis A vaccination** (Havrix, Vaqta) are recommended for infants or toddlers.
- **Haemophilus influenzae type B** (ActHIB) is recommended as part of routine childhood vaccinations.
- **Meningococcal vaccinations** defend against certain types of bacterial meningitis. The two different forms available in the US have different age recommendations (MenACWY for children 11–16 and MenB for children 16–18).
- **Measles, mumps, and rubella (MMR) vaccination** is recommended as part of routine childhood vaccinations, with one dose at 12–15 months and the second at 4–6 years.
- **Varicella (chicken pox) vaccination** (Varivax) is now routine for all children aged 12–15 months, and a booster is given at 4–6 years of age. This can also be given in conjunction with the measles, mumps, and rubella vaccination (MMRV).
- **Human papillomavirus vaccination** (Gardasil) helps protect against a common sexually transmitted disease that causes cervical cancer. Vaccination is recommended for males and females from ages 9–12.

ADULT VACCINATIONS

Adult vaccination recommendations per CDC guidelines are as follows:

- The annual **influenza vaccine** (Afluria, Flulaval, Fluzone, Fluarix) is recommended for all adults, especially those with a medical condition that puts them at increased risk for flu complications.
- **TDaP vaccine** protects against tetanus, diphtheria, and pertussis (whooping cough). Although initially administered during childhood, adults should receive a booster shot every 10 years as well as during pregnancy.
- **Hepatitis B vaccination** (Engerix-B, Recombivax HB) is recommended for all adults ages 19–59 and **hepatitis A vaccination** (Havrix, Vaqta) is only recommended to patients who are at high risk.
- **Meningococcal vaccination** (Menactra, Menveo, Trumenba, Bexsero) should be given to patients at high risk for exposure, including military service members, college students, travelers, and patients with a compromised immune system.
- **Pneumococcal vaccines** protect against various strains of Streptococcus pneumoniae bacteria. Patients over the age of 65 should receive both pneumococcal vaccines, Pneumovax-23 and Prevnar-13, spaced 1 year apart.
- **Herpes zoster vaccines** (Shingrix) protect against shingles, a painful condition in which the virus attacks the nerves. It usually occurs in elderly patients or those who are immunocompromised. Shingles is caused by the same varicella virus that causes chicken pox, but it presents with different symptoms once it is reactivated. Vaccination is recommended in adults over the age of 50 and patients with reduced immunity.

VACCINES

Vaccinations work by taking advantage of our body's acquired immune system. After exposure to a pathogen (a harmful virus or bacteria), our body remembers that specific pathogen and produces specific cells that fight off the infection quickly if we encounter that same pathogen again. A vaccination is the first exposure that signals the body to produce immune cells against the pathogen and prevents us from getting ill from that pathogen in the future. Common side effects of vaccines include redness, swelling, and pain at the injection site. Patients may also experience fever and soreness at the site of injection.

- **Live vaccines** contain the actual pathogen, but it has been attenuated or made to be less harmful. Most patients do not get ill from live vaccines, but patients who have a compromised immune system might. Therefore, live vaccines should not be administered to certain groups of patients: pregnant women, patients receiving chemotherapy, patients who have had an organ transplant in the past, patients taking medications that lower their immune response, and HIV patients. Vaccinations that are live include Varivax, Zostavax, MMR, yellow fever vaccine, and typhoid vaccine.
- **Inactivated vaccines** contain parts of a pathogen, which are not disease-causing. Immunocompromised patients can receive inactivated vaccines.

CARDIOVASCULAR DRUGS

Cardiovascular medications are among the most commonly prescribed drugs. They are used to treat hypertension (high blood pressure), hyperlipidemia (high cholesterol), blood clots, angina (chest pain), and heart arrhythmias.

Generic Name	Brand Name
Antihypertensives	
Lisinopril	Zestril
Lisinopril/hydrochlorothiazide	Zestoretic
Metoprolol	Lopressor
Amlodipine	Norvasc
Furosemide	Lasix
Atenolol	Tenormin
Carvedilol	Coreg
Losartan	Cozaar
Losartan/hydrochlorothiazide	Hyzaar
Tamsulosin	Flomax
Propranolol	Inderal
Spironolactone	Aldactone
Triamterene/hydrochlorothiazide	Maxzide
Valsartan	Diovan
Valsartan/hydrochlorothiazide	Diovan HCT
Antihypertensives	
Enalapril	Vasotec
Amlodipine/benazepril	Lotrel
Benazepril	Lotensin
Clonidine	Catapres
Hydralazine	Apresoline
Ramipril	Altace
Nifedipine	Procardia XL

Generic Name	Brand Name
Olmesartan	Benicar
Nebivolol	Bystolic
Doxazosin	Cardura
Irbesartan	Avapro
Terazosin	APO-Terazosin
Chlorthalidone	Thalitone
Guanfacine	Intuniv
Antihyperlipidemics	
Atorvastatin	Lipitor
Simvastatin	Zocor
Rosuvastatin	Crestor
Lovastatin	Altoprev
Fenofibrate	Tricor
Ezetimibe	Zetia
Gemfibrozil	Lopid
Omega-3 acid	Lovaza
Blood Thinners (Antiplatelets and Anticoagulants)	
Aspirin	Bayer
Clopidogrel	Plavix
Warfarin	Coumadin
Rivaroxaban	Xarelto
Apixaban	Eliquis
Enoxaparin	Lovenox
Angina Drugs (Nitrates and Calcium Channel Blockers)	
Nitroglycerin	Nitrostat
Isosorbide mononitrate	Imdur
Diltiazem	Cardizem
Verapamil	Calan SR
Antiarrhythmics	
Amiodarone	Nexterone

MEDICATIONS FOR ENDOCRINE SYSTEM DISORDERS

Endocrine system disorder drugs include antihyperglycemic treatments for diabetes, contraceptives, hormone replacement therapies, hormonal cancer treatments, treatments for thyroid disorders, and corticosteroid hormones that are used to treat a wide range of inflammatory conditions. The brand names and generic names of the top medications used to treat **endocrine system disorders**:

Generic Name	Brand Name
Antihyperglycemics	
Metformin	Glucophage
Glipizide	Glucotrol
Glimepiride	Amaryl
Sitagliptin	Januvia
Sitagliptin/metformin	Janumet
Glyburide	Glynase
Pioglitazone	Actos

Generic Name	Brand Name
Canagliflozin	Invokana
Insulin lispro	Humalog
Insulin glargine	Lantus
Insulin detemir	Levemir
Insulin aspart	Novolog
Insulin regular	Humulin
Liraglutide	Victoza
Corticosteroid Hormones (Anti-inflammatory, Bronchodilators)	
Fluticasone inhaler	Flovent
Budesonide inhaler	Pulmicort
Fluticasone/salmeterol inhaler	Advair
Budesonide/formoterol inhaler	Symbicort
Methylprednisolone	Solu-Medrol, Medrol
Prednisone	Prednisone Intensol, Rayos
Prednisolone	Millpred
Hydrocortisone	Cortef
Clobetasol propionate cream	Clobex
Triamcinolone cream	Kenalog
Mometasone nasal spray	Propel
Contraceptives (Birth Control)	
Ethinyl estradiol/norethindrone	Estrostep. Loestrin
Ethinyl estradiol/levonorgestrel	Altavera, Levonest
Ethinyl estradiol/drospirenone	Ocella, Yasmin
Ethinyl estradiol/norgestimate	Mili, Monolinyah
Ethinyl estradiol/desogestrel	Apri
Ethinyl estradiol/etonogestrel vaginal ring	NuvaRing
Postmenopausal Hormone Replacement Therapy	
Estradiol vaginal ring	Estring
Conjugated estrogens	Premarin
Hormonal Anticancer Drugs	
Anastrozole	Arimidex
Male Hormone Replacement Therapy	
Testosterone	Andriol, Androgel
Antiandrogens (to Treat Prostate Enlargement and Pattern Baldness)	
Finasteride	Proscar
Thyroid Hormone Replacements	
Levothyroxine	Synthroid, Levoxyl

MEDICATIONS FOR NEUROLOGICAL DISORDERS

The top medications used to treat neurological disorders:

Generic Name	Brand Name
Antidepressants	
Sertraline	Zoloft
Fluoxetine	Prozac
Citalopram	Celexa
Trazodone	APO-Trazadone, TEVA-Trazodone

Generic Name	Brand Name
Bupropion	Wellbutrin
Escitalopram	Lexapro
Duloxetine	Cymbalta
Venlafaxine	Effexor
Paroxetine	Paxil
Amitriptyline	Elavil
Mirtazapine	Remeron
Antipsychotics	
Quetiapine	Seroquel
Divalproex	Depakote
Risperidone	Risperdal
Aripiprazole	Abilify
Lithium	Lithobid
ADHD Treatments	
Dextroamphetamine and amphetamine	Adderall
Methylphenidate	Ritalin
Lisdexamfetamine	Vyvanse
Atomoxetine	Strattera
Stimulants Used for Weight Loss	
Phentermine	Lomaira, Adipex-P
Muscle Relaxers	
Cyclobenzaprine	Amrix, Fexmid
Tizanidine	Zanaflex
Baclofen	Lioresal
Carisoprodol	Soma
Methocarbamol	Robaxin
Antiparkinsonian drugs	
Ropinirole	Requip
Pramipexole	Mirapex ER
Antiepileptics	
Gabapentin	Neurontin
Lamotrigine	Lamictal
Topiramate	Topamax
Pregabalin	Lyrica
Levetiracetam	Keppra
Phenytoin	Dilantin
Oxcarbazepine	Trileptal
Divalproex	Depakote
Sedatives/Antianxiety Drugs	
Alprazolam	Xanax
Clonazepam	Klonopin
Zolpidem	Ambien
Lorazepam	Ativan
Diazepam	Valium
Buspirone	Buspar
Temazepam	Restoril

Generic Name	Brand Name
Alzheimer's Drugs	
Memantine	Namenda
Donepezil	Aricept
Analgesics	
Acetaminophen	Tylenol
Acetaminophen/hydrocodone	Lortab
Tramadol	Conzip, Qdolo
Ibuprofen	Motrin, Advil
Meloxicam	Anjeso
Oxycodone	Oxycontin
Naproxen	Aleve
Hydrocodone	Hysingla ER
Diclofenac	Cambia
Celecoxib	Celebrex
Morphine	Duramorph, Infumorph
Lidocaine	Xylocaine
Migraine Treatments	
Sumatriptan	Imitrex

Analgesics are pain relievers. These include Tylenol, NSAIDs, and opioids. Many antiepileptic drugs can also be used as analgesics to relieve nerve pain.

DRUGS FOR INFECTIONS AND RESPIRATORY DISORDERS

The top drugs used to treat infections and respiratory disorders:

Generic Name	Brand Name
Antibiotics	
Amoxicillin	APO-Amoxi, Novamoxin
Azithromycin	Zithromax
Sulfamethoxazole/trimethoprim	Bactrim
Amoxicillin/clavulanate potassium	Augmentin
Bacitracin/neomycin/polymyxin B cream	Neosporin
Ciprofloxacin	Cipro
Cephalexin	(None currently on the market)
Doxycycline	Doryx
Clindamycin	Cleocin
Levofloxacin	Levaquin
Metronidazole	Flagyl
Nitrofurantoin	Macrobid
Antivirals	
Acyclovir	(None currently on the market)
Valacyclovir	Valtrex
Antifungals	
Fluconazole	Diflucan
Bronchodilators	
Albuterol inhaler	Ventolin, ProAir, Proventil
Tiotropium inhaler	Spiriva
Albuterol/ipratropium nebulized, inhaled	Combivent

Generic Name	Brand Name
Fluticasone/salmeterol inhaler	Advair
Budesonide/formoterol inhaler	Symbicort
Oral Antiasthma Drugs	
Montelukast	Singulair
Antihistamines	
Loratadine	Claritin
Cetirizine	Zyrtec
Hydroxyzine	Vistaril
Promethazine	Phenergan
Meclizine	Bonine
Antitussives	
Benzonatate	(None currently on the market)

Anti-infectives include antibiotics, antivirals, and antifungals. Bronchodilators are used to treat asthma and COPD. Antihistamines can be used to relieve the respiratory symptoms of respiratory illnesses and seasonal allergies, such as runny nose, congestion, watery eyes, and nasal congestion. Some antihistamines, such as meclizine, can also be used to relieve nausea and vomiting. Antitussives are used to relieve cough.

> **Review Video: Antibiotics: An Overview**
> Visit mometrix.com/academy and enter code: 165628

DRUGS FOR ULCERATIVE COLITIS, URINARY INCONTINENCE, AND IRRITABLE BOWEL SYNDROME

The most common vitamins/supplements and drugs used to treat gastrointestinal and urinary conditions:

Generic Name	Brand Name
Ulcerative Colitis Drugs	
Mesalamine	Pentasa
Urinary Incontinence Drugs	
Oxybutynin	Ditropan
Solifenacin	Vesicare
Irritable Bowel Syndrome Drugs	
Dicyclomine	Bentyl

Urinary incontinence drugs relax the bladder muscles and treat urinary urgency. Drugs used to treat irritable bowel syndrome help reduce stomach cramping by relaxing the muscles in the intestines.

DIURETIC MEDICATIONS

Diuretics are medications that promote the excretion of water from the body in the urine. They are used to treat high blood pressure (hypertension) and edema (swelling). There are three main classes of diuretics: thiazide diuretics, loop diuretics, and potassium-sparing diuretics.

- **Thiazide diuretics** promote the excretion of sodium and water by the kidney, allowing more water to leave the body in the urine. Thiazide diuretics are not very potent, but they can be combined with other diuretics for an additive effect. The most commonly prescribed thiazide diuretic is hydrochlorothiazide.

- **Loop diuretics** also promote the excretion of sodium and water in the urine, but they act on a different part of the kidney than thiazide diuretics. Loop diuretics act quickly and are far more potent than thiazide diuretics. Commonly prescribed loop diuretics include furosemide (Lasix) and bumetanide (Bumex).
- Because diuretics promote the excretion of water and electrolytes from the body, one of their main side effects is hypokalemia (low potassium). **Potassium-sparing diuretics** do not cause hypokalemia like other diuretics do, so they are often used in combination with another class of diuretic to help prevent low potassium levels. Potassium-sparing diuretics include amiloride, triamterene (Dyrenium), and spironolactone (Aldactone).

Review Video: Diuretics
Visit mometrix.com/academy and enter code: 373276

Therapeutic Equivalence

Therapeutic equivalence means that a medication is equivalent to or substitutable for another. Equivalent medications have the same active ingredients, the same efficacy, and the same safety profile. These medications must also be equivalent in their dosage form (e.g., tablet, cream, patch, injection) and the way in which the body is able to absorb it (bioavailability).

A pharmaceutical example of therapeutic equivalence is generic substitution. If the doctor prescribes a branded product for a patient, the patient can choose to have any of the cheaper generic versions dispensed instead. In order to legally substitute the product, the medications must be determined to be therapeutically equivalent and must be approved by the FDA. The FDA's *Approved Drug Products with Therapeutic Equivalence Evaluations* (commonly known as the *Orange Book*) contains an official list of therapeutically equivalent products, although the pharmacy computer system will alert you if you try to substitute a product that is not therapeutically equivalent.

For example, Lasix 40 mg tablets (brand name) is equivalent to furosemide 40 mg tablets made by any generic manufacturer. The generic versions of diltiazem solution for injection in the picture are therapeutically equivalent.

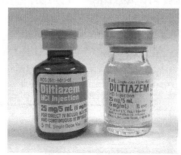

Common and Life-Threatening Drug Interactions and Contraindications

Common drug interactions include:

Interaction	Description	Example
Drug-disease	A drug interacts with or interferes with an existing medical condition.	Pseudoephedrine increases blood pressure and is not recommended in patients who have high blood pressure (aka hypertension).
Drug-drug	The effects of one drug are changed when taken in combination with another drug.	Enalapril and amlodipine are both antihypertensive medications. When taken together, the patient's blood pressure will be lower than if the medications were taken separately.
Drug-supplement	A supplement or vitamin interferes with the way a drug acts or is absorbed.	Calcium supplements decrease the absorption of many medications, such as tetracycline. Potassium supplements reduce the effectiveness of the blood thinner warfarin.
Drug-food	The effects of a drug are changed when taken in combination with a particular food.	Grapefruit juice decreases the ability of statin drugs to be metabolized (broken down).
Drug-nutrient	A drug affects the way that the body absorbs, uses, or excretes a nutrient.	Diuretics, such as furosemide, increase the amount of potassium excreted in the urine.
Drug-laboratory	A drug alters the results of a laboratory test.	Corticosteroids, such as prednisone and dexamethasone, can elevate blood glucose levels.

ANTICOAGULANTS AND ANTIPLATELETS

Because blood thinners prevent blood clotting, their main side effect is bleeding. Combining multiple blood thinners increases bleeding risk and should be avoided. Patients should watch for stomach pain or black tarry stools, which indicate gastrointestinal bleeding. Signs and symptoms of a head bleed would be sudden headache, nausea, vomiting, blurred vision, weakness or numbness on one side of the body, or difficulty speaking. Patients taking blood thinners are also at a higher risk of having nosebleeds and excessive bleeding from minor scrapes and bruises.

Patients taking a blood thinner should avoid OTC aspirin and NSAIDs (ibuprofen, naproxen) because these medications can also thin the blood. The pharmacist should examine the patient's profile for any drug interactions that may put them at a higher risk for bleeding. Particular caution should be taken when dispensing warfarin because it is involved in many drug interactions that can increase the patient's risk of bleeding. Warfarin interacts with many antibiotics, antifungals, antiarrhythmics, statins, and antiepileptic medications. Patients taking warfarin should also avoid eating a lot of green leafy vegetables that are high in vitamin K.

ANTIEPILEPTIC MEDICATIONS

Common side effects of antiepileptic drugs include anxiety, suicidal thoughts, memory and concentration impairment, blurred vision, nausea, vomiting, dry mouth, skin rashes, headache, fatigue, drowsiness, and dizziness. Carbamazepine and oxcarbazepine can cause a rare but serious side effect called neutropenia, which hinders the body's ability to fight infection. Divalproex and valproic acid are teratogenic, meaning that if they are taken during pregnancy, they can cause birth defects. Some anticonvulsants, such as ezogabine, increase the risk of heart arrythmias. Gabapentin, pregabalin, and levetiracetam are associated with fewer adverse effects and fewer drug interactions.

Common drug interactions include diuretics, metformin, lithium, blood thinners, rifampin, digoxin, antidepressants, statins, and other antiepileptics. Carbamazepine, phenytoin, fosphenytoin, primidone, and phenobarbital tend to speed up the metabolism of other medications and reduce their effectiveness. This is of particular concern when used in combination with warfarin, lithium, digoxin, and other antiepileptic medications. Many seizure medications reduce the effectiveness of hormonal birth control, so a nonhormonal birth control method, such as an IUD, should be recommended instead.

ANALGESICS

Analgesics include acetaminophen, NSAIDs, and opioids.

- **Acetaminophen** is metabolized in the liver and therefore should be used judiciously in individuals with hepatic disease or a compromised liver.
- **NSAIDs** can thin the blood and increase bleeding risk. Therefore, they should not be administered to patients with stomach ulcers or patients taking other anticoagulants. NSAIDs can worsen asthma symptoms and should be avoided in asthmatic patients. They can also worsen renal failure and cause fluid retention, so patients with renal failure or heart failure should avoid NSAIDs. NSAIDs interact with diuretics, blood thinners, ACE inhibitors, methotrexate, and lithium.
- **Opioids** relax the bowel muscles and slow digestion. Therefore, they are contraindicated in patients with intestinal disorders or infection, including ulcerative colitis and *Clostridium difficile*. Opioids work on the nervous system and cause central nervous system (CNS) depression. Therefore, they interact with other nervous system drugs, including antipsychotics and alcohol. If used in combination, adverse effects such as sedation and confusion can be made worse. Elderly patients should be more cautious because they are more prone to the sedative effects.

CARDIOVASCULAR DRUGS

Drug interactions associated with common cardiovascular drugs include:

- **Beta-blockers** are contraindicated in patients with asthma because these drugs can cause airway constriction. They should also be avoided in diabetics because they can mask the symptoms of hypoglycemia. Beta-blockers should also be avoided during pregnancy. Drug interactions include verapamil, diltiazem, amiodarone, clonidine, and digoxin.
- **Angiotensin-converting enzyme (ACE) inhibitors** are contraindicated in pregnant women and patients with severe renal impairment. NSAIDs also cause renal impairment, so avoid using both drugs together. Because ACE inhibitors can raise potassium levels (hyperkalemia), they interact with other medications that raise potassium levels, including some diuretics.
- **Calcium channel blockers** should be avoided during pregnancy. They interact with digoxin, cyclosporine, and grapefruit juice. Verapamil and diltiazem should be avoided in heart failure, and they interact with beta-blockers and statins.

- **Diuretics** enhance the excretion of water and electrolytes in the urine. Therefore, they can cause electrolyte imbalances. They should be avoided in patients with gout. They interact with lithium, digoxin, NSAIDs, ACE inhibitors, and diabetes drugs. Triamterene interacts with methotrexate and phenytoin.
- **Nitrates**, such as nitroglycerin, interact with erectile dysfunction drugs, such as sildenafil (Viagra). Both medications lower blood pressure, so combined used can cause severe hypotension.

STATINS

HMG CoA reductase inhibitors, more commonly known as statins, are used to treat high cholesterol. They should be avoided in pregnant women as well as in patients with liver failure because they are broken down in the liver.

Statins interact with warfarin, fibrates, HIV antivirals, cyclosporine, and macrolide antibiotics. Statin drugs can increase the effects of the anticoagulant warfarin and increase the risk of bleeding. More frequent warfarin monitoring and blood tests should be done when patients are taking both drugs together. Gemfibrozil and fenofibrate (fibrate drugs also used to treat high cholesterol) can increase the levels of statin drugs in the body and increase the risk of getting muscle symptoms (myopathy). HIV antivirals, cyclosporine, and macrolide antibiotics also increase statin levels and increase the risk of myopathy. Statin drugs should be withheld while completing a course of treatment with macrolide antibiotics because the risk outweighs the benefits. The statin can be resumed once the short course of antibiotics is completed.

Statins are also involved in a drug-food interaction with grapefruit juice that increases the risk of myopathy. Grapefruit juice should be avoided in patients taking statins.

ANTIBIOTICS

A thorough allergy history should be taken before dispensing antibiotics to a patient. If a patient has a penicillin allergy, they should avoid penicillin antibiotics as well as cephalosporins and carbapenem antibiotics due to a high risk of cross-reactivity.

Many antibiotics are contraindicated during pregnancy: vancomycin, tetracyclines, gentamicin, Bactrim, and metronidazole. Quinolone antibiotics (e.g., ciprofloxacin, levofloxacin) are contraindicated in epilepsy. Tetracyclines should not be given to children. Alcohol use should be avoided with any antibiotic, but it is particularly important to avoid alcohol when taking metronidazole to avoid a serious adverse effect.

Most antibiotics increase the effects of warfarin, so extra monitoring is required throughout the course of antibiotic use. Antibiotics can also reduce the effectiveness of contraceptives, so another birth control method should be used during antibiotic use. Some antibiotics, including tetracyclines and quinolones, cannot be taken with milk, antacids, or vitamins. Vancomycin and gentamicin interact with furosemide and cyclosporine. Macrolide antibiotics, such as erythromycin and clarithromycin, interact with statins. The statin drug should be withheld during antibiotic treatment. Bactrim should be avoided in patients taking methotrexate or phenytoin. The tuberculosis treatment rifampicin interacts with and reduces the effectiveness of many other drugs.

ANTIVIRALS AND ANTIFUNGALS

Most antiviral and antifungal drugs are metabolized in the liver, so they require dosage adjustments or avoidance in patients with liver impairment.

HIV antiviral drugs are involved in numerous significant drug interactions. Most antivirals increase the actions of other medications, making patients more prone to adverse effects. Some medications involved in this interaction include antihistamines, benzodiazepines, calcium channel blockers, antiepileptics, corticosteroids, statins, warfarin, and macrolide antibiotics. In contrast, protease antivirals (e.g., ritonavir) reduce the effectiveness of hormonal birth control, so women should be advised to use condoms or an IUD instead.

Antifungal drugs are also metabolized in the liver and are contraindicated in liver failure. Many antifungals increase the effects of other medications, making patients more prone to adverse effects. Ketoconazole should not be taken with antacids or alcohol. Amphotericin is a potent intravenous (IV) antifungal that can cause electrolyte imbalances, so caution should be taken when it is used in combination with diuretics, corticosteroids, or digoxin.

DIABETES TREATMENTS

Diet has a huge impact on diabetes and blood glucose levels. Most diabetics are well trained on what foods to avoid and how to alter their insulin injections according to the carbohydrates they eat. Diabetics should also be counseled on the effects of alcohol on insulin. Alcohol increases the effects of insulin and lowers blood glucose levels, putting the patient at greater risk of hypoglycemia (blood sugar levels that are too low). Diabetics should avoid alcohol, but if they do drink, they should inject less insulin or eat more carbohydrates.

Insulin interacts with oral sulfonylurea antidiabetic drugs, so this combination should be avoided. The effects of insulin and oral antidiabetic drugs are reduced by corticosteroids and diuretics. Most oral antidiabetic medications should be avoided in pregnancy and severe hepatic impairment. The glitazones can worsen heart failure and should be avoided in patients with cardiac issues. Metformin should be avoided in renal impairment, and it interacts with other drugs that cause kidney impairment (e.g., NSAIDs).

PARKINSON'S DISEASE AND ALZHEIMER'S DISEASE TREATMENTS

Parkinson's disease (PD) is defined by low dopamine levels, so most treatment options aim to boost dopamine levels. Antipsychotic drugs do the opposite. They lower dopamine levels to prevent the symptoms of psychosis that are associated with high levels of dopamine. Therefore, antipsychotic medications should not be given to patients with PD. Anticholinergic medications are indicated in the treatment of Parkinsonian tremors by blocking acetylcholine. Metoclopramide, an anti-nausea medication, should be avoided in Parkinson's disease as it can worsen Parkinsonian tremors. Most PD drugs lower blood pressure, so they enhance the effects of antihypertensive medications. Caution should be used in patients with cardiac disease and elderly patients who are more prone to falls.

Alzheimer's disease (AD) drugs aim to increase acetylcholine levels. Therefore, they interact with anticholinergic medications that block acetylcholine. TCAs, antipsychotics, antiepileptics, irritable bowel syndrome drugs, and drugs used to treat urinary incontinence are anticholinergic and interact with AD treatments. If taken in combination, these medications can increase confusion, dizziness, fall risk, and the risk of cardiac symptoms.

ANXIETY AND INSOMNIA TREATMENTS

All psychological drugs interact with alcohol, opioids, and antihistamines. Profound sedation occurs when these drugs are combined, and elderly patients are particularly sensitive to these interactions.

- **Antidepressants** increase the risk of seizure, so they should be avoided in epilepsy or with antiepileptic drugs. Additionally, antidepressants are contraindicated in cardiac disease because they can cause significant hypotension and increase the risk of arrhythmias. Antidepressants should be avoided in patients with bipolar disorder. Monoamine oxidase inhibitors are a class of antidepressant that are rarely used today because they are involved in a wide range of drug-drug and drug-food interactions.
- **Antipsychotics** should be avoided in patients with cardiac arrhythmias, liver impairment, epilepsy, PD, and hypotension. They interact with anti-Parkinson's drugs, antihypertensives, antiepileptics, antidepressants, and lithium.
- **Sedatives** include the benzodiazepines and Z-drugs used to treat anxiety and insomnia. Tolerance develops quickly with these schedule IV medications, and the potential for abuse is high. They should only be used short-term or for sporadic use.

INHALED MEDICATIONS FOR ASTHMA AND COPD

Asthma and chronic obstructive pulmonary disease (COPD) are respiratory conditions in which the airway is inflamed, constricted, and blocked. Treatments for these conditions are similar and involve using inhalers and nebulizers to deliver drugs locally into the lungs. Drug classes used in inhaled treatments include bronchodilators (beta-agonists and antimuscarinics) to open the airway and corticosteroids to reduce inflammation. Although these drugs are delivered to the lungs, some systemic effects are possible.

Beta agonists stimulate the sympathetic immune system, so they can raise blood pressure, raise heart rate, and cause arrhythmias. Caution should be taken in patients with cardiac disease. Drug interactions include antihypertensives, antiarrhythmics, and sympathomimetics (e.g., pseudoephedrine).

Antimuscarinic bronchodilators have anticholinergic effects that can be enhanced when combined with other anticholinergic drugs, such as urinary incontinence drugs. In the treatment of respiratory disorders, the use of multiple antimuscarinic drugs should be avoided.

Asthmatic patients should avoid the use of NSAIDs (e.g., ibuprofen) because it can worsen asthma symptoms.

THERAPEUTIC CONTRAINDICATION

A therapeutic contraindication is a specific situation or condition in which a drug should not be administered because it may increase the risk of causing harm to the patient. A contraindication is usually a disease state, patient group, or medical diagnosis. For example, if a drug is contraindicated in hypertension, that means that patients with hypertension (high blood pressure) should not use that drug.

Many drugs are contraindicated in pregnancy, including tetracyclines, vancomycin, ACE inhibitors, NSAIDs, and lithium. Another common contraindication is advanced age (elderly patients). Extra caution should be taken when antidepressants, antihistamines, antipsychotics, and sedatives are used in elderly patients because they are at increased risk of experiencing side effects. Other examples of common contraindications to drug treatments include alcohol use, liver (hepatic) impairment, kidney(renal) impairment, hypertension, asthma, cardiac arrhythmias, epilepsy, PD, childhood, electrolyte imbalances, immune disorders, and active infection.

MEDICATIONS THAT ARE CONTRAINDICATED IN ELDERLY PATIENTS

Elderly patients have a reduced ability to metabolize (break down) medications and are generally more susceptible to adverse effects. Many elderly patients have a reduced ability to excrete drugs via the kidneys, which can increase the risk of toxicity and kidney damage. Drugs that cause sedation can lead to delirium and confusion in elderly patients as well as increase their risk of falling and fracturing a bone.

The different types of medications that are contraindicated in elderly patients:

Drug Classification	Examples	Concern
Antihistamines	Benadryl, hydroxyzine, promethazine	Increased sedation can lead to delirium and falls.
Antispasmodics/ Anticholinergics	Dicyclomine, oxybutynin	
TCAs	Amitriptyline, nortriptyline, doxepin	
Muscle relaxants	Cyclobenzaprine, carisoprodol, methocarbamol	
Benzodiazepines	Alprazolam, lorazepam, diazepam	
Hypnotics (Z-drugs)	Zolpidem, zaleplon, zopiclone	
Antipsychotics	Haloperidol, olanzapine, quetiapine, risperidone	Increased risk of stroke.
Antihypertensives (alpha-blockers and centrally acting agents)	Doxazosin, prazosin, terazosin, clonidine	Increased risk of hypotension and orthostatic hypotension, which may lead to falls.
Cardiac glycosides	Digoxin	Increased risk of toxicity.
NSAIDs	Ibuprofen, naproxen, aspirin	Increased bleeding risk. Increased risk of kidney damage.

TERATOGENICITY AND MEDICATIONS THAT ARE CONTRAINDICATED IN PREGNANT WOMEN

Teratogenicity is the ability of a drug to be toxic to a fetus/embryo and lead to birth defects. Teratogenicity is an adverse effect of some medications that are contraindicated in pregnancy.

The following types of medications can be teratogenic: isotretinoin, thalidomide and its derivatives, ACE inhibitors, anticoagulants (e.g., warfarin), estrogens, androgens (e.g., testosterone), antiepileptics drugs (e.g., carbamazepine, phenytoin, phenobarbital, sodium valproate), medications used to treat hyperthyroidism (e.g., methimazole, carbimazole, radioactive iodine), lithium, NSAIDs, tetracycline antibiotics, sulfa antibiotics (e.g., Bactrim), ciprofloxacin, anticancer agents (e.g., cyclophosphamide, methotrexate), some oral antidiabetic drugs, vitamin A supplements, and alcohol.

Isotretinoin (Accutane) and thalidomide derivatives (Thalomid) have particularly profound birth defects when used during pregnancy. Because of their teratogenicity, these drugs are required by the FDA to participate in a Risk Evaluation and Mitigation Strategy (REMS) program. These REMS programs require documentation of at least two contraceptive methods and monthly pregnancy testing for women of childbearing potential.

Dosage Forms and Routes of Administration

DOSAGE FORMS OF MEDICATIONS

Medications come in a variety of forms making them available and distributed throughout the body at different rates:

- **Tablets**: A compressed powder is administered orally (swallowed).
- **Sublingual or orally dissolving tablets**: A compressed powder tablet is placed under the tongue and left to dissolve (NOT swallowed).
- **Capsules:** A powder or liquid within a gelatin coating (capsules) is administered orally (swallowed).
- **Solutions**: Medication is dissolved in a water-based liquid and administered orally (swallowed).
- **Suspensions:** Medication is suspended in a liquid (NOT dissolved) and must be shaken before use to get an accurate dose. It is administered orally (swallowed).
- **Transdermal patches**: A patch is placed on the skin, and medication diffuses through the patch and the skin and into the bloodstream.
- **Suppositories**: Medication is incorporated into a waxy solid capsule that dissolves when exposed to body temperature. Can be inserted into the rectum, vagina, or urethra.
- **Ointments**: Oily semisolid preparation containing medication. They are applied topically.
- **Creams**: Water-based semisolid preparation containing medication. They are applied topically.
- **Inhalations:** Medication is either dissolved in a liquid and sprayed into the mouth (metered-dose inhalers), or the medication is compressed into powder particles and inhaled (dry powder inhalers [DPIs]).
- **Injections:** Medication is dissolved in a sterile (no bacteria), water-based liquid and can be injected into the body.

ORAL MEDICATION ADMINISTRATION

Most medications are administered orally because it is convenient and relatively inexpensive. However, oral absorption of a drug can take a long time because it must pass through the digestive tract. Absorption can also be unpredictable and is dependent upon what is in the digestive tract (drug-food interactions). Some medications are absorbed better on an empty stomach, whereas others are absorbed better after a meal. One way to speed up oral absorption is to leave the tablet in the mouth instead of swallowing it so that it is absorbed directly into the veins in the mouth, bypassing the digestive tract. This is the idea behind sublingual and buccal tablets. Sublingual tablets dissolve on or under the tongue, whereas buccal tablets are placed on the inside of the cheek. Sublingual or buccal tablets may also be easier for patients with nausea or vomiting to tolerate.

- **Tablet examples** (most common): enalapril, Senna, amlodipine, atenolol, warfarin
- **Capsule examples:** doxycycline, Advil Liqui-Gels, omeprazole, ergocalciferol (vitamin D)
- **Sublingual examples:** Zofran ODT, Claritin RediTabs, Tylenol Meltaways, Maxalt-MLT, Prevacid SoluTab, Nitrostat
- **Buccal examples** (not as common): prochlorperazine buccal tablets, Nicorette lozenge

ROUTES OF ADMINISTRATION FOR PARENTERAL (INJECTABLE) MEDICATIONS

Types of parenteral (injectable) medications include the following:

- **Subcutaneous (SC, SubQ)** medications are injected under the skin ("sub" means under, and "cutaneous" means skin). The skin near the injection site is pinched, and a needle is inserted into the fatty tissue beneath the skin. Most self-administered injectables, such as insulin, are administered subcutaneously.
- **Intramuscular (IM)** medications are injected into the muscle. The advantages of IM administration are that larger volumes of medication can be administered and longer acting formulations can be used. Most IM injections are administered into the deltoid muscle of the upper arm, but some are injected into the buttocks. Examples of IM medications include most vaccines, the Depo-Provera contraceptive, and most antipsychotic injections.
- **Intravenous (IV)** medications are injected directly into a vein. IV is the quickest way to get medication through your system, but administration requires medical training and is usually limited to hospital settings. Many oral medications are also available in IV form, such as nitroglycerin, verapamil, potassium, and sodium.
- **Intrathecal (IT)** means injecting a medication directly into the space around the spinal cord. This route of administration is rare and dangerous and is generally reserved for chemotherapy medications, such as methotrexate.

OTIC AND OPTIC DROPS

Otic (ear) drops

- Examples: Ciprodex, ofloxacin, Cortisporin (polymyxin, neomycin, hydrocortisone)

Optic (eye) drops

- Examples: GoodSense Eye Drops, Restasis (single-use vials), latanoprost, sodium cromoglycate, Optilast
- Otic and optic drops are solutions manufactured in small-volume package sizes, such as 1, 5, 8, 10, or 15 mL dropper bottles. Drops are usually in multidose bottles that expire 28 days after opening, but some manufacturers offer single-use packaging. Some ophthalmic drugs are formulated as gels or ointments instead of liquids so they last longer. They do not need to be applied as often, but they can cause temporary blurred vision in the patient. Both otic and optic dosage forms are considered topical because they are applied directly to their site of action and do NOT have significant systemic (widespread) effects.

Optic drops must be sterilized during manufacturing because the eye is an environment that is free of bacteria. Otic drops are manufactured in a clean environment, but they do not necessarily need to be sterile. For this reason, it is permissible to use an optic drop in the ear, but it is NOT permissible to use an otic drop in the eye.

INHALED ROUTES OF ADMINISTRATION

Inhaled medications are designed to work specifically in the lungs rather than systemically (throughout the whole body). However, small amounts of inhaled medications can be absorbed into the body and can cause side effects.

- **Metered-dose inhalers (MDIs)** contain a drug solution within a canister. When the patient presses down on the canister, a propellant (e.g., hydrofluoroalkane [HFA]) helps spray a set amount of drug solution into the patient's mouth to be inhaled. Examples of MDIs include Proair HFA, Ventolin HFA, Proventil HFA, Flovent HFA, Atrovent HFA, Advair HFA, and QVAR RediHaler.
- **Dry powder inhalers (DPIs)** contain a drug within small granules of powder. Before inhaling, the patient must prep the device. Then, the patient must inhale deeply to draw the powder into their lungs. Examples of DPIs include Advair Diskus, Spiriva HandiHaler, and Symbicort Turbuhaler.
- **Nebulizer solutions** are small vials/ampoules of drug solution that are designed to be inserted into a nebulizer machine. Nebulizers aerosolize the solution into small particles that can be inhaled into the lungs more quickly and efficiently than with inhalers. Examples include albuterol sulfate nebulization solution 2.5 mg/3 mL, sodium chloride inhalation solution, and tobramycin inhalation solution.

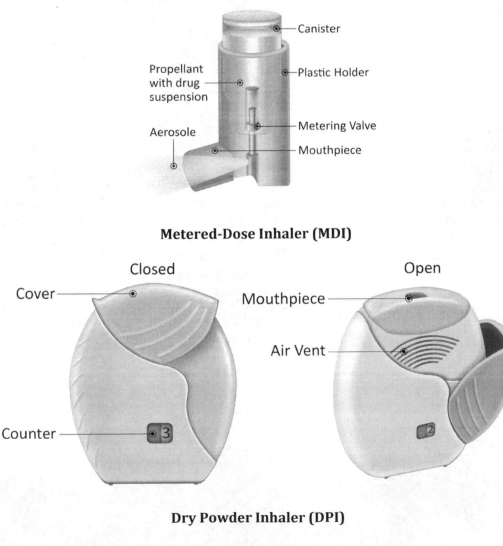

Metered-Dose Inhaler (MDI)

Dry Powder Inhaler (DPI)

STORAGE REQUIREMENTS FOR MEDICATIONS

Most medications can be stored at room temperature, which is defined as 20 °C to 25 °C or 59 °F to 77 °F. This includes most tablets, capsules, liquid solutions, creams, inhalers, and patches.

Some medications require refrigeration between 2 °C and 8 °C, or 36 °F and 46 °F. Medications that usually require refrigeration include injectables, vaccines, and antibiotic suspensions.

Controlled medications are usually kept in a locked cupboard, but not all states require them to be locked away.

Hazardous substances should be kept separately from regular pharmacy stock. Examples of hazardous substances include chemotherapy agents, including methotrexate. Pharmacy personnel who are handling hazardous substances should wear gloves. Some hazardous substances recommend that two layers of gloves (double gloving) should be worn. A separate counting tray should be used to count hazardous substances.

Hazardous wastes should also be stored separately from the rest of the pharmacy stock. Hazardous wastes include expired medications, recalled medications, damaged products, and incorrectly compounded products. These products should be put in designated bins and labeled as hazardous.

ADMINISTERING EYE DROPS

Eye drops are administered into the eye to treat eye conditions or infections. The eye is sterile (no bacteria are present), and it must remain that way in order to prevent infection. Therefore, eye drops should be administered carefully to prevent contamination or infection.

- Step 1: Wash your hands before applying eye drops or eye ointments.
- Step 2: Tilt your head backwards while sitting, standing, or lying down.
- Step 3: Place your index finger on the soft spot of skin just under the lower eyelid, and gently pull the eyelid downward to form a pocket.
- Step 4: While looking up, squeeze one drop into the pocket formed in the lower eyelid. Ensure that you do not allow the eyedropper to touch the eye or face.
- Step 5: Close your eye for approximately 3 minutes. Do not blink or rub/wipe your eyes.

If multiple eye drops need to be applied, wait 5 minutes between applications. If using an eye ointment, apply this last and use it at bedtime because ointments can cause blurred vision.

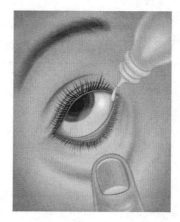

MEDICATIONS INTENDED FOR SHORT- AND LONG-TERM USE

The duration of treatment is the amount of time that the patient is expected to take a medication in order to treat their condition. Some medications are intended for short-term use, whereas others are intended to be taken for the long term.

Medications that are intended for short-term use are generally used to treat an acute (sudden or temporary) illness. Examples of acute indications include infections, electrolyte imbalances, perioperative treatment (around the time of surgery), bone fracture, trauma, headaches/migraines, gastrointestinal disturbances (nausea, vomiting, and diarrhea), and treatment of poisoning. For acute conditions, medication treatments will be stopped once symptoms have improved.

Medications that are intended for long-term use are generally used to treat a chronic (persistent, recurrent) illness. Examples of chronic illnesses that require long-term drug therapy include hypertension, diabetes, rheumatoid arthritis, hypothyroidism, epilepsy, asthma, hypercholesterolemia, psychosis, inflammatory bowel disease, PD, and glaucoma. Medication for chronic conditions will be prescribed for a long period of time, if not indefinitely.

Common and Severe Medication Side Effects, Adverse Effects, and Allergies

ADVERSE EFFECT AND SIDE EFFECT

An adverse effect is an unintended or undesired effect of a drug. A side effect is an unintended secondary effect of a medication. An adverse effect is different from a side effect because side effects may be desired or wanted, whereas an adverse effect is undesired or harmful. Adverse effects may be local (e.g., rash) or systemic (e.g., raised blood pressure). Local effects remain in one area of the body, whereas systemic effects are spread throughout the body. Adverse effects can range from mild (e.g., nausea) to severe (e.g., kidney failure).

Types of adverse effects: allergies, gastrointestinal effects (e.g., nausea, vomiting, diarrhea, abdominal pain), central nervous system (CNS) effects (drug dependence, tolerance, drowsiness), hematological effects (blood clotting, bleeding), nephrotoxicity (kidney[renal] impairment), hepatotoxicity (liver impairment), ototoxicity (causes damage to the ear), immunosuppression (reduces the ability to fight infection), carcinogenicity (ability to cause cancer), and teratogenicity (the ability to harm the fetus or cause birth defects in pregnant women).

> **Review Video: Mnemonics for Drug Side Effects**
> Visit mometrix.com/academy and enter code: 452450

ALLERGIES

An allergy occurs when the body's own immune system reacts to the presence of a foreign substance (e.g., a drug) and causes an adverse effect. Allergic reactions can range in severity from a mild rash to anaphylactic shock. Anaphylactic shock is a life-threatening reaction that results from dangerously low blood pressure and shortness of breath. Anaphylaxis should be treated immediately with epinephrine (e.g., EpiPen).

It is important to get a thorough allergy history before dispensing for a patient. However, patients who have not yet been exposed to a medication will not know if they are allergic to it, so they should be cautioned on the warning signs. A rash is a sign of minor allergy and usually goes away on its own after the medication course is complete. Signs of a more severe allergy include swelling of the face, tongue, or throat and difficulty breathing. These symptoms require immediate medical attention and discontinuation of the medication. Fortunately, rashes are far more common than anaphylactic allergies. Many patients also report an allergy to a drug because they experienced a side effect, so be sure to document the details of the allergy in the patient profile if known.

Drugs That Commonly Cause Allergies

A patient can be allergic to any medication, but medication allergies are more common in some drug classes than in others. Antibiotics are a common culprit, particularly older classes of antibiotics including penicillins, cephalosporins, and sulfa drugs (e.g., Bactrim). Up to 10% of the population reports being allergic to penicillin, but most patients only experience a minor rash. Only about 1% of the population experiences a true anaphylactic allergy to penicillin. Cephalosporin antibiotics are structurally related to penicillins, so some patients who are allergic to penicillin are also allergic to cephalosporins. The chance of cross-reactivity is thought to be about 10%.

Antifungals and antiviral drugs are also among the commonly reported allergies. Chemotherapy drugs, NSAIDs, insulin, antiepileptic drugs, and biologic injections are also common culprits of drug allergies. An allergy is far more likely with injectable medications compared to the oral route. Certain injectable medications require test doses and allergy monitoring as part of their infusion protocol.

Antihyperlipidemic and Antihypertensive Medications

The most common class of antihyperlipidemic medications is the HMG CoA reductase inhibitors, commonly referred to as **statins**. Common side effects of statins include headache, nausea, abdominal pain, drowsiness, dizziness, and muscle aches. Many patients experience minor muscle aches with statin use, but some patients may experience more serious muscle side effects called myopathy or rhabdomyolysis. Patients should be referred to their doctor if they experience any muscle pains while taking a statin. Some other antihyperlipidemic medications act in the digestive tract, including bile acid binders (e.g., cholestyramine and colestipol). These medications are usually well tolerated, but some patients experience abdominal cramping, constipation, nausea, or vomiting.

Antihypertensives have the following known side effects:

- **Beta-blockers and alpha-blockers** commonly cause fatigue (tiredness), cold hands, upset stomach, constipation, dizziness, shortness of breath, low blood pressure (hypotension), low heart rate (bradycardia), and fainting.
- **Calcium channel blockers** can cause adverse effects such as dizziness, swelling, blurred vision, fatigue, and weight gain.
- **ACE inhibitors** are known for causing an unproductive dry cough, high potassium levels (hyperkalemia), nausea, and loss of appetite.
- **Diuretics** can lead to adverse effects such as dry mouth, weakness, loss of appetite, muscle twitching, upset stomach, and electrolyte imbalances.

Antibiotics

Antibiotics are used to treat bacterial or microbial infections. All antibiotics have the potential to cause nausea, vomiting, diarrhea, stomach upset, and abdominal pain. Antibiotics can also kill the normal flora (good bacteria) in the body and lead to secondary infections, such as thrush or intestinal infection (colitis, *Clostridium difficile*). This is more common with broad-spectrum (less specific) antibiotics and longer courses of treatment. Patients can take a probiotic to help prevent this side effect.

69

The potential adverse effects associated with antibiotics:

Antibiotic Classification	Drug Examples	Potential Side Effects
Penicillins	Amoxicillin, penicillin	Allergy in 1–10% of patients. Anaphylaxis (a rare but serious form of allergy). Skin rash (a common, less severe form of allergy).
Cephalosporins	Cefaclor, cefixime	Allergy: About 10% of patients with a penicillin allergy are also allergic to cephalosporins.
Tetracyclines	Tetracycline, doxycycline, minocycline	Sensitivity to sunlight. Tooth staining, so avoid in children.
Macrolides	Erythromycin, clarithromycin	Arrhythmias. Ototoxicity (ear problems) with high doses.
Quinolones	Ciprofloxacin, levofloxacin	Arrhythmias. Muscle tendon rupture. Increased seizure risk.
Sulfonamides (sulfa drugs)	Sulfamethoxazole-trimethoprim (Bactrim)	Allergy — anaphylaxis or skin rash.

> **Review Video: Antibiotics: An Overview**
> Visit mometrix.com/academy and enter code: 165628

ANTINEOPLASTIC AGENTS

Most antineoplastic agents have the same classic chemotherapy side effects. These include hair loss, increased risk of infection (immunosuppression), low red blood cell count (anemia), bruising or bleeding easily, skin rashes (especially at the site of injection), fatigue, nausea, vomiting, diarrhea, constipation, gastrointestinal ulcers, mouth sores, and weight loss. Most of these side effects are due to the fact that antineoplastic agents are so good at killing cells that they kill normal body cells in addition to cancer cells. Some of the newer cancer medications are better at targeting cancer cells and have fewer side effects.

Hormonal anticancer therapies are among the targeted antineoplastic agents. Because they target cancer cells and avoid killing healthy body cells, hormonal therapies have fewer of the classic chemotherapy side effects. However, they do cause hormone-related side effects in the patient. For instance, tamoxifen causes menopause-like symptoms in women because it blocks estrogen. These symptoms include hot flashes, mood swings, depression, headache, hair thinning, loss of libido (sex drive), and fatigue. Bicalutamide also causes menopause-like side effects when taken by men because it blocks androgens (male sex hormones). Side effects include hot flashes, breast tenderness, weight changes, headaches, and difficulty sleeping.

ORAL ANTIHYPERGLYCEMIC DRUGS

Oral antihyperglycemic drugs have various side effects:

- **Metformin** is a first-line drug for treating type 2 diabetes mellitus because it has fewer side effects than many of the other antihyperglycemic drugs. It commonly causes nausea and stomach pains, but it does not cause hypoglycemia (too-low blood sugar) or weight gain like many other agents.
- **Sulfonylureas** are very effective at lowering blood glucose and are commonly used as an addition to metformin. However, they are associated with an increased risk of hypoglycemia and weight gain.
- **Thiazolidinediones** are no longer commonly used because there were found to be associated with an increased risk of cardiovascular disease and heart failure. They also cause weight gain and edema (swelling).
- **Acarbose** is rarely used because it often causes abdominal discomfort.
- **DPP-4 inhibitors** are well tolerated by patients and have few side effects. They do not cause weight gain or hypoglycemia like many of the other antidiabetic medications, but they are newer and more expensive.
- **SGLT-2 inhibitors** are becoming popular because instead of causing weight gain, they can help diabetic patients lose weight. This is beneficial to diabetics because they are already susceptible to weight gain. Unfortunately, they do increase the risk of genital and urinary tract infections.

DRUGS USED TO TREAT PARKINSON'S DISEASE AND ALZHEIMER'S DISEASE

Side effects of Parkinson's disease (PD) drugs include:

- **Dopaminergic drugs** commonly cause nausea, vomiting, agitation, confusion, depression, psychosis, dyskinesias (involuntary muscle movements), compulsive disorders (e.g., gambling), and orthostatic hypotension (dizziness upon standing).
- **MAO-B inhibitors** also cause a number of adverse effects that are similar to those of dopaminergic drugs. The common side effects for MAO-B inhibitors include nausea, vomiting, agitation, confusion, dizziness, dyskinesias, insomnia, lack of appetite, depression, anxiety, and psychosis.
- **Anticholinergic drugs** used for PD cause adverse effects similar to those of other anticholinergics that are used to treat urinary retention. Anticholinergic side effects include dry mouth, blurred vision, constipation, urinary retention, confusion, agitation, and psychosis.

Side effects of Alzheimer's disease (AD) drugs include:

- **Cholinesterase inhibitors** have an opposite effect to that of anticholinergic drugs. They increase acetylcholine levels by blocking the enzyme acetylcholinesterase, which is responsible for breaking down acetylcholine. Common side effects of cholinesterase inhibitors include nausea, vomiting, upset stomach, and weight loss. Starting at a low dose and gradually titrating the dose up to the intended maintenance dose helps minimize gastrointestinal adverse side effects.
- **NMDA receptor antagonists (blockers)** are used to treat moderate to severe cases of AD. NMDA blockers commonly cause dizziness, headache, drowsiness, high blood pressure, and restlessness.

STIMULANT MEDICATIONS

Attention-deficit/hyperactivity disorder (ADHD) is treated using stimulants, such as amphetamines, that excite the brain and help with focus, concentration, and motivation. Common side effects of stimulants include restlessness, nervousness, insomnia, mood swings, headache, raised blood pressure, loss of appetite, stomachaches, headaches, and weight loss. The stimulants used to treat ADHD are schedule II controlled substances and are prone to abuse. Some noncontrolled nonstimulant medications, such as Strattera, are now used to treat more resistant forms of ADHD. The adverse effects of these nonstimulants include dry mouth, nausea, upset stomach, weight loss, and insomnia.

The side effects of appetite loss and weight loss have made stimulants a target for weight loss treatments. Phentermine is a schedule IV drug prescribed to assist in weight loss in patients who have not responded to diet and exercise alone. In addition to its ability to improve attention and wakefulness, caffeine is also available as an OTC medication in tablet form as a weight loss supplement. The OTC nasal decongestant pseudoephedrine also has stimulant effects and similar side effects to ADHD stimulants. They should be avoided in patients with hypertension because of their effects on blood pressure.

SEIZURES

Epilepsy is a disorder in which a patient has seizures. Epilepsy is complex to diagnose because not every patient that has a seizure is diagnosed with a seizure disorder. Some patients have recurrent seizures, whereas others have had one seizure caused by an acute illness or a drug therapy.

Some forms of epilepsy have genetic links and run in families. Other seizure disorders may be linked to another medical issue, such as a birth defect, head injury, tumor, stroke, electrolyte imbalance (e.g., low sodium), hypoglycemia (low glucose), fever, or infection.

Certain medications can also increase a patient's risk of having a seizure. Recreational substances, including alcohol and cocaine, can cause seizures. Prescription medications can also increase seizure risk: narcotic pain medications (e.g., tramadol, meperidine), methylphenidate (used to treat ADHD), anesthesia drugs, metoclopramide, some antidepressants, and some antibiotics. Paradoxically, anticonvulsants that are used to treat epilepsy are also known to cause seizures. This adverse effect is of most concern when anticonvulsants are being used to treat a different disorder, such as migraines or bipolar disorder.

OPIOID PAIN MEDICATIONS

Opioids are central nervous system (CNS) depressants used to treat pain. One of the main adverse effects is a high risk of dependence and addiction, and there are many widely seen advertisements warning of the potentially addictive properties of opioids. Prescription opioids are one of the main culprits of the current opioid epidemic alongside other illegal opioids, including heroin and cocaine. Patients receiving a prescription for an opioid should be warned about this potential adverse effect and encouraged to only use these medications on an as-needed basis. Some state laws require additional warning stickers for opioid bottles or restrict the quantity of opioids that can be dispensed at a time.

Opioids can also cause nausea and vomiting in many patients. They also commonly cause constipation. Opioids slow down the movement of the digestive tract and can lead to reduced bowel movements.

In addition to slowing the digestive system, opioids also slow down respiration or breathing. This adverse effect is exploited by using opioids to suppress coughing, such as with Phenergan with

Codeine cough syrup. However, high doses of more potent opioids, such as oxycodone or morphine, can reduce the respiration rate to dangerous levels.

INHALED MEDICATIONS

Inhaled dosage forms include MDIs, DPIs, and nebulizer solutions. Nebulization delivers higher doses of medication to the body compared to inhalers, so it is associated with a higher risk of side effects. Inhaled medications used to treat asthma and COPD include bronchodilators, such as beta agonists and muscarinic antagonists, and anti-inflammatory corticosteroids.

- **Beta agonists** can cause tachycardia (a fast heart rate), cardiac arrhythmias, and tremors. They are also known to cause hypokalemia (low potassium levels). Examples of inhaled beta agonists include albuterol, levalbuterol, terbutaline, salmeterol, and formoterol.
- **Muscarinic antagonists** are selective and act locally, so they rarely cause significant adverse effects. However, they can potentially cause dry mouth, blurred vision, difficulty urinating, and glaucoma. The patient's eyes should be protected when administering nebulizers. Examples of inhaled muscarinic antagonists include ipratropium and tiotropium.
- **Inhaled corticosteroids** provide localized actions, so they do not cause as many adverse effects as oral steroids. However, they still have the potential to cause fluid retention, weight gain, hyperglycemia (high blood glucose), and hypokalemia (low potassium). Because corticosteroids reduce the body's immune response, patients frequently get a localized infection called thrush, a fungal infection in the mouth or throat.

OSTEOPOROSIS MEDICATIONS

There are two main types of medications used to prevent or treat osteoporosis: calcium with vitamin D supplements and bisphosphonates.

- Adverse effects associated with calcium and vitamin D supplements are uncommon. In rare cases, they can cause hypercalcemia (high blood calcium levels). Signs of hypercalcemia include nausea, vomiting, and thirst. High doses of vitamin D are contraindicated in pregnancy.
- Bisphosphonates used to treat osteoporosis include alendronate (Fosamax), risedronate (Actonel), and zoledronate (Reclast). The main side effects of bisphosphonates include hypocalcemia (low blood calcium levels) and gastrointestinal ulceration. These medications irritate the esophagus, so they should be taken with a full glass of water and the patient should not lay down for at least 30 minutes after taking the medication in order to avoid irritation to the esophagus. Bisphosphonates are contraindicated in patients with gastrointestinal ulcers, patients with moderate to severe renal impairment, and pregnant women.

HERBAL SUPPLEMENTS

An herbal supplement is a product derived from a plant that is used to treat an illness, condition, or disorder. Herbal supplements can be purchased as OTC formulas. Although they are regulated by the FDA, they are not monitored as closely as drugs.

Supplement	Indication
Aloe vera	Used topically for burns, cuts, scrapes, and psoriasis; taken orally for constipation and other gastrointestinal disorders
Coenzyme Q10	Hypertension, heart failure, and to reduce the muscle aches associated with statins

73

Echinacea	Respiratory infections
Evening primrose oil	Eczema/dermatitis
Fish oil	Hypercholesterolemia, hypertension, coronary artery disease, prevention of cardiovascular disease, and rheumatoid arthritis
Garlic	Hypercholesterolemia and prevention of cardiovascular disease
Ginger	Nausea, vomiting
Ginkgo biloba	Enhancement of memory/cognition, dementia, anxiety disorders, and schizophrenia
Ginseng	Improvement of immune function and mental performance
Glucosamine and chondroitin	Osteoarthritis
Green tea	Performance enhancement, prevention of cardiovascular disease, and prevention of cancer
Melatonin	Sleep disorders
Probiotics	Antibiotic-induced diarrhea, gastrointestinal disorders, and dermatitis
St. John's wort (*Hypericum perforatum*)	Depression, anxiety

VITAMINS AND MINERALS

A vitamin is an organic molecule that is required for the normal growth and function of the human body.

Vitamin	Indication(s)
Vitamin D (ergocalciferol, calcitriol, alfacalcidol)	Dietary deficiency, hypoparathyroidism, renal failure, prevention of osteoporosis, and topical treatment of psoriasis
Vitamin K (menadiol, phytomenadione)	Treatment of neonatal vitamin K deficiency, overtreatment with warfarin, dietary malabsorption, drug-induced malabsorption (e.g., cholestyramine), and hepatic cirrhosis induced clotting disorders
Vitamin B_{12} (hydroxocobalamin, cyanocobalamin)	Treatment and prevention of deficiency, especially following gastric bypass surgery
Folic acid (vitamin B_9)	Prevention and treatment of folate deficiency, prevention of neural tube defects during pregnancy, and reduction of bone marrow toxicity in patients taking methotrexate

Minerals, such as iron and magnesium, are inorganic substances that are essential for normal body functions.

Mineral	Indication(s)
Calcium	Low calcium levels, high potassium levels (renal impairment), osteoporosis
Magnesium	Low magnesium levels, cardiac arrhythmias, severe asthma
Potassium	Low potassium levels (e.g., due to diuretic or corticosteroid use)
Iron	Treatment and prevention of deficiency, anemia

INDICATIONS FOR MEDICATIONS

An indication is a condition, disease state, or reason for using a medication, device, or medical treatment. The chart below denotes some of the common medications or medical treatments and their indications or reasons for use.

Treatment	Indication
Antihypertensive medications	Hypertension (high blood pressure)
Antidepressant medications	Clinical depression
Thyroidectomy (surgical removal of the thyroid gland)	Hyperthyroidism, thyroid cancer
Antacids	Heartburn (gastroesophageal reflux)
Antiemetic medications	Nausea/vomiting
Vasodilators/nitrate drugs	Angina (chest pain)
Anticoagulant medications	Blood clot, stroke, heart attack, prevention of blood clots following surgery
Diuretic medications	Edema (fluid buildup), hypertension
Inhaled corticosteroids	Asthma, COPD
Pseudoephedrine	Nasal/sinus congestion
Ibuprofen (Motrin)	Headache, joint pain, inflammation, swelling
Doxylamine (Unisom)	Insomnia (difficulty sleeping)
Anticonvulsant medications	Epilepsy/seizure disorders
Antipsychotic drugs	Psychosis, schizophrenia, bipolar disorder
Antibiotics	Bacterial infection
Insulin	Diabetes mellitus
Metformin	Diabetes mellitus
DMARDs	Rheumatoid arthritis
Bisphosphonates (e.g., alendronate)	Osteoporosis, fragile bones
Chemotherapy treatments	Cancer/malignancy
Dopamine agonists	Parkinson's Disease

NONPRESCRIPTION MEDICATIONS AND DIETARY SUPPLEMENTS

Nonprescription, or over-the-counter (OTC), medications are drugs that are preapproved by the Food and Drug Administration (FDA) for sale to patients without a prescription. The product packaging must contain complete product information and a drug facts panel that includes directions for use, warnings, active and inactive ingredients, and a telephone number to call with questions. OTC drugs must go through the same drug approval process as prescription drugs and must be proven to be safe and effective.

Dietary supplements, such as vitamins, minerals, and medical foods, are still regulated by the FDA, but regulations are not as strict as they are for drugs. The FDA ensures that dietary supplements are manufactured using good manufacturing practices, but no proof of safety or efficacy is required. The packaging must state the name and quantity of each ingredient, but no other information is required. Dietary supplements cannot advertise that the product can cure, diagnose, or prevent any disease. However, dietary supplements can claim that they improve general structures or functions in the body. If a dietary supplement wants to claim that it can be used to treat or prevent a disease or condition, this claim must first be preapproved by the FDA.

MUSCLE RELAXANTS

Muscle relaxants, also known as spasmolytics, are used to treat muscle spasms, muscle cramps, and muscle pains. They do this by reducing muscle tone and relaxing the muscles. Muscle relaxers may be used to treat a variety of muscle conditions, including lower back pain, neck pain, fibromyalgia, multiple sclerosis, cerebral palsy, and amyotrophic lateral sclerosis. Most muscle relaxers are centrally acting, so they lead to significant drowsiness. Some benzodiazepines that are used to treat anxiety can also be used as muscle relaxers, such as diazepam. Muscle relaxers are generally only used in the short term because they can lead to dependence or addiction. For this reason, some of the muscle relaxants are schedule IV controlled medications, including diazepam and carisoprodol.

Generic Name	Brand Name
Carisoprodol	Soma
Cyclobenzaprine	Amrix, Fexmid
Metaxalone	(None currently on the market)
Methocarbamol	Robaxin
Tizanidine	Zanaflex
Baclofen	Lioresal
Dantrolene	Dantrium
Diazepam	Valium

Drug Stability

Drug stability is the ability of a drug to maintain its original physical and chemical properties. When a drug begins to degrade or change its properties and become unstable, it is adulterated and can no longer be used.

Changes in pH, exposure to light, and high temperatures are common culprits in drug instability. This is why some drugs must be stored in a refrigerator or in dark-colored packaging to prevent light exposure. The material that a drug is packaged in can also react with a medication and cause it to become unstable. If removing a drug from its original packaging, the drug must be compatible with the new packaging. This is particularly relevant when compounding or preparing IV medications because some medications cannot be packaged in polyvinyl chloride (PVC) IV bags. Additionally, some medications must be diluted prior to use (e.g., IV solutions, vaccines, antibiotic suspensions). Only diluents approved by the manufacturer should be used to prevent instability issues. Combining medications can also lead to instability, so it is best for nurses to check with a pharmacist before administering multiple medications in the same infusion.

SIGNS OF DRUG DEGRADATION OR INSTABILITY IN DOSAGE FORMS

For tablets and capsules, signs of instability include discoloration (e.g., yellowing of white tablets) and changes in hardness. Ointments, creams, and gels also become discolored, but they can also go through changes in consistency (e.g., dryness, grittiness) and uniformity (liquid separates from solid). Liquid dosage forms can become discolored, acquire a foul odor, and undergo gas buildup (pressure upon opening the container). Unstable liquid dosage forms may also form precipitates (solid particles) and undergo phase separation. Phase separation occurs when the solid particles or oil droplets in a liquid mixture separate from the aqueous (watery) parts of a liquid, similar to expired milk becoming chunky. Emulsions and suspensions are particularly prone to phase separation because they contain solids or oils suspended in a watery liquid. Caking, creaming, and difficulty resuspending are signs of phase separation. Powder formulations (e.g., amoxicillin suspension) that are unstable can become discolored or smelly, and they can begin to cake or clump together.

SOLUTIONS, SUSPENSIONS, AND RECONSTITUTABLE FORMULATIONS

A solution is an oral liquid in which a solid drug is uniformly dissolved. Because the drug is dissolved in the solution, a uniform dose is easily obtained, and no shaking or mixing is required prior to use.

A suspension is an oral liquid in which particles of solid drug are dispersed, but not dissolved. The drug particles settle to the bottom of the container when stored, so the medication must be shaken well before use in order to redistribute the particles to obtain a uniform dose. Because the drug is not dissolved in the liquid, the taste of the drug is masked. Therefore, suspensions are useful for formulating drugs that have an unpleasant taste.

A reconstitutable drug is an oral liquid that is formulated as a fine powder that requires water to be added to it (reconstitution) prior to dispensing. After reconstitution, the powder and liquid form a suspension. Most liquid antibiotics are formulated this way due to stability issues between the drug and water.

Narrow-Therapeutic-Index Medications

The therapeutic index is a ratio of the dose of a drug that causes a toxic effect versus the dose of a drug that causes a therapeutic or beneficial effect. A numerical value can be given to the therapeutic index by dividing the toxic dose in 50% of the population (TD_{50}) by the therapeutic/effective dose in 50% of the population (ED_{50}).

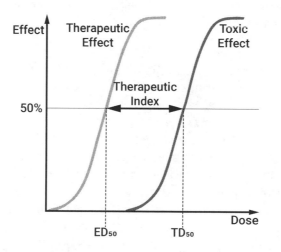

Medications that have a **narrow therapeutic index** do not have a very wide range between the effective dose and a toxic dose. This narrow dosage range means that small changes in the dose can lead to toxic effects. Therefore, medication levels need to be monitored very closely for these medications. Many drugs with a narrow therapeutic index require therapeutic drug monitoring, in which laboratory testing is used to determine drug levels in the patient.

Examples of medications with a narrow therapeutic index: lithium, warfarin, digoxin, phenytoin, theophylline, cyclosporine, tacrolimus, and many chemotherapy agents

Incompatibilities Related to Nonsterile Compounding and Reconstitution

DRUG INCOMPATIBILITY

Drug incompatibility is an undesirable reaction between two drugs, a drug and a solution, or a drug and its packaging. Drug incompatibilities can lead to drug degradation or instability and may lead to adverse reactions in the patient. Compounded drugs are particularly susceptible to incompatibilities because multiple ingredients are being combined.

During reconstitution, liquid is added to a powder to form a suspension.

Most antibiotic suspensions (e.g., amoxicillin) require reconstitution prior to dispensing. Antibiotics are formulated this way because they degrade quickly in water and have a short shelf life. Once reconstituted, most antibiotics must be stored in a refrigerator, and they expire 14 days after reconstitution. Some medications may require dilution, mixing, or compounding prior to dispensing to a patient. It is important to reconstitute or dilute a product based on the instructions in the package insert or manufacturer's instructions so that the correct type and amount of diluent are used. Using the incorrect diluent can lead to incompatibility reactions.

COMPOUNDING PROCESSES MAKING PRODUCTS MORE SUSCEPTIBLE TO DRUG INCOMPATIBILITIES

Drug incompatibility occurs when a drug interacts with another ingredient in its formulation or packaging. This leads to potential degradation of the drugs and adverse reactions in the patient. Compounded drugs are particularly susceptible to incompatibilities because multiple ingredients are being combined.

Chemical complexation occurs when two drugs combine to form another drug, leading to altered effects or adverse reactions. Incompatibility can also occur when the incorrect diluent (liquid being added to a powder or solution) is added to a drug. For medications that require dilution or reconstitution, the package insert or container will include directions on how to prepare the product and what diluent to use. Compounded medications must also be packaged in materials approved by the manufacturer. Some drugs are incompatible with certain types of plastic packaging. Incompatibilities can also occur during administration. Sometimes, nurses want to administer multiple medications at the same time. Some drugs are incompatible and cannot be administered together; refer to a pharmacist for questions regarding compatibility issues.

Proper Storage of Medications

POISON PREVENTION PACKAGING ACT OF 1970

The Poison Prevention Packaging Act of 1970 requires that medications be packaged in a child-proof container that 80% of children younger than 5 years old cannot open, but 90% of adults can open. Patients can request (oral or written) that non-safety caps be used for all of their medications, whereas prescribers can only request non-safety caps on behalf of a patient for each specific prescription.

Certain products are exempt from this law and are not required to be packaged or dispensed with a child-proof cap:

- Topical creams/lotions/ointments (except lidocaine, dibucaine, and minoxidil)
- Sublingual nitroglycerin

- Isosorbide dinitrate ≤10 mg
- Cholestyramine/colestipol powder
- Oral contraceptives and medroxyprogesterone
- Unit dose potassium <50 mEq
- Erythromycin tablets ≤16 mg/package or suspension ≤8 g/package
- Effervescent tablets of aspirin or acetaminophen
- One package size of an OTC product if the label states "this package is for households without young children" (the same product must also be available in child-proof packaging)
- Drugs administered on site at a hospital or nursing home
- Lozenges
- Inhalers
- Pancrelipase
- Sucrose
- Mebendazole ≤600 mg/package
- Dental products (except products with >264 mg sodium fluoride)
- Steroid dose packs: methylprednisolone <84 mg, betamethasone <12.6 mg

STORAGE OF ORAL POWDERS FOR RECONSTITUTION

Most liquid antibiotics are formulated as a powder that requires reconstitution (mixing) with water prior to dispensing. The packaging contains instructions on how to reconstitute the product and how much water to add. Prior to reconstitution, powders for reconstitution are stored at room temperature. After reconstitution, most liquid antibiotics have a shortened expiration date and must be kept refrigerated. Cipro, Suprax, and Zithromax are not required to be refrigerated after reconstitution, but they may be stored in a refrigerator to improve their taste.

Trimethoprim-sulfamethoxazole (Septra) is an antibiotic suspension that is already in liquid form and does not require reconstitution. It should be stored at room temperature.

Brand Name	Generic Name
Amoxil suspension	Amoxicillin
Augmentin suspension	Amoxicillin/clavulanic acid
APO-Cefaclor suspension	Cefaclor
Ceftin suspension	Cefuroxime
APO-Cefprozil suspension	Cefprozil
Cipro suspension	Ciprofloxacin
APO-Cefadroxil suspension	Cefadroxil
None currently on the market	Cephalexin
Suprax suspension	Cefixime
Tamiflu suspension	Oseltamivir
None currently on the market	Penicillin V
Zithromax suspension	Azithromycin

PRESCRIBED PRODUCTS THAT REQUIRE REFRIGERATION

Most injectable medications, biologics, blood factors, and vaccines require refrigeration. Oral antibiotic liquids that require reconstitution usually require refrigeration after mixing. There are also a few eye drops, inhalers, gels, and nasal sprays that must be stored in the refrigerator.

Brand Name	Generic Name
Acanya	Clindamycin/benzoyl peroxide

Brand Name	Generic Name
ActHIB	*Haemophilus influenzae* type B vaccine
Adacel	TDaP vaccine
Apidra	Insulin glulisine
Benzamycin gel (reconstituted)	Erythromycin/benzoyl peroxide
Byetta	Exenatide
CombiPatch	Estradiol/norethindrone
Enbrel	Etanercept
Engerix-B	Hepatitis B vaccine
Epogen	Epoetin alfa
Forteo	Teriparatide
Havrix	Hepatitis A vaccine
Humalog	Insulin lispro
Humira	Adalimumab
Humulin N	NPH insulin
Humulin R	Regular insulin
Lactinex	A blend of *Lactobacillus acidophilus* and *Lactobacillus helveticus* (*bulgaricus*)
Lantus	Insulin glargine
Levemir	Insulin detemir
Leukeran	Chlorambucil
Miacalcin nasal spray	Calcitonin
MMR II	Measles, mumps, and rubella vaccine
Neulasta	Pegfilgrastim
Neupogen	Filgrastim
Novolin N	NPH insulin
Novolin R	Regular insulin
Novolog	Insulin aspart
NovoSeven	Coagulation factor VII
NuvaRing	Etonogestrel/ethinyl estradiol
Perforomist	Formoterol
Phenergan suppositories	Promethazine
Pneumovax 23 Prevnar 13	Pneumococcal vaccine
Procrit	Epoetin alfa
Risperdal Consta	Risperidone
Sandostatin	Octreotide
Victoza	Liraglutide
Xalatan eye drops	Latanoprost

STORAGE REQUIREMENTS OF INJECTABLE MEDICATIONS

Some injectable medications should be stored at room temperature, whereas others must be stored in the refrigerator. It is important to read the storage information on the packaging or in the package insert if you are unsure of how to store a medication.

Most vaccines must be stored in a refrigerator, although there are a few that should be stored in a freezer or at room temperature. Insulin products should be stored in a refrigerator, although they can be stored at controlled room temperature for up to 28 days once dispensed. Most single-use injection solutions packaged in vials or IV bags can be kept at room temperature, although there are some exceptions. Most sterile compounded products must be stored in a refrigerator and have a short beyond-use date; however, there are a few products that should not be stored in the fridge, so refer to the preparation instructions or a pharmacist if you are not sure of how to store a medication.

Storage Requirements of Vaccinations

Most vaccinations must be stored in a refrigerator between 2°C and 8°C (36°F and 46°F). If the vaccine is stored outside of this temperature range or becomes frozen, it must be discarded. Some vaccines are formulated as powders for reconstitution. If a diluent is provided in the packaging, the diluent must also be stored in the refrigerator and cannot become frozen. Varivax and Zostavax must be stored in a freezer and maintained between −58°F and 5°F. They can be kept in a refrigerator for up to 72 hours prior to use. Note that one brand of the herpes zoster vaccine must be refrigerated, and the other brand must be frozen.

- **Vaccines that should be refrigerated:** influenza vaccine (Flulaval, Fluzone, Fluarix); TDaP vaccine (Adacel, Boostrix); hepatitis B vaccination (Engerix-B, Recombivax HB); hepatitis A vaccination (Havrix, Vaqta); *Haemophilus influenzae* type B (Pentacel, Vaxelis); meningococcal vaccinations (Menactra, Menveo, Menquadfi); MMR vaccination; human papillomavirus vaccination (Gardasil, Cervarix); pneumococcal vaccines (Pneumovax-23, Prevnar-13); and herpes zoster vaccine (Shingrix)
- **Vaccines that should be frozen:** varicella (chicken pox) vaccination (Varivax, Proquad); herpes zoster vaccines (Zostavax)

Light-Sensitive Pharmaceutical Products

Some medications are sensitive to light and become unstable and adulterated if exposed to bright lights. Light-sensitive medications must be stored in amber or brown packaging to minimize their exposure to light, even if the drug is being transported within the pharmacy or hospital. There is a long list of medications that are sensitive to light, so if you are not sure whether a medication needs to be protected from light, refer to the manufacturer's information or the guidelines at your pharmacy. In time, you will become familiar with the medications that your pharmacy commonly dispenses.

Light-sensitive medications: aminophylline, amiodarone, amphotericin B, bupivacaine/epinephrine, cefepime, cefotaxime, cefazolin, chlorpheniramine, chlorpromazine, cisplatin, dacarbazine, diazepam, digoxin, diphenhydramine, dopamine, doxorubicin, doxycycline, epinephrine, fluorouracil, folic acid, furosemide, haloperidol, hydrocortisone, hydromorphone, iron (iron sucrose and ferrous gluconate), isoproterenol, methadone, morphine, nicardipine, nitroglycerine, nitroprusside, norepinephrine, phenylephrine, prochlorperazine, promethazine, propranolol, terbutaline, testosterone, thiamine, vincristine, vitamin B complex, vitamin K (menadiol and phytonadione), and vitamin B_{12} (cyanocobalamin)

Storage Requirements for Medications in Pharmacy

For the specific storage requirements of a medication, refer to the label and package instructions from the manufacturer. Most medications can be stored in a cool, dry place with a room temperature between 68°F and 77°F and a humidity of <40%. The room temperature and humidity of the pharmacy should be monitored and recorded daily. Some medications must be stored in a refrigerator, at temperatures between 36°F and 46°F. Pharmacy refrigerator temperatures should be checked and recorded at least twice daily. Occasionally, you may encounter a medication that must be kept frozen (e.g., Zostavax vaccine) between −13°F and 14°F.

Medications should always be stored away from light or heat sources. Some medications (e.g., nitroglycerin) are particularly sensitive to light and should be packaged in amber vials or dark-colored packaging to prevent light exposure.

Hazardous wastes, including expired medications and damaged/defective products, must be stored in designated bins labeled "Hazardous Wastes."

For error prevention, look-alike/sound-alike (LASA) medications should be separated or stored on different shelves and labeled with warning stickers. Stock should be rotated (older bottles should be placed in front of newer bottles) to prevent medications from expiring.

RESTRICTING ACCESS TO PHARMACY STOCK

All prescription-only medications must be stored in the pharmacy or pharmacy department. The doors to the pharmacy department must remain locked regardless of whether the pharmacy is open or closed. Only authorized staff members should be allowed access to the pharmacy department. The pharmacy should install an alarm system that safeguards against theft. The alarm system must be activated when the pharmacy is closed. Only authorized pharmacists should have access to the pharmacy alarm code. Anyone who has been convicted of a felony offense relating to controlled substances is not allowed to be employed in the pharmacy department or have access to controlled substances. A criminal background check is a routine part of licensure for pharmacy technicians and pharmacists. Schedules III–V medications can be stored with regular noncontrolled pharmacy stock. Schedule II medications are usually kept in a locked safe but can legally be dispersed among regular pharmacy stock in such a manner as to obstruct theft or diversion.

Chapter Quiz

Ready to see how well you retained what you just read? Scan the QR code to go directly to the chapter quiz interface for this study guide. If you're using a computer, simply visit the bonus page at **mometrix.com/bonus948/ptcb** and click the Chapter Quizzes link.

Federal Requirements

Transform passive reading into active learning! After immersing yourself in this chapter, put your comprehension to the test by taking a quiz. The insights you gained will stay with you longer this way. Scan the QR code to go directly to the chapter quiz interface for this study guide. If you're using a computer, simply visit the bonus page at **mometrix.com/bonus948/ptcb** and click the Chapter Quizzes link.

Handling and Disposal of Pharmaceutical Substances and Waste

ENVIRONMENT IN WHICH HAZARDOUS DRUGS SHOULD BE COMPOUNDED

Hazardous medications should always be handled with extra caution, especially by women of childbearing potential. Pharmacy personnel should always wear gloves when handling any hazardous medications, such as when counting out tablets during the dispensing process. Some hazardous chemotherapy agents' manufacturers recommend that two layers of gloves (double gloving) are worn.

Preparing sterile compounds requires extra precautions to protect the compounder and the product. Personal protective equipment (PPE), including a gown, face mask, hair cover, shoe covers, and two layers of sterile chemotherapy gloves must be worn by the preparer. Tablets should not be cut, and capsules should not be opened when working with any hazardous substance. Hazardous substances should be prepared in a negative pressure isolator, which ensures that hazardous particles are directed away from the preparer. Alternatively, a 0.2 micron hydrophobic filter can be used to prepare the product.

The most up-to-date list of hazardous medications can be found on the Centers for Disease Control and Prevention (CDC)'s website.

INFORMATION REQUIRED ON PRESCRIPTION MEDICATION LABELS

A label is defined as the written or printed text and graphics upon the immediate container of a drug. The term "labeling" expands this definition to include other written or printed text and graphics upon or contained within the wrappers or external packaging of the product, such as package inserts.

When a pharmacy dispenses a medication to a patient, it is required to attach its own dispensing label that includes the following information:

- Date of fill
- Name and address of filling pharmacy
- Name of prescriber
- Name and strength of the drug or device
- Expiration date of the drug (OR 1 year from the date of dispensing, whichever is sooner)
- Prescription number
- Name of the patient
- Directions for use

- Generic drug name and name of the manufacturer (if a generic drug is dispensed)
- For controlled substances, the phrase "Caution: federal law prohibits transfer of this drug to any person other than the patient to whom it was prescribed" in >6 pt font

There are a few exceptions in which dispensing labels are not required. Labels are NOT required for drugs or devices dispensed to an inpatient at an institution, in an emergency scenario, or for drug samples or starter packs dispensed by an authorized prescriber.

ADULTERATION

Adulteration is when a drug product or device is contaminated, impure, or is not of the advertised strength. Adulteration can occur if the product is prepared, packaged, or stored under unsanitary conditions. Products that require refrigeration, such as insulin, become adulterated if they are stored outside of a refrigerator. Products can also be adulterated if they are manufactured, processed, packaged, or stored in a facility that does not comply with good manufacturing practices or refuses FDA inspection. For example, if a drug warehouse is shut down by the FDA for unsanitary conditions, the medications that are stored there are considered adulterated. Adulterated products also include banned devices and the use of unapproved color additives. Products can become adulterated if stored inappropriately or if mixed or packaged so as to reduce quality or purity. For example, IV products that have been mixed with an incompatible diluent (e.g., dextrose 5% instead or normal saline) or that have been packaged in an IV bag that the drug is not compatible with are considered adulterated.

MISBRANDING

Misbranding occurs when a drug product is associated with false or misleading labeling or advertising. Labeling issues occur when the label contains incorrect information or is missing information that is required by law. Misbranded labels may omit or falsely identify the brand or generic drug name, quantity or proportion of active ingredients, directions for use, address and phone number for reporting adverse drug reactions, storage requirements, or the "R-Only" phrase. Misbranding also occurs when a product is the exact imitation of another product (i.e., a counterfeit medication). Intentional falsification of a prescription, false or misleading advertising, or promotion of a drug for off-label use is also considered misbranding. Misbranding at the pharmacy level includes dispensing an R-only drug without a prescription, improper labeling or dispensing (i.e., a dispensing error), failure to comply with Risk Evaluation and mitigation Strategy (REMS), selling an item labeled "Not for resale," or failure to provide child-resistant packaging in accordance with the law.

Examples: The actual strength differs from the labeled strength, the label is missing the name and address of the manufacturer, a refrigerated product is missing the "Store in a refrigerator" statement, or a product that claims to be Xanax does not contain the active ingredient alprazolam.

INFORMATION REQUIRED ON OTC MEDICATIONS

The following information is required to be on the package or label of an OTC medication:

- For each active ingredient, the name and general pharmacological category (e.g., antihistamine) of the drug must be listed
- List of inactive ingredients in alphabetical order
- Name and address of the manufacturer, packager, or distributor
- Net quantity in the package
- Drug facts panel, which includes the following: directions for use, indications, side effects, dosages, administration route(s), contraindications, and other warnings or precautions

- Any required preparation for use (e.g., shake well)
- Lot number and expiration date
- Phone number for questions and comments
- Cautions and warnings: "For external use only," "For rectal/vaginal use only," "Do not use in...," or "Ask a doctor or pharmacist before use if you have certain conditions"
- Special storage instruction (e.g., "Keep in a refrigerator")
- Note: The National Drug Code (NDC) number is NOT mandatory on OTC medication labels

A sample OTC packaging label is shown, showing the information that is typically included on the label.

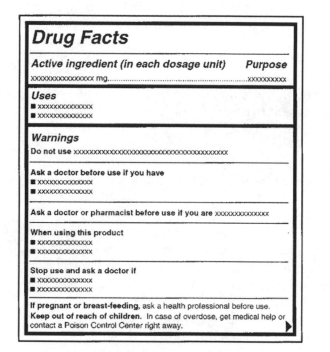

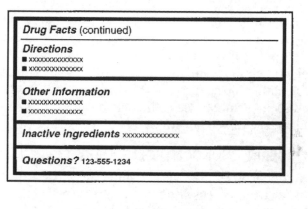

INFORMATION REQUIRED ON NEW NONCONTROLLED SUBSTANCE PRESCRIPTION ORDER

For noncontrolled substances, prescriptions may be accepted by written hard copy, electronic transmission, facsimile transmission, verbal telephone order, or verbal voicemail telephone message. Electronic prescriptions ARE permitted if the sender and the receiver have an approved prescription decryption software. There are no limits on the number of refills allowed for noncontrolled substance prescriptions, but federal law states that the prescription expires 12 months from the date written. Certain states have stricter laws indicating the time frame in which the first fill must be dispensed.

The following information is required to be on the prescription order:

- Date issued/written
- Name of the patient
    - The patient's address is only required for controlled medications
- Drug name, dosage form, and strength
- Total quantity of drug prescribed
- Directions for use

- Name and address of the prescriber
  - The prescriber's Drug Enforcement Administration (DEA) number is only required for controlled medications
- Prescriber's signature (digital signatures are acceptable for electronic prescriptions)

The number of refills allowed is not a required element of a prescription. If no refill number is listed, it can be assumed that the prescription is not refillable.

LOSS OR THEFT OF PHARMACY STOCK

If a theft occurs in the pharmacy department or stock is lost or missing, this occurrence should be reported to local police. If only noncontrolled substances are stolen or missing, the pharmacy is not required to notify the DEA. If controlled substances in any schedule are missing or stolen, the pharmacy must notify the DEA of the theft. The nearest DEA Diversion Field Office should be the first point of contact. The pharmacy must also fill out a DEA Form 106, which may be the written or electronic version. This form provides an estimate of what is known to be stolen or missing. This form must be sent to the DEA within 1 business day of the discovery of the theft or loss of controlled substances. The original copy of the form is sent to the DEA, and a copy must be kept on file at the pharmacy for at least 2 years.

ORDERING NONCONTROLLED SUBSTANCES

Any pharmacy that has obtained the proper licensure requirements in their state is authorized to order and possess controlled substances. Pharmacies should also register with the DEA in order to be able to order, possess, and dispense controlled substances. The DEA will assign each pharmacy/facility that is authorized to possess controlled substances a DEA number. These state and federal registrations allow the pharmacy to order prescription medications from wholesalers or distributors. With today's advances in technology, most pharmacy orders are automatically completed by the pharmacy dispensing software using current inventory counts and set par levels. However, pharmacy technicians are usually responsible for reviewing these orders and ensuring that adequate stock levels are maintained. Most wholesalers have electronic databases that allow pharmacy personnel to log in, review orders, place orders, and request returns. Order reviews allow pharmacy technicians the opportunity to check that owed medications are on the order and to resolve out-of-stock issues, brand preferences, and ordering errors. Schedules III, IV, and V controlled substances are ordered in the same manner as noncontrolled prescription items and OTC medications. Schedule II substances are the only medications that technicians are usually not involved in ordering.

RETURNING NONCONTROLLED MEDICATIONS

Occasionally, you will receive an item in the order from your wholesaler that is damaged or ordered in error. In these cases, you will want to return the item. Each wholesaler has different policies on medication returns. Most wholesalers do not allow refrigerated items or controlled substances to be returned. However, exceptions are possible if the ordering error or the damage to the medication is the fault of the wholesaler. Many wholesalers allow returns to be requested using their online portal. Once a return request is approved, a return authorization form will be sent to the pharmacy either electronically, by mail, or with the next medication delivery. A return authorization will require a signature of a pharmacy employee and will provide details of how to package the return. During the next medication delivery, the delivery driver will pick up the tote containing the return and review the return authorization paperwork. Once the return has been processed, the pharmacy will receive an invoice for the account credit.

INVESTIGATIONAL DRUGS

Investigational or clinical trial drugs should be secured and **stored** in a separate room or separate storage area in the pharmacy. Only those pharmacy staff members that are delegated or authorized to work with investigational drugs should have access. Products should be stored under the storage conditions (e.g., temperature, humidity) specified by the manufacturer or study sponsor. Documentation of proper storage is important for validation of the trial.

Before investigational drugs can be ordered and received, the pharmacy must be approved by the study sponsor to participate in the trial. Once the study is ready to begin, the clinical protocol will specify how to **order and receive** the investigational product. When the products are shipped to the pharmacy, they should be clearly labeled as investigational drug products.

If an investigational drug product is **lost or stolen**, the sponsor of the trial should be notified immediately. For suspected thefts, the local police should also be notified. If the stolen medication is a controlled substance, the DEA should be notified using DEA Form 106.

When **dispensing** investigational drugs, handling requirements set out in the study protocol should be adhered to. Partial or empty vials of investigational drugs that are **returned** by patients/participants should be returned to the pharmacy's investigational drug team. Some study protocols require pharmacy staff to receive, count, and document drugs that are returned by patients. Patient returns, empty containers, and expired investigational drugs that are no longer dispensable must be stored in a separate, limited-access area until they can be destroyed or returned to the manufacturer/sponsor.

The immediate package or container for every investigational drug must contain the statement "Caution: New Drug — Limited by federal (or United States) law to investigational use." The pharmacy dispensing label for investigational drugs also requires additional information. The following information is required to be on the pharmacy label in addition to standard labeling requirements:

- Name of the investigational drug product (for blinded trials, the product name should read "[Drug product name] or placebo")
- Product strength or concentration (unless blinded)
- Quantity
- Lot number, container number, or kit number
- Expiration date, retest date, or period of use
- Manufacturer/sponsor name and address
- Clinical research protocol number

STORING AND DISPOSING HAZARDOUS AND NONHAZARDOUS WASTES

Pharmaceutical wastes include expired drugs, patient returned drugs, damaged drugs, partially used vials of single-use injection solutions, empty vials or containers of hazardous substances, syringes contaminated with hazardous substances, and any other items contaminated with hazardous substances or body fluids. Hazardous substances should be separated from other pharmacy stock and placed in leak-proof bags or bins labeled as hazardous waste. Sharps contaminated with a hazardous substance should be placed in a sharps bin labeled as hazardous.

Expired, damaged, or patient-returned medications can usually be sent to a reverse distributor for a credit. Items received from a wholesaler or distributor that are already damaged can usually be returned for a credit. Any other pharmaceutical hazardous wastes cannot be sent back to wholesalers or distributors for credit. Instead, they must be disposed of properly. A pharmaceutical waste management service, such as Stericycle, is usually contracted to periodically pick up waste from the pharmacy and dispose of it.

HAZARDOUS PHARMACEUTICAL PRODUCTS

Hazardous substances are those that can cause potential harm to pharmacy personnel who are handling or dispensing them. Nearly all chemotherapy drugs used to treat cancer are hazardous substances. There are hundreds of hazardous chemotherapy agents, but a few of the more commonly dispensed substances are listed in the table below. Many immune modulators used to treat transplant rejection, inflammatory bowel diseases, and rheumatoid arthritis are also hazardous. Some antiviral drugs and hormone modulators are also potentially hazardous. These substances should be handled with extra caution, including wearing gloves during dispensing.

Brand Name	Generic Name
Anticancer Drugs	
Efudex	Fluorouracil
Trexall, Rheumatrex	Methotrexate
Cytoxan	Cyclophosphamide
Ellence	Epirubicin
Taxol	Paclitaxel
Vincasar	Vincristine
Xeloda	Capecitabine
Afinitor	Everolimus
Revlimid	Lenalidomide
Purinethol	Mercaptopurine
Pomalyst	Pomalidomide
Temodar	Temozolomide
Thalomid	Thalidomide
Immune Modulators	
Imuran	Azathioprine
Sandimmune, Neoral	Cyclosporine
Prograf	Tacrolimus
CellCept, Myfortic	Mycophenolate
Hydrea	Hydroxyurea
Antivirals	
Cytovene	Ganciclovir
Rebetol	Ribavirin
Valcyte	Valganciclovir
Retrovir	Zidovudine
Hormone Modulators	
Casodex	Bicalutamide
Propecia, Proscar	Finasteride
Retinoids	
Accutane	Isotretinoin
Retin-A	Tretinoin (topical)
Vesanoid	Tretinoin (oral)

The most up-to-date list of hazardous medications can be found on the CDC website.

DRUG TAKE-BACK PROGRAM

Medications that are not disposed of properly pose risks to the environment as well as to the public. Controlled medications, such as oxycodone and morphine, are particularly susceptible to abuse by others if not disposed of properly by the patient. A drug take-back program allows patients to return any expired or unused medications to an authorized medication collection site for proper disposal. Some drug take-back collection sites are in operation year-round. Many hospital outpatient pharmacies and police stations have self-serve collection receptacles in which patients can drop off any unwanted medications. These receptacles are locked at the end of the business day and are emptied periodically. Twice every year, the DEA also sponsors a National Drug Take Back Day when many temporary collection sites are available to promote the safe disposal of medications. The only types of medications that are not accepted at collection sites are illicit drugs (e.g., heroin, cocaine, marijuana), inhalers, and needles/sharps. Sharps should be disposed of in a sharps bin and mailed to the address of the sharps disposal service listed on the container.

NONPRESCRIPTION AND PRESCRIPTION-ONLY MEDICATIONS

Prescription and nonprescription (OTC) drugs must be preapproved by the FDA for sale to patients. They undergo the same drug approval process through the FDA and must be proven to be safe and effective.

Nonprescription medications have been proven to be safe enough for patients to purchase without a prescription when they are used according to the directions on the label. The product packaging must contain complete product information and a drug facts panel that includes directions for use, warnings, active and inactive ingredients, and a telephone number to call with questions. Drug advertising for OTC medications is regulated by the Federal Trade Commission.

Prescription-only medications require a prescription from a prescriber in order for patients to purchase them. The manufacturer's label must contain the statement "R Only" or "Caution: Federal law prohibits dispensing without a prescription." The manufacturer's packaging must also contain a drug package insert that contains adequate information for use by prescribers and dispensers. The dispensing label must contain adequate directions for use. Drug advertising regulations for prescription-only medications are stricter than for OTC medications and are enforced by the FDA.

Controlled Substance Prescriptions and DEA Controlled Substance Schedules

CLASSES OR SCHEDULES OF CONTROLLED SUBSTANCES

Schedule I — Drugs that have a high potential for abuse and no medical purpose. These cannot be obtained without a special license and are usually only used for research.

- Examples: heroin, illicit drugs

Schedule II — Drugs that have a high potential for abuse but have accepted medical uses.

- Examples: most opioids (oxycodone, morphine, hydrocodone), methadone, cocaine

Schedule III — Drugs that have less potential for abuse than schedule II drugs but can still cause low to moderate physical or psychological dependence. These drugs have accepted medical uses.

- Examples: anabolic steroids, ketamine

Schedule IV — Drugs that have less potential for abuse than schedule III drugs but can still lead to limited physical or psychological dependence. These drugs have accepted medical uses.

- Examples: benzodiazepines (alprazolam, clonazepam), sleeping tablets (zolpidem), propoxyphene

Schedule V — Drugs that have some potential for abuse but can still cause limited physical or psychological dependence. These drugs have accepted medical uses. In some states, certain schedule V medications can be sold OTC.

- Examples: diphenoxylate, pregabalin, promethazine with codeine cough syrup

REFILLING CONTROLLED SUBSTANCE PRESCRIPTION

Schedule II substance prescriptions cannot be refilled. However, they can be partially filled if the remaining quantity is dispensed within 72 hours. For patients in long-term-care facilities or those who are terminally ill, the law allows schedule II prescriptions to be partially filled an unlimited number of times for up to 60 days after the date that the prescription is written.

Schedules III and IV prescriptions may be refilled up to five times within 6 months (controlled substance prescriptions expire 6 months after the date written). There is no limit on the number of times that a schedule III or IV prescription may be partially filled so long as the total quantity prescribed is not exceeded and refills are not issued after the 6-month expiration date.

Schedule V and noncontrolled medications have no federal restrictions on the number of times that they can be refilled, although many state laws set stricter requirements for refills and expiration dates. Most states follow the schedules III and IV rules for schedule V refills, allowing up to five refills and a 6-month expiration date. For noncontrolled substances, many states set an expiration date of 12 months from the date that the prescription is written.

INFORMATION REQUIRED ON CONTROLLED SUBSTANCE PRESCRIPTIONS

Listed below are the federal requirements for controlled substance prescriptions. Be sure to check the state laws where you will be working because many states have additional requirements for controlled substance prescriptions.

- Date issued/written
- Full name and address of the patient
- Drug name, dosage form, strength, and quantity
- Directions for use
- Name, address, and DEA number of the prescriber
- The prescriber's signature must be hand-written in indelible ink (digital signatures are acceptable for electronic prescriptions)

Each controlled substance should be written on a separate prescription form. The pharmacist may rewrite the prescriptions onto two separate forms in order to make them valid. Electronic prescriptions ARE permitted for controlled substances if the sender and receiver are each using an approved prescription decryption software. Some states require controlled substances to be prescribed electronically or on special prescription paper.

"For office use" prescriptions from prescribers are NOT permissible. A DEA Form 222 (for schedule II substances) or a valid order form (for schedules III–V) must be filled out by the prescriber in order to obtain controlled substances for office use.

REFILL AND TRANSFER REQUIREMENTS FOR CONTROLLED AND NONCONTROLLED MEDICATIONS

Schedule II controlled substances are NOT refillable and CANNOT be transferred between pharmacies.

Schedules III–IV controlled substances can be refilled up to five times (total of six fills). The refills must be issued within 6 months of the date the prescription is written. If refills remain after the 6-month period, they are no longer valid because the prescription has expired. Schedules III–IV prescriptions may be transferred between pharmacies only ONE time. Chain pharmacies that share a common database can transfer prescriptions an unlimited amount of times.

Schedule V controlled substances may be refilled without limits.

Noncontrolled-substance prescriptions do not have a legal limit on the number of refills that can be prescribed. However, the prescription expires 12 months from the date it was written, and refills cannot be issued after the prescription has expired. Noncontrolled prescriptions do not have any restrictions on prescriptions transfers and can be transferred between pharmacies an unlimited number of times. However, certain states' laws and insurance regulations may limit the number of times that a prescription can be transferred.

HANDLING HAZARDOUS SUBSTANCE EXPOSURES AND SPILLS

Immediately after **exposure to a hazardous substance**, a supervisor must be notified, and someone should be designated to call for medical help if required. The substance's Material Safety Data Sheet (MSDS) should be consulted on what to do in the event of an exposure.

- **Skin exposures** can cause burns, blisters, rashes, sores, or irritation. Remove clothing around the affected skin area, and wash the area with cool water for 15 minutes.
- **Eye exposures** require flushing the eyes for 15 minutes. Contact lenses should be removed prior to the eye wash. Instructions for eye wash stations may vary, so check with your manager on how to locate and use the eye wash station at your pharmacy.

In the event of a **hazardous substance spill**, every pharmacy should have a spill kit available. Notify your supervisor and coworkers of the spill, and evacuate the area if necessary. Check the MSDS for any special precautions or PPE required prior to cleaning up the spill. Use the spill kit to absorb the chemicals, and then place them in a chemical spill bag for disposal. Wash the area with water and detergent. For large spills, call a poison control center for assistance with cleaning up the spill.

OSHA STANDARDS FOR REDUCING RISK OF BLOODBORNE PATHOGEN EXPOSURE

OSHA is the Occupational Safety and Health Administration, a government agency that helps protect employees and healthcare workers from exposure to potentially hazardous substances and chemicals. In 2000, OSHA developed the Needlestick Safety and Prevention Act to provide employers with standards for preventing the transmission of bloodborne pathogens. OSHA recommendations for reducing the risk of bloodborne pathogen transmission include the following:

- Require bloodborne pathogen training for all at-risk employees.
- Wear PPE whenever there is a reasonable risk of exposure.
- Wash hands prior to and after patient care, after removal of PPE, and after contact with blood or potentially infectious material.
- Use safer or needleless devices to reduce needlestick injuries or sharps exposures.

- Avoid splashing, spraying, or spattering body fluids.
- Use properly labeled biohazard containers or red bags labeled "Infectious Waste" for the transfer or disposal of contaminated materials.
- Use approved disinfectants on contaminated items and equipment before reuse.
- Offer hepatitis B vaccination to all employees that are at potential risk of exposure.
- Prohibit eating and drinking in work areas in which there is a risk of exposure.
- Ensure that a postexposure evaluation and a follow-up plan are in place to address exposures.

NEEDLESTICK INJURIES AND BLOODBORNE PATHOGEN EXPOSURES

A bloodborne pathogen exposure occurs when a healthcare worker or employee is exposed to human blood or any other potentially infectious material or body fluid. Body fluids other than blood that can carry infectious pathogens include cerebrospinal fluid, synovial joint fluid, pleural fluid, amniotic fluid, pericardial fluid, peritoneal fluid, semen, vaginal secretions, saliva, and fluids from tissues or body organs. All body fluids should be assumed to be infected even if the patient is not known to carry any infectious diseases. Standard precautions and exposure prevention procedures should be followed regardless of the patient being treated.

A needlestick injury results from piercing the skin or mucous membrane with a needle. If the needle was exposed to potentially infectious material prior to piercing the skin of the healthcare worker, then there is also a bloodborne pathogen exposure. Although needlestick injuries are a common type of bloodborne pathogen exposure, other common ways to be exposed to infectious material include contact with the eyes, nose, mouth, or broken/cut skin.

STEPS TO FOLLOW AFTER EXPOSURE TO BLOOD OR POTENTIALLY INFECTIOUS MATERIAL

The OSHA standards and procedures for preventing bloodborne pathogen exposures should be followed by all healthcare workers. Despite our best efforts to prevent exposures, there will always be bloodborne pathogen and needlestick incidents. Therefore, we need to know how to react in the event of an exposure to blood or other potentially infectious material or body fluid. The following steps indicate the recommended procedure to follow immediately following a bloodborne pathogen exposure:

1. Wash or irrigate the site of exposure:
   a. For needlestick injuries, wash the puncture site with soap and water.
   b. For skin exposures, wash the exposure site with soap and water.
   c. For exposure into the nose or mouth, flush the area with water.
   d. For eye exposures, irrigate the eyes with clean water, saline, or sterile irrigation fluid. If your department has an eye wash station, this is the best source for irrigation.
2. Report the exposure to your instructor, preceptor, or supervisor.
3. Seek medical evaluation as soon as possible. Postexposure prophylaxis treatments help prevent infection and are more effective if administered as soon as possible after exposure.

DISPOSAL OF USED SHARPS

Sharp objects that require disposal, such as needles and syringes, must be place in a sharps bin. Sharps bins are usually plastic containers that have a one-way opening for the disposal of sharps that also prevent removal of objects from the container. After using a needle, lancet, syringe, or other sharp, place it in a sharps bin as soon as possible. Needles should NOT be recapped because the recapping process increases the risk of needlestick injury. Additionally, capped needles may be mistaken for new needles and may be used again. Do not attempt to remove the needles at the end of a syringe because this increases the risk of needlestick injury. Discard any used sharp along with whatever it is attached to without trying to remove it. Chemotherapy and other hazardous substances should be disposed of in a separate sharps bin labeled as hazardous. If a patient does not have a sharps container, they should dispose of their sharps in a hard, sealable container, such as a laundry detergent bottle.

Controlled Substances

DEA FORMS

DEA Form 222 — used to order, sell, or transfer schedule I or II controlled substances

- Three carbon copies: Copy 1 (brown) is kept by the supplier/distributor/wholesaler; copy 2 (green) is sent to the DEA by the supplier at the end of the month; copy 3 (blue) is kept by the purchaser/pharmacy.
- Only the registrant and those authorized by power of attorney on behalf of the registrant can complete this form.
- Orders may be partially filled by the supplier, but the remaining quantity must be shipped within 60 days.
- Forms must be stored at the pharmacy for 2 years from the date of execution.
- Forms must be written in indelible ink or typewritten (may be electronic), and no changes or erasures are permitted.

DEA Form 224 — controlled substance registration for manufacturers, distributors, or dispensers that wish to handle controlled substances

DEA Form 41 — controlled substance destruction/disposal

DEA Form 106 — to report theft or loss of controlled substances

All DEA forms must be kept on file at the pharmacy for a minimum of 2 years.

FILING PRESCRIPTIONS

The three different ways in which prescriptions can be filed with reference to their controlled drug schedule are as follows:

- Three separate prescriptions files
  - Schedule II substances
  - Schedules III, IV, and V substances
  - All noncontrolled drugs
- Two separate prescription files:
  - Schedule II substances
  - All other drugs dispensed*
- Electronic Prescription Records
  - All records of prescriptions created, signed, transmitted, and received electronically must be retained for 2 years from the date of creation or receipt OR in accordance with (present or future) federal or state laws requiring longer retention periods
  - Electronic records must be easily read
  - Records for controlled substances should be retrievable from all other records

*If schedules III–V prescriptions are mixed with noncontrolled drugs (as in the option with 2 files), a ≥1-inch red letter C must be used in all schedule III–V prescriptions to identify them from the rest of the prescriptions in that file. The only exception to this rule is if the pharmacy has a computer system that can adequately differentiate and retrieve those prescriptions.

Inventories and ordering forms (DEA Form 222) for schedule II drugs must be kept separate from other records. All records for any controlled substance must be kept on file for at least 2 years according to federal laws, but most state laws and insurance regulations require records to be kept for longer. Prescription records can be kept at a central storage location so long as the DEA is notified beforehand, and the records remain retrievable within 2 business days. Certain records, such as inventories and executed DEA Forms 222, must be kept at the pharmacy and cannot be sent to a central location.

ACCEPTING CONTROLLED SUBSTANCE PRESCRIPTIONS VIA FAX

Schedules III–V controlled medications CAN be accepted by facsimile transmission.

- Schedule II controlled medications are generally NOT allowed to be accepted by facsimile transmission, except when the patient is a resident of a long-term-care facility.
- The patient is enrolled in a hospice care program licensed by the state or certified by Medicare. The prescriber must note on the R, "Hospice Patient."
- A narcotic pain therapy drug is prescribed for a terminally ill patient (e.g., home infusion/IV pain therapy).
- The medication is a parenteral, IV, IM, SC, or intraspinal infusion that is going to be compounded for direct administration to a patient.
- The prescriber, patient, or patient's agent faxes a valid, signed prescription to the pharmacy in order to expedite pre-dispensing preparations. The original prescription must be received by the pharmacy prior to actual dispensing.

ACCEPTING VERBAL ORDERS FOR CONTROLLED SUBSTANCES

Schedules III–V controlled medications CAN be accepted by verbal order or voicemail.

Verbal orders for schedule II controlled substances are ONLY permitted in emergency situations under the following conditions:

- The drug is required for immediate administration.
- No alternative drug that is NOT a schedule II substance will be effective.
- The prescriber is unable to provide a written prescription.
- The pharmacist must verify the authenticity of the prescriber issuing the verbal order.
- The quantity prescribed in the verbal order should cover the emergency period only.
- The information given in the verbal order must be immediately reduced to writing by the pharmacist (verbal orders cannot be taken by pharmacy technicians).
- An original hard-copy prescription must be postmarked or delivered to the pharmacy within 7 days of the verbal order. The hard-copy prescription from the prescriber must be signed in indelible ink, state "Authorization for emergency dispensing," and include the date of the verbal order. Prescribers are responsible for sending a hard copy of the prescription to the pharmacy within the required time frame. If the prescription is not received or postmarked within 7 days, the pharmacy must notify the DEA.

PARTIALLY FILLING CONTROLLED MEDICATION PRESCRIPTIONS

Schedules III–V controlled substances CAN be partially filled so long as the maximum quantity prescribed is never exceeded. Any refills or partial fills cannot be dispensed beyond 6 months after the date that the prescription was written.

The law allows schedule II medications to be partially filled so long as the remaining balance is supplied within 72 hours. This means that the patient must pick up the partial balance within 72 hours, so most retail pharmacies find this service too risky to offer. If the partial fill is not supplied within 72 hours, the remaining balance on the prescription must be voided and the prescriber must be notified.

There are certain exceptions to this rule that allow prescriptions to be partially filled for up to 60 days from the date of issuance of the prescription. These exceptions include patients in long-term-care facilities and patients who are terminally ill. In these cases, the prescription must indicate either "LTCF" or "Terminally ill," respectively. The prescription can be partially filled an unlimited number of times within the 60-day period so long as the pharmacist records the date, quantity dispensed, remaining quantity authorized, and dispensing pharmacist's name for each fill.

ACCOMMODATIONS FOR PATIENTS WITH PHYSICAL LIMITATIONS

The Poison Prevention Packaging Act of 1970 requires that medications be packaged in child-proof containers. However, patients with arthritis or other physical limitations may not be able to open these child-proof containers to access their medications. Patients can request (orally or in writing) that non-safety caps be used for all of their medications. Additionally, prescribers can request non-safety caps on behalf of a patient, but this would apply only for that specific prescription. Pharmacy technicians can document these requests in the patient's medical record to ensure that their medications are packaged accordingly.

For patients with visual impairments, most pharmacy computer systems allow prescription labels to be printed in large font sizes to accommodate these patients. Unfortunately, most computer systems cannot print labels in braille, but there are a few text-to-speech technologies available that can assist with this challenge (e.g., ScripTalk).

Hearing-impaired patients do not need any special accommodations when it comes to their medication labels, but counseling these patients can be tricky. The pharmacist should provide them with written information about their medication.

INFORMATION RECORDED WHEN CONTROLLED SUBSTANCE IS RECEIVED AND DISPENSED

A continuous inventory is not required for schedules III–V controlled substances, but it is required for schedule II substances. In a controlled substance log, the pharmacy must keep a record of the current inventory, drugs received, and drugs dispensed for each NDC of schedule II substance kept in the pharmacy.

When schedule II drugs are received from an order, the following information must be recorded in the controlled substance log: the name of the substance; dosage form; strength of the substance; number of dosage units or volume in the container; number of containers received; date of receipt; and name, address, and registration number of the supplier. All controlled substance (schedules II–V) invoices must be kept, and schedule II invoices must be kept separate from schedules III–V invoices.

When schedule II drugs are dispensed to patients, the following information must be recorded in the controlled substance log: name of the drug dispensed, date of dispensing, whether the drug was administered or dispensed to the patient, name of the patient to whom the drug was dispensed, and quantity of drug dispensed. Similar entries must be made when controlled substances are distributed to another pharmacy or practitioner, lost/stolen, or destroyed/disposed of.

DISPOSAL OF CONTROLLED SUBSTANCES

A DEA Form 41 must be used to document the destruction of controlled substances. The form should include the name, address, phone number, and DEA number of the pharmacy/facility; name, strength, form, NDC number, and quantity of each controlled substance destroyed; date, location, and method of destruction; and signatures of two authorized witnesses. There are three main options for disposing of controlled substances:

1. They can be transferred or returned to a reverse distributor authorized to possess controlled substances. The reverse distributor will issue a DEA Form 222 for the transfer/return of schedule II drugs.
2. They may be destroyed in the presence of an authorized member of the DEA Drug Control Division or law enforcement. A DEA Form 41 detailing the controlled substances disposed of must be filled out and sent to the DEA.
3. Hospitals or facilities that are licensed to administer medications may obtain a blanket authorization from the DEA to immediately destroy controlled substances on site in the presence of two authorized employees. A record of the destruction should be recorded using a DEA Form 41, and the form should be submitted to the DEA Drug Control Division within 10 days of the destruction.

ORDERING CONTROLLED SUBSTANCES

Schedules III–V controlled substances can be ordered with other noncontrolled medications.

Schedule II controlled substances must be ordered using either an electronic or written version of DEA Form 222. DEA Form 222 must be typewritten or filled out in ink by a person authorized by the DEA. In most pharmacies, only one pharmacist is authorized by the DEA to place schedule II substance orders. Other pharmacists may place orders on their behalf if they obtain power of attorney. Strikethroughs, scratch-outs, or other alterations are not allowed on DEA Form 222. If a mistake is made, one must start over with a new form.

Paper DEA Forms 222 are triplicates consisting of three copies. Copy 3 (blue) should be kept by the pharmacy or ordering facility. Copies 1 (brown) and 2 (green) are submitted to the wholesaler when placing an order. The wholesaler will keep copy 1 and send copy 2 to the DEA at the end of each month. Upon receiving the order, the pharmacy will complete copy 3 of the form with the actual quantities of medication received and keep the form on file at the pharmacy for at least 2 years.

SCHEDULE II CONTROLLED SUBSTANCES

Schedule II controlled substances have a high potential for abuse and usually are kept locked up in the pharmacy safe. Schedule II substances must adhere to stricter prescription requirements. Only valid paper or electronic prescriptions are accepted, no refills are permitted, no prescription transfers are permitted, and prescriptions expire after 6 months. Substances that are classified as schedule II include opioid pain medications, CNS stimulants used to treat ADHD, and barbiturates used for sedation and to treat seizures. Codeine is only classified as a schedule II substance when it is not used in combination with another noncontrolled substance or if each dosage unit contains

96

more than 90 mg of codeine. Diphenoxylate, a component of the laxative Lomotil, is a schedule II substance when not used in combination with another product.

Brand Name	Generic Name
Codeine	Codeine
Vicodin, Norco, Lortab	Hydrocodone
Dilaudid	Hydromorphone
MS Contin, Roxanol, Kadian	Morphine
Oxycontin, Percocet	Oxycodone
Opana	Oxymorphone
Panlor	Dihydrocodeine
Duragesic, Sublimaze	Fentanyl
Dolophine	Methadone
Demerol	Meperidine
Adderall, Vyvanse	Amphetamine
Desoxyn	Methamphetamine
Ritalin, Concerta, Metadate	Methylphenidate
Pentasol	Pentobarbital

SCHEDULE III CONTROLLED SUBSTANCES

Some CNS stimulants used for weight loss are classified as schedule III substances, including benzphetamine and chlorphentermine.

Synthetic cannabinoids (marijuana derivatives), such as dronabinol (Marinol) are also schedule III.

Anabolic steroids are also schedule III substances, including testosterone (Depo-Testosterone, AndroGel) and dihydrotestosterone (Andractim).

Some barbiturates used to treat seizures that are normally classified as schedule II substances are classified as schedule III substances when formulated as a suppository or in combination with another noncontrolled substance. Pentobarbital and secobarbital suppositories are schedule III medications.

Ketamine (Ketalar), which is used for pain and sedation, is a schedule III substance.

Some opioid pain medications are also classified as schedule III substances, including buprenorphine (Suboxone, Subutex, Zubsolv). Codeine and dihydrocodeine are considered schedule III substances when the product contains ≤90 mg per dosage unit or ≤1.8 g per 100 mL of solution when used in combination with another noncontrolled substance. Morphine is a schedule III substance if it is used in combination with a noncontrolled substance and the product contains ≤50 mg per 100 mL or 100 g.

SCHEDULE IV CONTROLLED SUBSTANCES

Most drugs in the schedule IV classification are benzodiazepines. Examples of benzodiazepines in this class include alprazolam (Xanax), chlordiazepoxide, clobazam, clonazepam (Klonopin), diazepam (Valium), flurazepam, loprazolam, lorazepam (Ativan), nitrazepam, oxazepam, temazepam, and triazolam. The Z-drugs used to treat insomnia are also schedule IV substances. Z-drugs include zaleplon (Sonata), zolpidem (Ambien), zopiclone (Imovane), and eszopiclone (Lunesta).

The opioid pain medication tramadol (Ultram) is also a schedule IV substance.

Some muscle relaxers are schedule IV controlled substances, including dextropropoxyphene (Darvon, Darvocet) and carisoprodol (Soma).

Many CNS stimulants used to aid in weight loss are classified as schedule IV controlled substances. This includes phentermine (Adipex-P), diethylpropion (Tenuate), and mazindol (Mazanor). Modafinil (Provigil), a stimulant used to treat sleep disorders, is also a schedule IV substance.

The CNS depressant phenobarbital, which is used to treat seizure disorders, is also a schedule IV medication.

SCHEDULE V CONTROLLED SUBSTANCES

Schedule V controlled substances are generally combination products that contain a schedule II, III, or IV controlled substance and at least one other noncontrolled substance.

Diphenoxylate, which is normally a schedule II controlled substance on its own, is classified as a schedule V substance when no more than 2.5 mg is combined with at least 25 mcg of atropine per dosage unit. Therefore, the medication Lomotil (2.5 mg diphenoxylate/0.025 mg atropine), used to treat diarrhea, is a schedule V substance.

The opiates codeine and dihydrocodeine may also be considered schedule V substances when combined in low concentrations with another noncontrolled ingredient. Products that contain ≤200 mg of codeine per 100 mL or 100 g of product are classified as schedule V substances. This includes Phenergan with Codeine syrup, which contains 6.25 mg promethazine and 10 mg codeine per teaspoonful (5 mL) of syrup, and Robitussin/Cheratussin AC, which contains 100 mg of guaifenesin and 10 mg of codeine per teaspoonful. Products that contain ≤100 mg of dihydrocodeine per 100 mL of 100 grams of product are also classified as schedule V substance. Many states allow some schedule V cough syrups to be sold OTC.

Restricted Drug Programs and Related Medication Processing

OTC PSEUDOEPHEDRINE

The 2005 Combat Methamphetamine Epidemic Act began restricting OTC sales of pseudoephedrine, ephedrine, and phenylpropanolamine. This law requires these medications to be kept behind a counter in a locked cabinet, and it places restrictions on the OTC sale of these products. Note that sales of these products pursuant to a valid prescription are not subject to the same restrictions. Pharmacies that sell pseudoephedrine products must submit a self-certification to the DEA annually confirming that they train their employees on the requirements and limits for sale of listed chemicals.

Requirements for OTC sale of pseudoephedrine:

- A maximum of 3.6 g per day or 9 g per month (7.5 g/month for mail order/online pharmacies) can be sold to the same customer.
- Customers must be 18 years or older to purchase and show a valid photo ID.
- Make electronic record of the sale: photo ID number; date and time of transaction; product name; quantity sold; purchaser's name, address, and date of birth; and purchaser's signature.
- Records of sale must be kept for 2 years from the date of last entry.

REMS Program

Before a medication can be marketed to patients, the FDA must first evaluate its safety and effectiveness. The FDA does not usually approve medications that pose serious safety risks, but sometimes the benefits outweigh the risks. The FDA can approve these medications conditional of participation in a postmarketing safety program. A Risk Evaluation and Mitigation Strategy (REMS) is a drug safety program required by the FDA for certain medications that pose serious safety concerns. REMS programs are designed to reinforce appropriate and safe use of a medication. REMS programs are specific to the medication but usually involve supplemental patient counseling, patient education, and laboratory monitoring (e.g., pregnancy testing). There may even be extra training or continuing education required for the prescriber and dispensing pharmacist.

The following are medications that require REMS: Accutane (isotretinoin), Clozaril (clozapine), Pomalyst (pomalidomide), Revlimid (lenalidomide), Thalomid (thalidomide).

DSCSA

The Drug Supply Chain Security Act (DSCSA) was enacted in 2013 as an effort to reduce the prevalence of counterfeit drugs. This act established a national tracing system for medications, known as a drug pedigree. These pedigrees track and record drug movement. Tracking begins at the manufacturing facility where the drug is produced. Any time a drug is relocated to a new location, such as a distribution facility or pharmacy, it is documented in the drug pedigree. The types of tracking information contained in the drug pedigree include the name, strength, and dosage of the product; NDC number; container size; number of containers; product lot numbers; transaction date; shipment date; name and address of the seller and purchaser; and transaction history. Pharmacies are required to obtain drug pedigree information and maintain drug pedigrees for 6 years.

In addition to establishing drug pedigree requirements, the DSCSA also established national licensing standards for wholesale distribution.

OSHA Requirements for Working with Hazardous Substances

OSHA regulates the use of hazardous substances in the workplace. OSHA requires every workplace to keep an MSDS book or binder that contains information on all the hazardous chemicals that are to be used in the workplace. In a pharmacy, the MSDS binder may contain information about cleaning products, isopropyl alcohol, and hazardous medications. MSDS sheets contain information on chemicals, their identifying characteristics, flammability, volatility, storage requirements, exposure prevention, and what to do in case of a spill or an exposure. Expired or damaged medications are also considered hazardous substances and should be stored in a designated bin or area of the pharmacy labeled "Hazardous waste" and kept separate from other medication stock.

When working with certain substances, employees are required to protect themselves by wearing PPE such as gloves, gowns, goggles, foot covers, hair covers, and masks. Most retail pharmacies do not work with any substances that require PPE to be worn, but if you will be working with chemotherapy agents, preparing compounded products, or preparing sterile IV products, you may be required to wear PPE.

Prescription-Only, Behind-the-Counter, and OTC Medications

Prescription-only medications, also known as legend drugs, cannot be obtained without a prescription. The label on the medication container must contain the phrase "R Only" or "Caution: Federal law prohibits dispensing without a prescription." These medications require approval from the FDA before they can be sold.

Over-the-counter (OTC) medications are still regulated by the FDA but do not require a prescription. The FDA has determined that these medications are safe enough for use by the general population without the need for consultation with a healthcare provider.

Behind-the-counter medications are OTC medications that must be kept behind the pharmacy counter or in a locked cabinet because of their potential for abuse. The purchaser must be at least 18 years old and show photo ID prior to purchasing. There are certain restrictions on the amount of behind-the-counter medications that can be sold to the same purchaser in a set time period. The most common example of a behind-the counter medication is pseudoephedrine (Sudafed). Some states also allow schedule V controlled substances, such as promethazine with codeine cough syrup, to be sold as a behind-the-counter medication.

RESTRICTIONS WITH DISPENSING ISOTRETINOIN

The dispensing of isotretinoin (Accutane) is restricted by the FDA through a REMS program called iPledge. The use of isotretinoin is restricted because it can cause serious fetal abnormalities or fetal death in women who are pregnant. All prescribers, pharmacies, and patients who deal with isotretinoin are required to register with the iPledge program. Adverse effects must be reported quarterly, and participating facilities are evaluated annually for program compliance.

Permitted prescriptions for isotretinoin may be via telephone, fax, or email, and dispensed to the patient within 7 days of a negative pregnancy test. A maximum of 30 days' supply can be dispensed at a time.

Patients who register with the iPledge program must receive medication counseling from a pharmacist and sign a consent form. Female patients must agree to monthly pregnancy testing and comply with using two methods of contraception throughout the duration of treatment and for 30 days after treatment.

FDA Requirements

DRUG VS. DEVICE

According to the FDA, a drug is any compound recognized in the official *United States Pharmacopeia* (USP), *National Formulary* (NF), or *The Homœopathic Pharmacopœia of the United States*. A device is an instrument, apparatus, implement, machine, contrivance, implant, in vitro reagent, or other component, part, or accessory that is recognized in the official NF or USP. Drugs and devices are both intended for the use in the diagnosis, cure, mitigation, treatment, or prevention of disease in humans or animals. Both drugs and devices affect the structure or function of the body, but drugs achieve this through chemical action whereas devices achieve this through physical action or presence. The differentiation between drugs and devices can get confusing because many products are devices that contain a drug (e.g., hormonal IUD). In most cases, when a product meets the definition of a drug and a device, the FDA classifies it as a device.

Examples of drugs include digoxin tablets, nitroglycerin tablets or patches, and erythromycin oral suspension.

Examples of devices include hearing aids, catheters, pacemakers, and Mirena.

DRUG RECALL CLASSES

If a medication causes adverse effects or if it is contaminated, damaged, or mislabeled, the FDA may require the manufacturer to recall the medication. The manufacturer will then have to supply distributors and pharmacies with information about the product that is being recalled (product name, lot number, package size, reason for the recall). This recall information sheet will also contain instructions on what the pharmacy should do with the affected products.

Class I — Drugs or devices that can cause serious adverse health consequences or death if administered. All of the affected medication in stock at the pharmacy must be isolated. A notice must also be issued to all patients to whom the drug has been dispensed asking the patients to return the medication to the pharmacy.

Class II — Drugs or devices that could cause temporary reversible effects or have a small chance of causing serious adverse effects if administered. All affected drug stocks at the pharmacy must be isolated, but a notice to patients is not usually required.

Class III — Drugs or devices that are unlikely to cause any adverse health effects if administered. Usually results from a packaging or labeling violation. These recalls are usually voluntary (not required).

OMNIBUS BUDGET RECONCILIATION ACT OF 1990

The Omnibus Budget Reconciliation Act of 1990 (OBRA-90) elevated the standards for drug therapy reviews and patient counseling in the pharmacy setting. Although OBRA-90 standards only apply to Medicaid patients, most states have passed similar regulations that apply to all pharmacy patients.

Under OBRA-90, a pharmacist must conduct a review of drug therapy prior to dispensing each prescription, which involves screening for therapeutic duplications, drug interactions, allergies, and contraindications. The pharmacist must also make a reasonable effort to obtain the following information for the patient's profile: name, address, telephone number, date of birth, gender, allergies, list of current medications, and relevant medical history.

OBRA-90 also requires pharmacists to offer each Medicaid patient counseling on their prescriptions. The law requires the pharmacist to counsel on information deemed significant by the pharmacist, such as the name and description of the medication, route of administration, directions for use, common side effects, proper storage, duration of treatment, and special precautions.

REGULATIONS GOVERNED BY STATE AND FEDERAL LAWS

Federal pharmacy laws are applicable in all 50 states. Applicable federal pharmacy laws can be found in the Code of Federal Regulations, Title 21. HIPAA privacy laws, standards for compounding, investigational drug regulations, drug packaging requirements, requirements for the sale of pseudoephedrine, and labeling requirements are all regulated by federal law. Most laws dealing with controlled substances are also part of federal law. Controlled-substance laws are enforced by the Drug Enforcement Agency (DEA).

State pharmacy laws are different depending on the state in which you are working. Some regulations vary greatly among states, whereas others are similar across all states. States regulate and enforce the licensing and regulation of pharmacies and facilities, pharmacists, and pharmacy technicians. Licensing requirements, required continuing education, license renewal periods, and renewal fees vary significantly among states. States are responsible for inspecting pharmacies and facilities, defining the role of pharmacy technicians, and regulating how long pharmacy records should be kept for.

HIPAA

The legislative requirements established by the Health Insurance Portability and Accountability Act of 1996 (HIPAA) are summarized below:

- Patient health information must be stored securely and disposed of properly.
- All healthcare providers are assigned a unique 10-digit National Provider Identifier (NPI) number that allows protected health information (PHI) to be transferred more securely.
- Patient authorization is required to disclose information for marketing and other disclosures not required for treatment. Patient authorization is not required for disclosures among healthcare providers that are necessary for patient treatment.
- Patients have a right to obtain a copy of their PHI. Patients themselves must sign and date an authorization form (good for up to 1 year), and the pharmacy must comply within 30 days.
- State laws or insurance company policies may require stricter privacy controls. For example, the Centers for Medicare and Medicaid Services (CMS) requires the use of tamper-resistant medications.
- Pharmacies must notify patients within 60 days of an information breach.
- A Notice of Privacy Practices must be posted in the pharmacy and must be made available to patients. This notice must include how the pharmacy intends to use, disclose, and protect the patient's health information as well as the patient's rights and information on how to file a complaint.

> **Review Video: HIPAA**
> Visit mometrix.com/academy and enter code: 412009

STORAGE AND DISPOSAL REQUIREMENTS FOR PHI

HIPAA placed restrictions on the storage, access, and transfer of electronic, paper, or oral patient health information. Protected health information (PHI) includes any document that contains a patient's name, address, date of birth, medical history, insurance information, or other identifying information. PHI that is stored or transmitted must have safeguards in place to prevent unauthorized access. Computer systems must be password protected and must be backed up daily to prevent data loss. Paper documents must be stored in a locked area.

PHI must be disposed of in a secure manner. Some smaller pharmacies shred all of their PHI. Most pharmacies accumulate too much PHI for this to be feasible. Retail pharmacies usually have a large trash bin where PHI is dumped. At regular intervals, a document shredding company will pick up the bin and dispose of its contents properly. Smaller PHI trash bins are usually scattered around the pharmacy, and then they are combined into a large PHI bin at the end of the day. Hospitals and large facilities have PHI information receptacles scattered around the facility. They usually look like gray boxes that have an opening for paper. A shredding or disposal service will collect these at regular intervals.

SCENARIOS IN WHICH PHI MAY BE DISCLOSED

All patients have a right to obtain their PHI. In hospitals, patients usually have to contact the medical records or health information services department. In retail pharmacies, pharmacy staff members generally have access to patient profile summaries and can print them for patients. Prior to obtaining PHI information, patients themselves must sign and date an authorization form (good for up to 1 year) and the pharmacy must comply within 30 days. Another family member or relative is NOT authorized to pick up a patient's medical records unless they are authorized by power of attorney to do so. If a child is younger than 18 years of age, their parent or legal guardian may obtain a copy of their PHI. Patient authorization is also required for disclosing PHI for any reason not related to treatment (e.g., marketing). PHI can be disclosed without patient authorization for refill reminders, disease management programs, communication with other healthcare providers in relation to treatment, communications to the patient, general health promotion, court orders or subpoenas, or for serious health threats (i.e., child abuse).

PPIs

Patient package inserts (PPIs), or medication guides, are informational leaflets designed to educate patients about a medication. PPIs have the following layout: table of contents, patient counseling information, highlights (boxed warnings, indications, usage, dosage, administration), recent changes to the leaflet, date of the initial drug approval, and toll-free phone number to report adverse drug reactions. These leaflets provide information about proper use of the medication, when the medication should not be used, and any serious adverse effects that may occur. PPIs must be approved by the FDA prior to use.

Certain medications require a PPI to be dispensed with it. These medications include oral contraceptives, IUDs, estrogen- or progesterone-containing products, and isoproterenol inhalations. Failure to provide a PPI for these medications is considered misbranding. For hospitalized patients, a PPI must be provided prior to the first administration, then every 30 days. For outpatients, a PPI must be provided for the first fill as well as each refill.

DEA Number

A DEA number is an identifier assigned to any healthcare provider that prescribes or dispenses controlled substances. This number helps identify and authenticate prescribers. A DEA number consists of two letters and seven numbers.

The first letter indicates the type of practitioner or facility.

- Medical doctors, doctors of osteopathy, veterinarians (doctors of veterinary medicine), dentists, podiatrists = A, B, or F.
- Midlevel practitioners (e.g., physician assistants, certified registered nurse practitioners) = M.
- Prescribers authorized to prescribe under a narcotic treatment program = X.

The second letter is the first letter of the prescriber's last name.

The numerical digits provide a mechanism for verifying the authenticity of a DEA number.

1. Add digits 1 + 3 + 5.
2. Add digits 2 + 4 + 6 and multiply this number by 2.
3. Calculate the total sum from steps 1 and 2.
4. The last digit of the total sum should equal the seventh digit of the DEA number.

DEA numbers can also be electronically verified on the DEA's website.

Recall Requirements for Drugs, Devices, Supplies, and Supplements

A recall is the voluntary removal or correction of a product that is on the market because it is adulterated, misbranded, or in violation of FDA approval. A recall can be initiated by the manufacturer or the FDA. Although voluntary, if a manufacturer does not comply with the recall requirements, they may face legal action and the FDA can seize the product.

The recall processes for prescription drugs, devices, supplies, OTC products, and supplements are very similar. In all cases, a recall is initiated and is assigned a class number that determines how quickly the pharmacy must act upon the recall. Class I recalls are the most urgent, whereas class III recalls are the least urgent. Although vitamins and supplements are regulated by the FDA, the regulations are not as strict as for drugs and devices. Therefore, vitamin and supplement recalls are rare. Medical device recalls are sometimes referred to as medical device safety alerts.

TRANSFERRING NONCONTROLLED SUBSTANCE PRESCRIPTION TO ANOTHER PHARMACY

Noncontrolled drugs can be transferred from pharmacy to pharmacy as many times as allowed by state laws so long as the maximum number of refills on the prescription is not exceeded.

The pharmacist transferring the prescription must give the following prescription information to the pharmacist at the receiving pharmacy: the prescription number, original date that the prescription was written, original number of refills authorized, date of first/initial dispensing, date of last refill, and number of valid refills remaining. The pharmacists should also exchange their names and information about their pharmacies, including the pharmacy name, address, and phone number.

Once the transfer is complete, the transferring pharmacist should transfer or void the prescription in the pharmacy computer system. Alternatively, the word "VOID" can be written on the face of the hard-copy prescription. The following information should be recorded in the pharmacy's computer system: the name and address of the pharmacy receiving the prescription, name of the receiving pharmacist, date of the transfer, and name of the transferring pharmacist.

RECEIVING NONCONTROLLED SUBSTANCE PRESCRIPTION TRANSFER FROM ANOTHER PHARMACY

In order to receive a noncontrolled substance prescription transfer from another pharmacy, the pharmacist must call the pharmacy in possession of the prescription and speak to another pharmacist.

The receiving pharmacist should obtain the following information from the transferring pharmacist: the prescription number, original date that the prescription was written, original number of refills authorized, date of first/initial dispensing, date of last refill, and number of valid refills remaining. The pharmacists should also exchange names and information about their pharmacies, including the pharmacy name, address, and phone number.

Once the transfer is complete, the pharmacist should reduce the prescription information to writing. The prescription information can be entered into the computer system by the pharmacist or a pharmacy technician. When entering the prescription information, the prescription origin must be marked as a pharmacy transfer, which will prompt the computer system to allow information about the transferring pharmacy and pharmacist to be entered.

Chapter Quiz

Ready to see how well you retained what you just read? Scan the QR code to go directly to the chapter quiz interface for this study guide. If you're using a computer, simply visit the bonus page at **mometrix.com/bonus948/ptcb** and click the Chapter Quizzes link.

Patient Safety and Quality Assurance

Transform passive reading into active learning! After immersing yourself in this chapter, put your comprehension to the test by taking a quiz. The insights you gained will stay with you longer this way. Scan the QR code to go directly to the chapter quiz interface for this study guide. If you're using a computer, simply visit the bonus page at **mometrix.com/bonus948/ptcb** and click the Chapter Quizzes link.

High-Alert/High-Risk and LASA Medications

LASA MEDICATIONS

Look-alike/sound-alike (LASA) medications are drugs with names that are either spelled similarly or sound similar when pronounced. Medications with similar names are prone to confusion and mix-up and can lead to medication errors.

LASA Medications	
Amlodipine	Amiloride
Alprazolam	Lorazepam
Bupropion	Buspirone
Ceftazidime	Ceftriaxone
Cefazolin	Cefoxitin
Celebrex	Celexa
Chlorpromazine	Chlordiazepoxide
Cisplatin	Carboplatin
Clobazam	Clonazepam
Clonidine	Klonopin, Clonazepam
Cyclosporine	Cycloserine
Dactinomycin	Daptomycin
Dobutamine	Dopamine
Docetaxel	Paclitaxel
Doxorubicin	Daunorubicin
Duloxetine	Fluoxetine
Epinephrine	Ephedrine
Flonase	Flovent
Fluoxetine	Fluvoxamine
Fluphenazine	Fluvoxamine
Glipizide	Glyburide
Guaifenesin	Guanfacine
Hydralazine	Hydroxyzine
Hydrocodone	Oxycodone
Hydromorphone	Oxymorphone
Humulin	Humalog
Infliximab	Rituximab
Isotretinoin	Tretinoin
Lamictal	Lamisil
Medroxyprogesterone	Methylprednisolone

Mifepristone	Misoprostol
Methimazole	Metolazone
Nifedipine	Nicardipine
Novolin	Novolog
Oxcarbazepine	Carbamazepine
Oxycodone	Oxymorphone
Paroxetine	Fluoxetine
Penicillin	Penicillamine
Phenobarbital	Pentobarbital
Prednisone	Prednisolone
Quinidine	Quinine
Rifaximin	Rifampin
Risperidone	Ropinirole
Sitagliptin	Saxagliptin
Sulfasalazine	Sulfadiazine
Tizanidine	Tiagabine
Tramadol	Trazodone
Valacyclovir	Valganciclovir
Vincristine	Vinblastine
Zyprexa	Zyrtec

HIGH-ALERT MEDICATION

High-alert medications are those that have the potential to cause significant harm if an error is made. Therefore, more caution and consideration must be taken when dispensing these medications.

High-Alert Medications		
IV adrenergic agonists (e.g., epinephrine)	Epidural administration of any medication	IV nitroprusside sodium
IV adrenergic antagonists (e.g., propranolol)	Oral hypoglycemic agents (e.g., glyburide, glimepiride, metformin)	Parenteral nutrition
Anesthetics (e.g., propofol)	IV inotropic agents (e.g., digoxin)	IV potassium chloride or potassium phosphate
IV antiarrhythmics (e.g., amiodarone)	Insulin	IV radiocontrast agents
Antithrombotic agents (e.g., warfarin, alteplase, apixaban)	Intrathecal administration of any medication	Sedation agents (e.g., chloral hydrate, midazolam, dexmedetomidine)
Chemotherapy agents (e.g., methotrexate)	Liposomal formulations (e.g., liposomal amphotericin B)	Sterile water for injection, inhalation, and irrigation in containers of ≥100 mL
Dextrose solutions ≥20% (hypertonic dextrose)	Narcotics/opioids (e.g., oxycodone, hydrocodone, hydromorphone)	IV sodium chloride >0.9% (hypertonic saline)
Dialysis solutions	Neuromuscular blocking agents (e.g., succinylcholine, rocuronium, vecuronium)	IV vasopressin

PHARMACEUTICAL BALANCE

A balance is used to weigh powders, liquids, and other ingredients during compound preparation. There are three main types of balances: class III torsion balances, electronic balances, and analytical balances. Class III torsion balances are commonly seen in pharmacies. Electronic balances are usually only used in pharmacies that do a significant amount of compounding. Analytical balances are very accurate and are used to weigh small amounts of material. They are typically only found in research facilities.

Balances should always be placed on a level surface. In order to calibrate the machine, a weighing paper should be placed on the scale (tare weight), then the scale should be calibrated to zero by pressing the zero or tare button. A spatula should be used to add or remove increments of the material being weighed until the correct amount is obtained. The scale and spatula should be cleaned after use to avoid cross contamination.

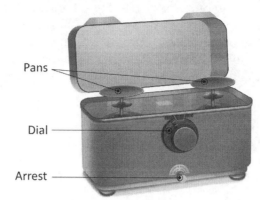

- Pans
- Dial
- Arrest

INFUSIONS PUMPS AND SYRINGE DRIVERS/PUMPS

Infusion pumps are used to deliver large volumes of bagged fluids to a patient, including IV fluids, IV medications, and total parenteral nutrition. Although they are most commonly used in hospitals or care facilities, some patients use infusion pumps at home. These pumps may also be referred to as volumetric infusion pumps because they move a set volume of fluid along the tubing using mechanical methods (e.g., rotary or linear mechanisms).

Syringe drivers/pumps deliver small volumes of fluid to a patient directly from a compatible disposable syringe. Unlike infusion pumps that are driven by volume, syringe pumps are calibrated to move the syringe plunger a set distance over time. Syringe pumps are used in hospitals and medical facilities to administer certain medications, including patient-controlled analgesia. They are also very convenient for administration of medications to patients at home (e.g., insulin, chemotherapy) because there are small portable syringe pumps available.

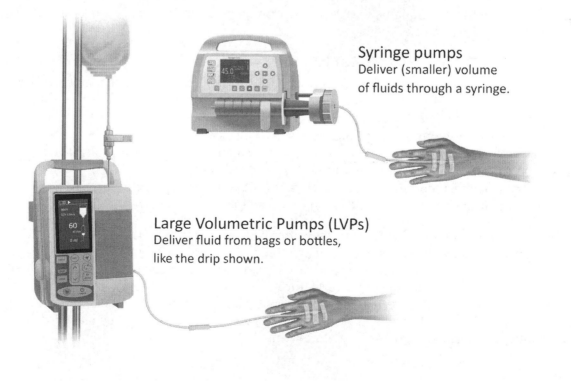

Syringe pumps
Deliver (smaller) volume
of fluids through a syringe.

Large Volumetric Pumps (LVPs)
Deliver fluid from bags or bottles,
like the drip shown.

INFUSION PUMPS

Infusion pumps are machines that are used by healthcare workers to administer set volumes of IV fluids to patients. Nurses use infusion pumps daily, but as a pharmacy technician, you will not deal with infusion pumps very often. However, you may receive questions or comments from nurses about infusion pumps and should be familiar with them. When maintained properly, these machines are very accurate and help improve patient care. However, each machine must undergo periodic maintenance and testing to ensure that it is performing its best.

Calibration and performance testing for infusion pumps are completed during an initial inspection when the machine is first purchased, after any repairs, and as part of their annual preventative maintenance. Hospital protocols or guidelines from the manufacturer are consulted to determine how to operate and calibrate the pump because there are many different types of pumps available on the market. Calibration involves verifying that it is administering the correct flow or volume that is stated.

ACCOMMODATIONS FOR DISABILITIES AND LANGUAGE BARRIERS

A disability includes any physical or mental disadvantage or impairment. Examples of commonly encountered disabilities include hearing impairments, visual impairments, learning disabilities, and physical disabilities. Patients with hearing impairments can be accommodated by receiving written drug information and counseling rather than verbal counseling. For patients with visual impairments, prescription labels can be printed in large font sizes or text-to-speech technologies (e.g., ScripTalk) can be used to assist with medication administration. Medication information leaflets must be written at or below a sixth-grade reading level to accommodate patients with learning or mental disabilities. Physical disabilities, such as arthritis, can be accommodated by offering the patient non-safety prescription bottle caps that are easier to open.

In today's diverse society, language barriers are becoming commonplace in pharmacies. Hospital pharmacies have translating services available to accommodate these patients. Although retail pharmacies do not usually offer translating services, most pharmacy computer systems can accommodate patients with language barriers by printing prescription labels and medication information leaflets in different languages.

ASSISTING PATIENTS WITH DRUG COST ISSUES

Socioeconomic status can be a major barrier to healthcare. Some patients have high copays or deductibles that leave them with high drug costs. Because insurance plans and formularies change often, it is best to contact the insurance company to obtain more information about the copay or deductible. The insurance company or pharmacist may also be able to recommend a cheaper alternative product. If the patient would like to use a cheaper alternative, the pharmacist can contact the prescriber to obtain authorization to amend the prescription accordingly. Cheaper alternatives can also be recommended for patients without insurance. Additionally, many free prescription discount cards (e.g., GoodR) can be offered to uninsured patients.

Manufacturers of branded medications usually offer copay assistance cards for patients with private insurance. Copay cards can usually be obtained quickly and easily through the drug manufacturer's website. Manufacturer copay cards are not allowed to be used for patients with government insurance, including Medicare, Medicaid, and Tricare. Alternatively, there are various copay assistance programs that can assist patients with drug costs. Information about these programs can usually be obtained on the drug manufacturer's website, but they usually require a lengthy application form and proof of patient income.

Error-Prevention Strategies

REPACKAGING BULK MEDICATIONS

Bulk medications can be repackaged by pharmacies into unit dose or individual packaging, provided that the integrity of the medication is not compromised, and a log is kept documenting the process. Repackaging is often performed in hospital pharmacies to create single-dose packaging for inpatients.

The repackaging log must contain the following information each time a medication is repackaged:

- Date of repackaging
- Drug name (including generic), strength, and dosage form
- Quantity of drug repackaged
- Manufacturer's name (e.g., Mylan)
- Lot number and manufacturer's expiration date
- Beyond-use date (expiration date of the medication now that it has been repackaged)
- Initials of the pharmacy technician who repackaged the product
- Initials of the pharmacist who checked or verified the repackaged product

Each repackaged medication must be labeled with the following information:

- Generic name of the drug
- Drug strength and dosage form
- Manufacturer's name (e.g., Sandoz) and lot number
- Expiration date of repackaged product
- Special handling instructions (e.g., refrigerate, shake well)

MEDICATION ERRORS

A medication error is any preventable medication event that has the potential to lead to medication misuse or patient harm. A near-miss is a medication error that is caught before the medication leaves the pharmacy. Medication error is a broad term that includes a variety of medication events including prescribing errors, computer entry errors, dispensing errors, labeling errors, and administration errors.

We are all human, and we all make mistakes. Making ourselves aware of the common causes of errors can help us reduce the number of errors that we make. Common causes of medication errors include look-alike medication names, sound-alike medication names, the use of error-prone abbreviations, alert fatigue, human error, distractions (noise, music, conversations), multitasking, and failure to use available barcode scanning technologies. Alert fatigue occurs when the computer system constantly prompts you with too many alerts, so you become less responsive to the alerts and miss an important one. Although multitasking may be helpful in some job roles, it is best to avoid working on multiple patient prescriptions at one time to avoid errors or mix-ups.

Listed below are some of the strategies used to prevent common types of medication errors:

- Verify patient identity using at least two patient identifiers (name, date of birth, address, etc.) during each encounter (drop-off and pick-up).
- Maintain up-to-date records of patient allergies, medications, and disease states (e.g., pregnancy) in the patient's medication profile.

- If any part of a prescription is unclear, alert the pharmacist and contact the prescriber's office to clarify.
- Verify the prescription information with the patient to ensure that what is prescribed is what is expected or intended.
- Only work on one patient's prescription at a time. Although pharmacies can get busy, it is quicker and safer to finish one patient's prescription before moving on to another.
- Use baskets to keep patient's prescription separate from each other.
- Keep pharmacy shelves neat and tidy, and separate LASA medications from each other.
- Check that the drug NDC number dispensed matches the NDC number on the label (use barcode technology if available).
- Avoid using error-prone abbreviations.
- Use tall-man lettering to help differentiate between look-alike and sound-alike medications. For example, NIFEdipine versus niCARdipine.

USING TECHNOLOGY TO REDUCE MEDICATION ERRORS

Pharmacy technology has come a long way in the past decade. Pharmacy computer systems have made significant advancements, and dispensing robots are now commonplace in large pharmacies. A popular English proverb tells us that to err is human. Therefore, we should use technology to try and reduce the number of errors that we make.

- Take notice of computerized alerts or warnings, and relay this information to a pharmacist prior to dispensing.
- Use barcode scanning technology every time you dispense a medication to ensure that the NDC number that is dispensed matches the NDC number on the label or in the computer system.
- If your pharmacy computer system allows you to prefill prescription information from an electronic prescription, use this feature to prevent manual typing errors.
- If available, use dispensing robots to dispense, count, and label prescriptions.
- Use a patient's electronic profile to document and identify allergy information, current medication information, and other medication information.
- Use the linking of Pyxis machines with pharmacy computer systems to monitor medication inventory and administration records to identify potential errors.

ERROR-PRONE ABBREVIATIONS

Abbreviation NOT to Use	Use Instead	Potential Error
U (for unit)	Unit	Mistaken for mL, cc., 0, or 4
IU (for international unit)	International unit	Mistaken for IV or 10
Q.D., QD, q.d., or qd	Daily	Mistaken for every other day, drops
Q.O.D., QOD, q.o.d., qod	Every other day	Mistaken for daily, four times a day
Chemical abbreviations (e.g., $MgSO_4$, NaCl, KCl)	Write out the full chemical/drug name	Easily confused for another drug
Drug name abbreviations (e.g., MS, HCTZ, NS)	Write out the full name of the medication (e.g., morphine sulfate, hydrochlorothiazide, normal saline)	Easily mistaken for another medication

Abbreviation NOT to Use	Use Instead	Potential Error
Trailing zero (e.g., 1.0 mg)	For whole numbers, do not put a decimal and a zero after the number	The decimal point may be missed, and an extra zero can be added to the dose. The patient could receive 10× the intended dose (e.g., 10 mg instead of 1 mg).
Lack of a leading zero (e.g., .5 mg)	For numbers less than 1, place a 0 in front of the decimal point (e.g., 0.5 mg)	The decimal point may be missed, and the number can be mistaken for a whole number. The patient may receive 10× the intended dose (e.g., 5 mg instead of 0.5 mg).

PACKAGING THAT PROTECTS PRODUCTS FROM LIGHT

Some products, such as nitroglycerin, furosemide, and doxycycline, are in dark-colored packaging because they are sensitive to light and are susceptible to instability and degradation if they are exposed to it. There are various packaging techniques that manufacturers use to prevent drugs from being exposed to light.

Most tablets today are packaged in white plastic bottles. White bottles contain the ingredient titanium dioxide that prevents light from entering the bottle; titanium dioxide is also an ingredient in sunscreens and cosmetics. Iron oxide is used to color medication bottles brown in order to prevent light from entering. Some products are packaged in brown plastic bottles or brown glass. The orange or amber vials that the pharmacy uses to dispense medications in also contain iron and are light-protective. Aluminum unit-dose blister packs can also be used for light protection. Secondary or outer packaging, such as cardboard boxes, also help protect products from light.

GLASS PACKAGING

Glass is used to package tablets, liquids, and solutions for injection (e.g., glass ampoules, glass vials). Glass is used less frequently than plastics due to cost, but it is still used to package medications that are incompatible with plastic. Glass is an excellent form of packaging because it is impervious (impenetrable) to water, oxygen, and carbon dioxide. Substances that react with and become unstable in the presence of water, oxygen, or carbon dioxide benefit from being packaged using glass. The weakest link for glass packing is the cap. Metal and plastic do not seal well against glass and may allow for the entry of contaminants. Rubber is often used in caps because it creates a more impenetrable seal and is tamper evident. However, penetration of the rubber seal for an injection solution (e.g., insulin vial) can cause rubber pieces to end up in the injection solution.

PLASTIC PACKAGING

Plastic is the most common material used in packaging pharmaceutical products. Tablets, eye drops, nebulizer solutions, bags of IV fluid, and solutions for injection are all packaged in plastic containers.

Polypropylene is a commonly used plastic because it is impervious (impenetrable) to water and gases. Therefore, it is useful for packaging products that react with and become unstable when exposed to water, oxygen, or carbon dioxide. Polypropylene is used in tablet bottles, eye drop bottles, and ear drop bottles. However, it is a rigid plastic and cannot be used to package bags of IV fluid.

Polyvinyl chloride (PVC) is used to package infusion fluids because it is lightweight and flexible. Compared to glass, it is lighter, easier to seal, and less expensive. PVC has the added benefits of being able to be frozen, then defrosted in the microwave. Therefore, it is useful in improving the shelf life of IV fluids. The downside to using PVC is that some medications are incompatible with this type of plastic. Polyethylene may be used as an alternative.

RECOMMENDATIONS FOR PREVENTING MEDICATION ERRORS

The National Coordinating Council for Medication Error Reporting and Preventing recommendations for preventing medication errors are summarized below:

- All prescriptions should be reviewed by a pharmacist prior to dispensing.
- Patient profiles should be current and complete. Reasonable attempts should be made to obtain information regarding allergies, current medications, and medical history.
- Attempts should be made to minimize distractions, such as reducing noise levels and avoiding personal interruption (e.g., cell phone use).
- Sufficient staffing should be provided.
- The pharmacy environment should be maintained at a comfortable temperature and should provide adequate lighting for staff.
- Medications storage should allow for products to be easily distinguished (e.g., signs, stickers, baskets, separators).
- Medications should be double-checked for accuracy before dispensing.
- Labels should be read at least three times: during product selection, during packaging/dispensing, and while being returned to the shelf.
- Pharmacists should counsel patients on the medication's indications for use, precautions/warnings, possible adverse effects, possible drug–drug or drug–food interactions, and storage requirements.
- Pharmacies should collect and analyze medication error data for quality improvement.
- Pharmacies should establish procedures for medication dispensing and provide initial and ongoing training for staff.

MEASURING PRODUCTIVITY AND EFFICIENCY

Because pharmacy staff members perform many different tasks, it can sometimes be difficult to measure productivity and efficiency. However, it is necessary to document and record pharmacy activity so management can provide the pharmacy with adequate resources and staff. One of the most popular ways to measure the productivity of a pharmacy is with prescription counts. Pharmacy computer systems will keep track of the number of prescriptions filled by the pharmacy on a daily basis, including a breakdown of how many prescriptions were new, refills, or transfers. Pharmacy staffing at many retail stores is based on the daily prescription count. Managers can also create staffing schedules more efficiently, knowing which shifts or days of the week are the busiest.

Other measures of productivity may include the time spent on receiving orders/shipments, time spent on patient counseling, number of vaccinations administered to patients, time spent on insurance billing, time spent on medication therapy management, and time spent on interventions. All of this information is used by pharmacy management to determine staffing needs, resource needs, and pharmacy efficiency.

MEASURING CUSTOMER SATISFACTION

Given the current growth and competition in the pharmacy business, pharmacies are becoming increasingly concerned with customer satisfaction. Additionally, many pharmacy accreditation organizations, such as The Joint Commission, require pharmacies to measure customer satisfaction.

Most pharmacies send out annual customer satisfaction surveys and allow patients to submit satisfaction surveys or complaints on their website. Customer satisfaction surveys ask patients to rate their pharmacy experience based on the friendliness of pharmacy staff, timeliness of prescription filling or delivery, convenience of the pharmacy location, ease of contacting pharmacy staff, quality of the services provided, and the range of services offered at the pharmacy.

In addition to sending customer satisfaction surveys to patients, many pharmacies also send surveys to prescribers and healthcare providers that they deal with regularly. After all, doctors and nurses are pharmacy customers as well. Pharmacies want to know how the staff at local doctors' offices perceive their services. These surveys are similar to those provided to patients, asking about the friendliness of pharmacy staff, the ease of contacting pharmacy staff, the quality of their interventions, and their dedication to patient care.

Issues That Require Pharmacist Intervention

QUALITY IMPROVEMENT PLANS

A quality improvement plan is a plan or set of standards developed by the management of an organization to improve processes and ensure high-quality patient care. Quality improvement plans set performance standards and goals related to adherence to standards of care, opportunities for improvement, identification and prevention of medication errors, processes for improving safety and efficiency, and strategies for effective teamwork and communication. The four main steps to a quality improvement plan are 1) plan, 2) do, 3) check, and 4) act.

Quality improvement plans in the pharmacy mainly aim to reduce medication errors and improve the quality of patient care. In order to obtain details about the quality and efficiency of pharmacy processes, management will need to obtain data from various sources. Some of the information sources commonly used include patient charts, patient medical records, electronic medical records, medication administration records (MAR charts), immunization records, and medication therapy management documentation.

PHARMACIST INTERVENTION

Pharmacy technicians perform many vital roles in the pharmacy, but there are some situations when a technician should involve a pharmacist. Pharmacy technicians are NOT legally allowed to perform the following roles in the pharmacy:

- Provide medical advice or OTC recommendations to patients
- Receive a new verbal or telephone prescription order
- Perform a clinical review of a prescription order or medication summary
- Discuss clinical interventions with the prescriber (e.g., drug interactions, prescription changes)
- Perform a drug utilization review
- Counsel a patient regarding an adverse event, drug interactions, or medication adherence
- Perform accuracy checks and final verifications or prescription orders
  - Some states are now allowing tech-check-tech programs in hospitals that allow technicians with specific training to check the dispensing of other technicians
- Administer immunizations
  - Some states are now allowing pharmacy technicians to administer immunizations after receiving proper training

- o Postimmunization follow-ups and immunization counseling must still be performed by a pharmacist
- Transfer prescriptions to another pharmacy
  - o Some states allow technicians to receive (but not give) prescription transfer information for noncontrolled medications

AUTOMATIC STOP ORDER

In hospitals or facilities, drugs are prescribed using medication orders rather than prescriptions. Orders are entered into a patient's chart in an online computer system that can be accessed by all healthcare personnel, including nurses, pharmacists, pharmacy technicians, and doctors. When the prescriber enters a medication order, they must fill in the usual required prescription fields, including the medication name, strength, dosage form, and directions for use. Medication orders may also have additional fields to fill out that are not required for normal prescriptions, such as the duration of therapy, days of treatment, total number of treatment doses, start date/time, stop date/time, and rate of infusion. Unlike prescriptions, medication orders do not include a set quantity to dispense. The nurses administer the medications on a dose-by-dose basis until the order is canceled or inactivated. An automatic stop order occurs when a prescriber does not specify a duration of therapy on the medication order. Instead, the order is automatically stopped or inactivated after a specified date/time, number of days, or number of doses.

Event Reporting Procedures

DOCUMENTING AND REPORTING MEDICATION ERRORS

All pharmacies should keep a medication error logbook in the pharmacy at all times, and all pharmacy staff members should know where it is located and how to document medication errors. Any time a dispensing error occurs, regardless of whether it reaches the patient or the pharmacist, the error should be recorded in the medication error log. Each pharmacy will have a policy that states who is responsible for reviewing medication errors and how often the error log should be reviewed. The types of information usually recorded in the error log includes the date the error occurred, the names of the medication(s) involved, the stage at which the error occurred, the stage at which the error was discovered, and the staff members that were involved. It is important to record as many details of the event as possible because this information will help during the review process. The idea of the logbook is not to place blame on specific employees, but to try and establish trends and come up with ideas for how to prevent the reoccurrence of common errors.

REPORTING ADVERSE EFFECTS OR ADVERSE REACTIONS

All drugs have the potential to cause adverse effects or reactions. For older medications that have been on the market for a while, the frequency and nature of commonly experienced adverse events are well known. However, less is known about the adverse effects associated with newer medications or rare adverse reactions. Therefore, it is important to report adverse drug events to MedWatch, the FDA's online voluntary reporting system for adverse drug reactions. Anyone can report an adverse drug event to MedWatch, including doctors, pharmacy technicians, pharmacists, patients, or caregivers. Reports can be made online, by phone, by mail, or by fax. The FDA's Adverse Event Reporting System database contains information about all the adverse events reported to the FDA through the MedWatch program. This database is especially useful in reporting severe reactions, rare reactions, or events related to drugs that have recently entered the market. The Vaccine Adverse Event Reporting System is an FDA program specifically designed to monitor adverse reactions associated with vaccinations.

The FDA's MedWatch program can be used to report adverse effects associated with any human drug (whether OTC or prescription-only), biologic (blood component, tissue-based products), medical device, vaccine, dietary supplement, infant formula, cosmetic, food, or beverage. MedWatch can even be used to report medication errors. Pharmacist and pharmacy technicians in practice rarely submit information on adverse drug reactions to the FDA because it is voluntary and time-consuming. However, the FDA encourages use of the MedWatch reporting system, even if you are not certain of all the details of the event.

Adverse event reporting through MedWatch is particularly encouraged for serious adverse reactions that involve hospitalization, involve a life-threatening reaction, result in disability or permanent damage, or result in death. The FDA also encourages the reporting of quality or safety concerns with a product, such as suspected contamination, suspected counterfeit products, defective products, inadequate packaging or labeling, or stability issues.

BAR-CODE AND DATA ENTRY TECHNOLOGIES

Each product has a unique scannable bar code that is linked to its National Drug Code (NDC) number. During the dispensing process, the bar code of each stock bottle is scanned to ensure that it matches the NDC number dispensed. Drug bar codes are also scanned when they are loaded into automated dispensing robots or cabinets (e.g., Pyxis machines). This helps ensure that the correct medication is loaded into the correct container, drawer, or pocket. When medications are loaded into or dispensed from an automated dispensing system, inventory levels are also updated. This helps ensure that the correct on-hand inventory for each medication is maintained in the computer system.

Data entry technologies are also used by pharmacies for quality assurance. Many pharmacy computer systems allow new prescriptions to be scanned into the system, and most of the prescription details are prefilled. In most hospitals, prescribers order medications using the same software that the pharmacy uses to dispense medications. Therefore, pharmacy technicians can pull prescription details from the computer system without manually entering the information. This reduces the risk of human error. Additionally, the computer system will usually automatically select preferred formulary products that are in stock at the pharmacy.

ROOT CAUSE ANALYSIS AND ANALYZING MEDICATION ERRORS

Root cause analysis is a problem-solving method used by pharmacies to determine the causes of medication errors and suggest methods for error prevention. Root cause analysis is triggered by a sentinel event, a medication error, or an undesirable event. Event analysis is not a simple 5-minute meeting. Analysis can take days to weeks to complete. Every pharmacy should have a multidisciplinary team in place that is trained on how to analyze sentinel events using root cause analysis.

The first step in root cause analysis is to collect data about the event and what happened. Data collection involves interviewing staff members, reviewing dispensing records, etc. Data collection can be time-consuming, but it is important to collect as much data as possible. Next, the team can brainstorm potential causes of the event. Then, a corrective action plan and report can be developed by the team. At a specified time period, the team should follow up with the action plan to ensure that it is effective and does not need to be revised.

Types of Prescription Errors

A prescription error is a mix-up or mistake that occurs any time during the prescribing, dispensing, or administration process and has the potential to cause patient harm. Near-misses are prescription errors that are caught before the medication reaches the patient. Prescription errors encompass a variety of different medication events:

- Dispensing the wrong drug, the wrong strength of drug, or the wrong formulation of drug (e.g., tablets instead of liquid)
- Dispensing a drug to the incorrect patient (patient name mix-ups)
- Dispensing the incorrect quantity of medication
- Refilling a prescription too early (which can lead to medication abuse or overdose)
- Incorrect labeling or directions
- Incorrect infusion rate information
- Compounding a medication incorrectly (e.g., adding too much or too little water)
- Preparing an IV admixture in an incompatible solution or in an incompatible bag
- Dispensing a drug to a patient with a known allergy or contraindication
- Dispensing a drug that interacts with another medication that the patient is taking
- Failure to provide adequate counseling or information to the patient
- Shipping a medication order to the incorrect address

Hygiene and Cleaning Standards

INFECTION CONTROL STANDARDS

The following are infection control standards used in pharmacies to prevent contamination:

- General Dispensing
  - Pharmacy personnel should wash their hands before and after patient interactions (e.g., gel-in, gel-out).
  - Equipment such as counting trays and spatulas should be cleaned and disinfected before and after use with 70% isopropyl alcohol.
  - Certain medications should be prepared using designated and labeled counting trays and spatulas. This includes antibiotics and other agents that have allergy potential, warfarin, chemotherapy agents, and other hazardous medications.

- Compounding
  - **Nonsterile compounding** follows the standards set by United States Pharmacopeia 795 (USP 795).
  - **Sterile compounding** follows the standards set by United States Pharmacopeia 797 (USP 797). Medications that are required to be compounded in a sterile environment include those administered through injection, IV infusion, intrathecal administration, or ocular administration.
  - **Hazardous medications** should be compounded using biological safety cabinets or laminar flow hoods. Hazardous materials should not be stocked or worked with in an area with positive pressure relative to the surrounding areas.

HANDWASHING

You have been washing your hands since you were a toddler, so it may seem childish to be taught how to wash your hands. However, any new job in healthcare will require you to receive some sort of training on handwashing and hand hygiene. Below are the correct steps for washing your hands.

1. Stand far enough away from the sink so that your clothing does not touch the sink.
2. Wet your hands and forearms.
3. Apply soap.

4. Rub the soap into all areas of the hands, including under the nails, as well as the wrists and arms (up to the elbow). Do this for 15–30 seconds.
5. Rinse soapy areas of the hands, wrists, and arms thoroughly with water.
6. Keep the faucet running while you dry the hands, wrists, and arms with a paper towel.
7. Use the paper towel to turn off the faucet.

Chapter Quiz

Ready to see how well you retained what you just read? Scan the QR code to go directly to the chapter quiz interface for this study guide. If you're using a computer, simply visit the bonus page at **mometrix.com/bonus948/ptcb** and click the Chapter Quizzes link.

Order Entry and Processing

Transform passive reading into active learning! After immersing yourself in this chapter, put your comprehension to the test by taking a quiz. The insights you gained will stay with you longer this way. Scan the QR code to go directly to the chapter quiz interface for this study guide. If you're using a computer, simply visit the bonus page at **mometrix.com/bonus948/ptcb** and click the Chapter Quizzes link.

Procedures to Compound Nonsterile Products

COMPOUNDING AND MANUFACTURING

Compounding is when a pharmacy makes or prepares small, reasonable quantities of a product in anticipation of receiving a prescription. Pharmacies are only allowed to compound a product if they have or expect to have a prescription for a specific patient. Compounds cannot be sold to another pharmacy, prescriber, or hospital unless that pharmacy has obtained a special outsourcing facility license. In order to compound a product, the pharmacy must only use FDA-approved ingredients. Compounding that occurs in pharmacies is only intended to be of a small scale, and the use of commercial-grade equipment is not allowed. The final product cannot duplicate a product that is commercially available for purchase, and the compound must not be a product that was withdrawn from the market for safety reasons.

Manufacturing happens when a facility that has been licensed, inspected, and approved by the FDA produces, repackages, or relabels drug products. Manufacturing facilities have a different license than a pharmacy does, which allows them to prepare products that are approved by the FDA. Unlike pharmacies, they must follow strict quality control measures and must follow current good manufacturing practices.

INSPECTING NONSTERILE COMPOUNDS DURING FINAL VERIFICATION

Once a nonsterile compounded product has been prepared, it must be checked and inspected before being dispensed to the patient. Verification of compounds is more involved than verifying other prescriptions because there are many different components to consider in addition to the physical inspection of the final product. The technician usually verified the ingredients prior to compounding, and a pharmacist inspects the final product after compounding.

All component ingredients should be verified to ensure that they are of the correct strength, the correct quantity was used, and that no expired ingredients were used. The label should be examined to ensure that the ingredients, quantity dispensed, storage instructions, directions for use, and beyond-use date are correct.

In addition to checking the ingredients, compounds must be physically examined for consistency, stability, and contamination issues. There should be no leaks or cracks in the packaging, and compatible packaging should be used. The product should have the clarity, color, odor, consistency, and volume that is expected, and there should not be any unexpected precipitates (clumps) or particulates.

COMPOUND ORAL SOLUTIONS

A solution is a liquid in which solid drug is dissolved. In order to dissolve a solid in a liquid, the solubility of the drug must be known. Solubility is defined as the maximum amount of solute (drug) that can be dissolved in a solvent (liquid). Solubility is given as an amount per volume (e.g., 1 mg/mL).

For example, if you want to produce a solution of amoxicillin and the solubility is 1 mg/mL, what is the maximum amount of amoxicillin that can be added to prepare 100 mL of the solution?

Solubility of amoxicillin = 1 mg/mL = 100 mg/100 mL

Therefore, 100 mg of amoxicillin should be added to prepare 100 mL of solution.

The concentration of the solution is 100 mg/100 mL = 5 mg/5 mL.

Preparation of a solution is very simple. The drug may be in powder, tablet, or capsule form. Powder can be weighed and added directly to the solution. Tablets must be crushed in a mortar and pestle, whereas capsules can be opened and crushed in a mortar and pestle before mixing into a solution.

PREPARING AN ORAL SUSPENSION

Suspensions contain finely ground solid drug dispersed within a liquid. Unlike solutions, the amount of drug added to the liquid is above the maximum solubility so the drug forms clumps or particles within the liquid. Suspensions often require thickening agents or flocculating agents to help keep these undissolved particles suspended within the liquid solvent. Levigating agents may also be required to reduce the size of the drug particles. In suspensions, the drug particles sink to the bottom of the container quickly, so the product must be shaken well prior to use.

Step 1: Solid drug is triturated (made into a fine powder) with a mortar and pestle. A levigating agent, such as mineral oil or glycerin, is added to form small clumps or particles of drug.

Step 2: A portion of the liquid solvent is added to the mortar, and the contents are mixed until uniform.

Step 3: The mixture is transferred into the final container. The remaining volume of solvent to be added is used to rinse the mortar and pestle and pour the remaining contents into the final container.

COMPOUNDING EMULSIONS

An emulsion is a mixture of two or more liquids that are immiscible (they do not mix). It is similar to a suspension, except the suspended particles are liquid instead of solid. An example would be adding vegetable oil to water. The two liquids do not mix and remain separated. In order to get oil and water to mix, an emulsifying agent (aka emulsifier, gum, or surfactant) must be added to help disperse droplets of one liquid in the other liquid. A common emulsifying agent used is sodium lauryl sulfate. Oil-in-water emulsions contain oil droplets dispersed in water, whereas water-in-oil emulsions contain water droplets suspended in oil.

1. Dry gum technique: The oil and emulsifier (gum) are mixed in a mortar and pestle. Then, the water is added and mixed until an emulsion is formed.
2. Wet gum technique: The water and emulsifier (gum) are mixed in a mortar and pestle. Then, oil is added and mixed in small portions at a time until all of the oil has been added.

CREAMS AND OINTMENTS

An ointment is composed of drug particles suspended in an oily base, whereas lotions and creams contain drug particles suspended in a watery emulsion. Ointments and creams are both topical preparations that are intended to be applied on the skin.

Preparation of an ointment begins by crushing the drug into a fine powder and mixing it with a levigating agent (e.g., mineral oil). This process is similar to preparing a suspension. The drug mixture can be added to the ointment base in small portions (geometric dilution) using a spatula and ointment slab until all ingredients are combined and uniformly mixed.

Creams are more similar to emulsions, so preparation begins by mixing the oil-soluble ingredients and water-soluble ingredients in separate beakers. Then, both beakers are heated using a hot plate. Once removed from the heat, the contents of both beakers are combined and stirred continuously until a uniform mixture is formed. For oil-in-water emulsions, the oil ingredients are added to the water ingredients. For water-in-oil emulsions, the water ingredients are added to the oil ingredients.

SUPPOSITORIES

Suppositories are tablets that are intended to be administered in the rectum. Most suppositories are composed of waxy substances that are designed to melt and disintegrate at body temperature once administered. Oil-based oleaginous suppositories are commonly prepared using cocoa butter or synthetic triglycerides. Water-based suppositories are composed of glycerinated glycerin or polyethylene glycol. These substances dissolve slowly and allow the suppository to have a prolonged duration of action.

Two main methods can be used to make suppositories. Fusion molding is the most popular method, in which the suppository base is melted using a hot plate and the active ingredients (drugs) are dissolved into the melted base. Then, the mixture is poured into a suppository mold and left to solidify. The compression molding method is used less commonly and involves pressing the suppository base and active ingredients into a compression mold.

PREPARING HAZARDOUS SUBSTANCES

Hazardous substances, such as chemotherapy, should be prepared in a biological safety cabinet or an isolator. Biological safety cabinets are workstations that contain air that has been filtered using a high-efficiency particulate air filter. Vents within the biological safety cabinets extract air from the cabinet to prevent hazardous substances from reaching the compounder. An isolator is a workstation that is enclosed and airtight. A set of built-in gloves allows the compounder access into the inside of the isolator. The environment inside the isolator is aseptic, meaning it is free from pathogens and contamination. Isolators and biological safety cabinets that are used to prepare hazardous substances should be at a negative pressure compared to the room. By maintaining the workstation at a lower pressure, any hazardous particles will remain inside the workstation rather than be pushed out into the room around it where they can potentially harm workers. Workers handling hazardous substances should wear gloves that are designed for handling hazardous substances. Tablets should not be cut, and capsules should not be opened when they contain any hazardous substance.

Formulas and Calculations

ABBREVIATIONS USED ON PRESCRIPTIONS

Prescribers commonly used medical abbreviations when writing prescriptions, especially within the prescription instructions or directions (also known as the sig). You should be familiar with commonly used abbreviations, but if any part of the prescription is unclear, you should call the prescriber's office to clarify.

Abbreviation	Meaning
po	By mouth, per oral route (e.g., tablets, capsules)
tab	Tablet
cap	Capsule
SR, XR, XL	Extended-release or slow-release
liq	Liquid
syr	Syrup
sol	Solution
susp	Suspension
SL	Sublingually (e.g., sublingual tablet)
ou	Each eye
os	Left eye
od	Right eye
bid	Twice a day
tid	Three times a day
qid	Four times a day
am	Morning
pm	Evening
hs	At bedtime
q	Every
top	Topically (e.g., patch, cream, lotion, ointment)
crm	Cream
oint, ung	Ointment
Pr	Per rectum, rectally (e.g., suppository)
inh	Inhalation (e.g., inhaler)
Per neb	By nebulizer
IV	Intravenously
SC, subc, subq	Subcutaneously
IM	Intramuscularly
au	Each ear
as	Left ear
ad	Right ear
UD	Use as directed
NR	No refills
DAW	Dispense as written (e.g., brand name requested)
w	With
w/o	Without
ac	Before food/meal
pc	After food/meal
stat	Immediately

Abbreviation	Meaning
prn	As needed

ABBREVIATIONS FOR DIFFERENT UNITS OF MEASURE

Abbreviation	Meaning
ss	One half, 1/2
L	Liter
mL	Milliliter
tsp	Teaspoon (5 mL)
tbsp	Tablespoon (15 mL)
Fl oz	Fluid once (30 mL)
gr	Grain
qs, qs ad	Dispense a sufficient quantity or add a sufficient quantity to make
aq	Water
ad	Up to
aa	Of each
gtt	Drop
G, g, gm	Gram
kg	Kilogram
mg	Milligram
mcg	Microgram
mEq	Milliequivalent
ds	Days' supply
lb	Pound
c	Cup

ROMAN NUMERALS

I	1	VI	6	L	50
II	2	VII	7	C	100
III	3	VIII	8	D	500
IV	4	IX	9	M	1000
V	5	X	10		

CONVERSION FACTORS

Conversion factors are used to change from one unit of measure to another. For instance, if a drug is prescribed in milliliters and the patient wants to know their dose in teaspoons, you will have to use a conversion factor.

Conversion Factors	
1 kg	2.2 lb
1 tsp	5 mL
1 tbsp	3 tsp (15 mL)
1 fl oz	29.57 mL (often rounded to 30 mL)
1 cup	8 oz
1 L	33.8 oz
1 gr	64.8 mg

ADDING AND SUBTRACTING FRACTIONS

In order to **add or subtract fractions**, you must first convert the fractions to an equivalent fraction so that both fractions have the same denominator (the number on the bottom of the fraction). An easy way of doing this is to multiply the two denominators together and multiply the numerators (the top number of the fraction) by the original denominator of the opposite fraction (cross-multiplication):

$$\frac{1}{4} + \frac{1}{6} =$$

Cross-multiply the numerators by the opposite denominator, and multiply the denominators to get a common denominator:

$$\frac{6}{24} + \frac{4}{24} =$$

Once the fractions are converted to have the same common denominator, the numerators (the numbers on the top of the fraction) can simply be added:

$$\frac{6}{24} + \frac{4}{24} = \frac{10}{24}$$

Reduce the fraction by converting it to its smallest possible form. Divide each part of the final fraction by a common whole number until the numbers cannot be divided any further:

$$\frac{10}{24} \div \frac{2}{2} = \frac{5}{12}$$

> **Review Video: Adding and Subtracting Fractions**
> Visit mometrix.com/academy and enter code: 378080

MULTIPLYING AND DIVIDING FRACTIONS

In order to **multiply fractions**, simply multiply the numerators (top numbers) and denominators (bottom numbers) separately. Then, reduce the final fraction to the smallest possible form by dividing the numerator and denominator by a common whole number until the numbers cannot be divided further.

Example:

$$\frac{1}{4} \times \frac{6}{8} = \frac{6}{32}$$

Reduce the fraction:

$$\frac{6}{32} \div \frac{2}{2} = \frac{3}{16}$$

In order to **divide fractions**, use the same process as multiplying fractions except flip the second fraction upside down. The mathematical term for a fraction that is flipped upside down is called the reciprocal. Then, reduce the fraction to its smallest possible form.

Example:

$$\frac{1}{4} \div \frac{6}{8} =$$

Flip the second fraction:

$$\frac{1}{4} \times \frac{8}{6} = \frac{8}{24}$$

Reduce the fraction:

$$\frac{8}{24} \div \frac{8}{8} = \frac{1}{3}$$

Review Video: <ins>Multiplying and Dividing Fractions</ins>
Visit mometrix.com/academy and enter code: 473632

DIMENSIONAL ANALYSIS

A useful method for solving problems involving unit conversions is **dimensional analysis**. In this method conversion factors (example: $\left(\frac{1\,g}{1,000\,mg}\right)$) or their reciprocals (example: $\left(\frac{1,000\,mg}{1\,g}\right)$) may be used to obtain the required unit. Consider this drip rate example:

$$\text{Drip rate} = \frac{25\,\text{mL}}{1\,\text{hour}} \times \frac{10\,\text{gtts}}{1\,\text{mL}} \times \frac{1\,\text{hour}}{60\,\text{min}} = \frac{250\,\text{gtts}}{60\,\text{min}} = 4.2\frac{\text{gtts}}{\text{min}}$$

In this example, the flow rate (25 mL/hour) was given, as was the conversion factor of 10 gtts (drops) per mL. Those values plus the conversion of 1 hour=60 minutes can be used to solve the problem.

One way to check that the problem was set up and solved correctly is to make sure the units cancel out across the problem to give the desired dimensions. This problem asked for drip rate, which is measured in drops (gtts) per unit of time (minutes in this problem). Below, the mL and hour in the numerator cancel out the mL and hour in the denominator because 1 hour ÷ 1 hour = 1 and 1 mL ÷ 1 mL = 1, so the resulting units match the units required for the answer.

$$\text{Drip rate} = \frac{25\,\cancel{\text{mL}}}{1\,\cancel{\text{hour}}} \times \frac{10\,\text{gtts}}{1\,\cancel{\text{mL}}} \times \frac{1\,\cancel{\text{hour}}}{60\,\text{min}} = \frac{250\,\text{gtts}}{60\,\text{min}} = 4.2\frac{\text{gtts}}{\text{min}}$$

DAYS' SUPPLY CALCULATIONS

Days' supply is the number of days that the prescribed quantity of drugs will last the patient when taken according to the prescribed directions. Insurance companies use days' supply to determine when a patient is ready for a prescription refill, so it is important to calculate it correctly. Most insurance companies will not allow a patient to refill their medication until they have ≤25% of medication left. If the days' supply is incorrectly calculated to be more than the true days' supply, it may lead to the insurance rejecting the claim stating that it is too soon to be refilled. If the days' supply is incorrectly calculated to be less than the true days' supply, it may allow the patient to refill too soon. This can lead to waste and potential medication abuse, particularly if the medication is a controlled substance.

General formula to calculate days' supply:

Total number of units prescribed ÷ number of units per dose ÷ number of doses per day

TABLETS, CAPSULES, AND ORAL LIQUIDS

Days' supply is the total number of days that a prescription will last if it is taken as prescribed. It is calculated by dividing the total quantity of product dispensed by the quantity used each day.

General formula:

$$\text{Days' supply} = \frac{\text{total \# of units prescribed}}{\text{total \# of units used per day}}$$

An alternative formula:

$$\text{Days' supply} = \text{total \# of units prescribed} \div \frac{\text{\# of units per dose}}{\text{\# of doses per day}}$$

Tablet/capsule example: A prescription written for #14 ciprofloxacin tablets with the sig, 1 BID:

$$14 \text{ tablets total} \div \frac{1 \text{ tablet per dose}}{2 \text{ doses per day}} = 7 \text{ days}$$

Oral liquid example: A prescription is written for promethazine with codeine syrup 6.25 mg–10 mg/5 mL, dispense #120 mL, take 1 tsp po q6h for cough:

$$1 \text{ tsp} = 5 \text{ mL}$$
$$24 \text{ hrs} \div 6 \text{ hrs} = 4 \text{ times per day}$$
$$120 \text{ mL dispensed} \div \left(\frac{5 \text{ mL}}{\text{dose}} \div \frac{4 \text{ doses}}{\text{day}} \right) = 6 \text{ days}$$
$$120 \text{ mL} \times \frac{1 \text{ dose}}{5 \text{ mL}} \times \frac{\text{day}}{4 \text{ doses}} = 6 \text{ days}$$

PRODUCTS DOSED IN DROPS

Some medications require very small amounts of liquid to be administered with each dose. Therefore, drops are used as the unit of measure for each dose. Eye drops, ear drops, and some oral liquids are dosed in drops. In order to calculate days' supply for these medications, it is necessary to know the conversion factor for drops to milliliters. Drop sizes can vary, but there are usually between 15 and 20 drops in each milliliter.

Eye drop example: A prescription is written for tobramycin 0.3% eye drops; instill 1–2 drops into the left eye every four hours for 5 days. The eye drops are only available in 3 mL and 5 mL bottles. The conversion factor is 15 drops/mL. What size bottle will the patient need?

For this problem, we need to work backward to solve for the quantity needed.

Up to two drops × one eye × six times a day (every 4 hours) × 5 days = 60 drops total

Covert drops to mL:

60 drops ÷ 15 drops/mL = 4 mL needed

Therefore, the patient will require a 5 mL bottle to complete the course.

Note: Don't forget to multiply by two eyes if drops are being applied to both eyes.

DECIMALS

To **multiply decimals**, first multiply the numbers as if there were no decimals present. Then, place a decimal point at the end of the number (to the right) and move the decimal place to the left the number of spaces equal to the total number of decimal places in the original numbers.

Example: 5.68 × 1.25

The total number of decimal places = 2 + 2 = 4

At first, multiply the numbers ignoring the decimal places: 568 × 125 = 71,000

Place a decimal place at the end of this number: 71,000

Move the decimal place to the left a total number of spaces equal to the total number of decimal places in the original numbers (in this case, four spaces): 7.1

To **convert a decimal to a percent**, move the decimal two places to the *right* and add a % sign.

Example: 0.30 = 30%

To **convert a percent to a decimal**, move the decimal point two places to the *left* and remove the % sign.

Example: 65% = 0.65

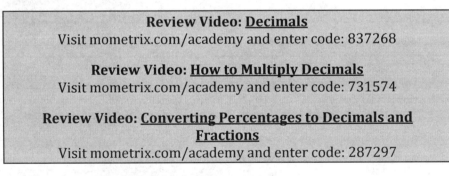

Review Video: Decimals
Visit mometrix.com/academy and enter code: 837268

Review Video: How to Multiply Decimals
Visit mometrix.com/academy and enter code: 731574

Review Video: Converting Percentages to Decimals and Fractions
Visit mometrix.com/academy and enter code: 287297

SAMPLE RATIO AND PROPORTION CALCULATION PROBLEM

You are to prepare an IV for a patient that contains potassium chloride 10 mEq in 500 mL. All you have in stock is potassium chloride 40 mEq/10 mL. How much of the stock solution should be added to the 500 mL IV bag in order to prepare the 10 mEq solution?

In order to solve this type of proportion problem, it is easiest to use cross multiplication. In cross multiplication, you summarize the information into two fractions where three values are known, and one value is unknown. Then, you cross-multiply to solve for the unknown value.

We know that the stock solution we have contains 40 mEq/10 mL, so this is our first fraction or proportion. We also know that we need to end with 10 mEq, but we don't know how much volume equates to 10 mEq. Therefore, our second fraction will be 10 mEq over an unknown volume:

$$\frac{10 \text{ mEq}}{? \text{ mL}} = \frac{40 \text{ mEq}}{10 \text{ mL}}$$

$$10 \text{ mEq} \times 10 \text{ mL} = 40 \text{ mEq} \times ? \text{ mL}$$

$$? \text{ mL} = \frac{(10 \times 10)}{40} \text{ mL}$$

$$= 2.5 \text{ mL}$$

The correct answer is 2.5 mL. This means that 2.5 mL of the 40 mEq/10 mL stock solution must be added to the 500 mL IV bag in order to prepare a 10 mEq/500 mL solution (although in reality the exact concentration would become 10 mEq/502.5 mL because nothing would be removed from the 500 mL IV bag when the 2.5 mL is added).

It's always a good idea to review your answer to ensure that it is reasonable. If the stock solution is 40 mEq/10 mL and we need 10mEq, that means that our answer will be one-fourth of 10 mL because 10 mEq is one-fourth of 40 mEq. Because 2.5 mL is one-fourth of 10 mEq, our answer is correct.

SAMPLE IV FLOW RATE/DRIP RATE PROBLEM

An IV antibiotic was prescribed for a patient to be administered at a rate of 25 mL/hour. What volume (in mL) of IV solution would be needed to last 8 hours? What is the drip rate if the IV is running through at a rate of 10 gtts/mL?

Flow rates can be expressed in mL/hour or mL/min depending upon what type of pump is being used to administer the IV:

$$\textbf{Flow rate} = \frac{\text{mL of IV solution}}{\text{hours or minutes}}$$

In this problem, the IV flow rate is given, and it is asking how many mL of solution are needed to run over an 8-hour time frame. In order to figure this out, the flow rate must be multiplied by the time period:

Flow rate (mL/hour) × hours = total mL administered

25 mL/hour × 8 hours = **200 mL** administered over 8 hours

The drip rate is the number of drops of IV solution that are administered per minute.

$$\textbf{Drip rate} = \frac{\text{gtts of IV solution}}{\text{minute}}$$

In order to calculate the drip rate from the flow rate, the mL of solution must be converted into drops (gtts). A conversion factor will be given for this. In this problem, the rate is 10 gtts/mL. If the flow rate is given in hours, then the time must be converted into minutes to calculate the drip rate.

$$\text{Drip rate} = \frac{25 \text{ mL}}{1 \text{ hour}} \times \frac{10 \text{ gtts}}{1 \text{ mL}} \times \frac{1 \text{ hour}}{60 \text{ min}} = \frac{250 \text{ gtts}}{60 \text{ min}} = 4.2 \frac{\text{gtts}}{\text{min}}$$

> **Review Video: Calculating IV Drip Rates**
> Visit mometrix.com/academy and enter code: 396112

SAMPLE AMOUNT OF GLUCOSE IN SOLUTION PROBLEM

How many grams of glucose are there in a 500 mL bag of glucose 5% solution? How many grams are contained in a 500 mL bag of glucose 0.5% solution?

A concentration is the amount of substance in a volume of solution. Concentrations can be expressed as weight to volume (g/100 mL), volume to volume (mL/100 mL) or weight to weight (g/100 g).

A percentage is the quantity of substance in 100. Because concentrations are also expressed as an amount per 100, no conversion or decimal place movement is required to convert the percentage into a concentration. To solve this problem, multiply the concentration of the solution by the volume of the bag to find the total amount of glucose contained within the bag:

$$\text{Glucose } 5\% = \frac{5 \text{ g}}{100 \text{ mL}} \times \frac{500 \text{ mL}}{\text{bag}} = \frac{(5 \times 500)}{100} = 25 \text{ g}$$

$$\text{Glucose } 0.5\% = \frac{0.5 \text{ g}}{100 \text{ mL}} \times \frac{500 \text{ mL}}{\text{bag}} = \frac{(0.5 \times 500)}{100} = 2.5 \text{ g}$$

Ensure that these answers are reasonable and make sense. If there is 5% glucose in a solution (5 g/100 mL), then a 500 mL bag will have five times as much as a 100 mL bag. Because 5 × 5 = 25, our answer of 25 g makes sense. For the 0.5% solution, move the decimal place to the left one place to find the answer in comparison to the answer for a 5% solution. Therefore, 2.5 g is a reasonable answer.

CALCULATIONS FOR PREPARING PARENTERAL NUTRITION ORDERS WITH STOCK SOLUTIONS

You are preparing a total parenteral nutrition order containing glycine 10% and dextrose 30% with a total volume of 500 mL. You have the following stock solutions: glycine 20%, dextrose 60%. What volume of the stock solutions are needed to prepare the total parenteral nutrition order?

When diluting a solution or dealing with stock solutions that contain a different concentration of substance than the solution being prepared, it is easiest to use the following equation for your calculations:

$$C_1 \times V_1 = C_2 \times V_2$$

C_1 is the concentration of the stock solution, V_1 is the volume of the stock solution needed to prepare the desired solution, C_2 is the concentration desired, and V_2 is the volume of the final/desired solution.

Because we are dealing with two different substances in this problem, we will have to use this equation twice.

$$Glycine\ 20\% \times (mL\ glycine\ 20\%\ needed) = glycine\ 10\% \times 500\ mL$$

$$\textbf{mL glycine 20\% needed} = (10 \times 500)/20 = \textbf{250 mL}$$

$$Dextrose\ 60\% \times (mL\ dextrose\ 60\%\ needed) = dextrose\ 30\% \times 500\ mL$$

$$\textbf{mL dextrose 60\% needed} = (30 \times 500)/60 = \textbf{250 mL}$$

In summary, we needed 250 mL of glycine 20% stock solution and 250 mL of dextrose 60% stock solution to prepare the 500 mL solution containing glycine 10% and dextrose 30%.

ALLIGATION

Explain how to use the alligation method (aka the tic-tac-toe method) to determine how many grams of 2% triamcinolone cream should be mixed with 5% triamcinolone cream to prepare a total of 20 g of 3% triamcinolone cream.

Alligation is used to calculate the quantity of each ingredient that is required when mixing two ingredients with different strengths to obtain a final product with a different strength.

Higher % ingredient		Desired % – lower % = number of parts of higher % ingredient required.
	Desired % of the final product	
Lower % ingredient		Higher % – desired % = number of parts of lower % ingredient required.
		Add the numbers in this column to determine the total number of parts.

The first two columns should be cross-subtracted to determine the number of parts of each ingredient to add. The total quantity of the final product desired must be divided by the total number of parts to determine the quantity in each part.

Example problem:

5% triamcinolone cream stock		1 part of 5% cream
	3% triamcinolone cream desired	
2% triamcinolone cream stock		2 parts of 2% cream
		3 parts total

The total quantity of 3% triamcinolone that we want to prepare is 20 g.

20 g ÷ 3 parts total = 6.7g per part

Because we need to add **1 part of 5% triamcinolone**, we need to add **6.7 g.**

Because we need to add **2 parts of 2% triamcinolone**, we need to add 6.7 g × 2 = **13.3 g.**

129

CALCULATING CHILD'S DOSE FROM ADULT'S DOSE OF DRUG

In most cases, the manufacturer's instructions will provide children's (pediatric) dosing for a medication. However, there are some instances in which pediatric dosing is not provided and must be calculated. The pharmacist is usually responsible for these calculations, but as a technician you should still be aware of these equations so that you can assist.

Clark's Rule:

$$\text{Child dose} = \frac{\text{weight of child in lbs.}}{150 \text{ lbs}} \times \text{adult dose}$$

Young's Rule:

$$\text{Child dose} = \frac{\text{age of child}}{\text{age of child} + 12} \times \text{adult dose}$$

Body Surface Area (BSA) Formula:

$$\text{Child dose} = \frac{\text{child BSA}}{\text{average adult BSA}} \times \text{adult dose}$$

BSA is also used in dosage calculations in some chemotherapy regimens.

Children are not the only patients who require dosing adjustments. Elderly (geriatric) patients also have a reduced ability to metabolize medications and may require dosage decreases. Geriatric dosage adjustments are usually listed in the manufacturer's instructions but can also be found in the *Geriatric Dosage Handbook*. Patient who are very frail or who have gastrointestinal diseases (e.g., Crohn's disease, ulcerative colitis) may also absorb and metabolize medications differently and may require dosage adjustments.

DETERMINING AMOUNT OF WATER FOR A CONCENTRATION PROBLEM

You are dispensing a 150 mL bottle of amoxicillin 250 mg/5 mL suspension to a patient and need to reconstitute it by adding 70 mL of water. However, the pharmacist explains that this patient requires the suspension to be reconstituted to a concentration of 165 mg/5 mL. What volume of water (total diluent volume) should be added to the stock bottle to prepare this concentration?

This problem can be solved many ways, but the easiest way for most students is to use the following equation:

$$\text{Final volume (FV)} = \text{volume of diluent (D)} + \text{powder volume (PV)}$$

Step 1: Determine the total quantity (mg) of drug in the stock bottle:

$$\frac{250 \text{ mg}}{5 \text{ mL}} \times 150 \text{ mL} = 7500 \text{ mg}$$

Step 2: Calculate the powder volume (PV) of the drug in the stock bottle using the following equations:

$$\text{FV} = \text{D} + \text{PV}$$
$$150 \text{ mL} = 70 \text{ mL} + \text{PV}$$
$$\text{PV} = 80 \text{ mL}$$

Step 3: Set up a cross-multiplication problem using the total quantity of drug in the stock bottle and the desired end concentration to solve for the final volume of the new suspension:

$$\frac{7500 \text{ mg}}{?\text{ mL}} = \frac{165 \text{ mg}}{5 \text{ mL}}$$
$$7500 \text{ mg} (5 \text{ mL}) = 165 \text{ mg} (?\text{ mL})$$
$$\text{FV} = 227.3 \text{ mL}$$

Step 4: Use the equation to solve for the volume of diluent needed to produce the new concentration:

$$\text{FV} = \text{D} + \text{PV}$$
$$227.3 \text{ mL} = \text{D} + 80 \text{ mL}$$
$$\text{Volume of diluent required (D)} = \mathbf{147.3 \text{ mL}}$$

CONVERTING BETWEEN GRAMS, KILOGRAMS, MILLIGRAMS, AND MICROGRAMS

A gram (g) is the basic metric unit of mass or weight. All other metric units of mass are centered around the gram. Metric units of measure can be easily converted from one form to another by moving the decimal place. A kilogram (kg) is 10^3 or 1000 times larger than a gram. Therefore, to convert grams to kilograms, the decimal place must be moved to the left three places. Milligrams (mg) and micrograms (mcg) are smaller than a gram. A milligram is 10^{-3} or 1000 times smaller than a gram, whereas a microgram is 10^{-6} or 1,000,000 times smaller than a gram. To convert grams to milligrams, the decimal place must be moved to the right three places. To convert grams to micrograms, the decimal place must be moved to the right six places.

Unit of Measure	Kilogram	Gram	Milligram	Microgram
Conversion factor	10^3	1	10^{-3}	10^{-6}
Sample conversion	0.008	8	8000	8,000,000

> **Review Video: Measurement Conversions**
> Visit mometrix.com/academy and enter code: 316703

INFORMATION DOCUMENTED IN ELECTRONIC PRESCRIPTION RECORD

An electronic prescription or medical record refers to a patient's profile within the pharmacy computer system or dispensing software. All records should include patient demographic information, including their name and address, telephone number, and date of birth. Some pharmacies also collect email information for patients as an alternative method of correspondence. Third-party billing or insurance plan information is also stored in the patient record. Patient preferences, including whether the patient opts out of child-proof safety caps, and notes are also part of the electronic record. Information regarding allergies and adverse reactions that the patient has experienced must be recorded in each patient's profile. The prescription fill history, refill information, and prescriptions on file are major components of a patient's prescription record. Hospital pharmacies or outpatient facilities may have extended access to a patient's medical record. Lab results, medication administration records, nursing orders, surgical notes, and prescriber interventions are examples of some of the types of information that are part of a patient's hospital medical record.

DOCUMENTATION REQUIREMENTS WITH COMPOUNDING

The master formulation is a recipe that details the information required to prepare the compound. A master formula contains a list of ingredients needed, equipment required, any calculations used, instructions for mixing, labeling requirements, compatibility/stability requirements, and storage requirements. The pharmacist or pharmacy technician should follow the procedure in the master formula when preparing a compound.

The compounding record is documentation of what happened or resulted during the compounding process. The compounding record contains the compounder's name, a reference to the master formula, a list of the products used, quantities of each product used, lot numbers and expiration dates for each product used, the beyond-use date of the compound, storage requirements, a copy of the label, and a description of the final product. Sometimes, multiple containers of the same compound are produced at the same time. This is called batch preparation. There will be one compounding record for each product or batch of products.

Compounding records should be kept on file for the same length of time as the prescription records. Federal law requires records to be kept for at least 2 years, but most state laws and company policies are more stringent.

Equipment/Supplies Required for Drug Administration

PRIORITIZING PHARMACY TASKS AND IMPROVING EFFICIENCY

Pharmacies are busy places and are constantly receiving new prescriptions or medication orders. Prioritizing the workload is important for ensuring patient safety and satisfaction.

In hospital pharmacies, dispensing queues will generally be coded with colors or symbols to designate the level of urgency of the prescription. Prescribers are often involved in marking the level of urgency of these orders, but pharmacy staff may also be involved in prioritizing orders. Stat orders (usually red) should be dealt with first, then urgent orders (usually orange or yellow), then nonurgent orders (usually green).

In retail or outpatient pharmacies, prescriptions generally come into the pharmacy through various systems. Patients who are physically present in the pharmacy generally have priority over electronic, faxed, and telephoned prescription orders. If a patient drops off a prescription, they should be asked if they are waiting and should be given an approximate wait time. Many pharmacies have a computer system that allows the pharmacy technician to mark prescriptions as waiting or urgent. Other pharmacies use colored baskets to let pharmacy staff know which prescriptions to prioritize. Red baskets are generally used to designate urgent prescriptions.

MAILING OR SHIPPING MEDICATIONS

Mail order pharmacies are becoming increasingly common in our online society. Pharmacies can mail any medication, including controlled substances and OTC products. The pharmacy should contact the patient prior to shipping the medication to verify the shipping address. The pharmacy is permitted to mail medications to the patient, a representative authorized by the patient, or the prescriber's office. The patient can have the medication delivered to a location of their choosing, which is not required to be their home address. Many patients choose to have medications delivered to their workplace so that they are not left unattended. However, medications do not require a delivery signature and can be delivered regardless of whether the patient is present.

Mailed medications should be packaged so that the contents of the package are not obvious. Because the patient is not picking the medication up at the pharmacy, important counseling points and information should be included in the package. This includes specific storage instruction, an information leaflet for each medication dispensed, and a toll-free number that the patient can call to contact the pharmacy with any questions.

REFRIGERATED MEDICATIONS

Disease-specific biological products are becoming increasingly prevalent as pharmaceutical technologies advance. Most of these biological products require refrigeration, so mailing of refrigerated pharmaceuticals is also becoming more common. Maintaining a refrigerated temperature range (36°F–46°F) throughout the process of transporting an item is referred to as the cold chain. There is a lack of legal regulation attached to mailing refrigerated medications, and there is no set process. Most pharmacies that mail refrigerated pharmaceuticals are members of an accreditation body, such as URAC (formerly the Utilization Review Accreditation Commission) or The Joint Commission, that establishes standards for cold chain validation.

Mailing refrigerated medications is not as simple as putting an ice pack in an insulated shipping box and hoping that it stays cold. Most accreditation bodies require pharmacies to validate or test their shipping methods and packaging prior to use and repeat the test at least twice a year. Testing requires shipping a temperature monitor to several locations using the same packaging techniques that would be used for refrigerated medications. When the temperature monitor is returned, the pharmacy staff can analyze the data to verify that the cold chain temperature range was maintained throughout the shipping process.

ACCESSORY SUPPLIES FOR ORAL MEDICATIONS

Oral liquids are administered in volumetric dosage units. This means that a patient must measure out a specific quantity of liquid to obtain each dose. Usually, doses are in increments of teaspoons (5 mL) or tablespoons (15 mL). Occasionally, patients will be required to measure a specific volume of liquid for each dose, such as 3.5 mL or 8 mL. You should ensure that the patient has the right tools and knowledge to administer the correct dose. Dosing spoons, oral syringes, or dosing cups should be dispensed with oral liquid for dose measurement. Depending upon the dosing device that is dispensed, the patient should be shown how to measure the correct dose.

Tablets and capsules usually have simple dosing instructions. However, some medications have complicated dosage regimens that may be confusing to the patient. For example, steroids are often prescribed as a tapering dose that involves taking many tablets initially and then decreasing the dose every few days. Manufacturers offer dose packs for some of these medications to make the directions clearer. Patients taking multiple medications may choose to have their medications packaged in weekly dosing trays to simplify administration.

SPACER

A spacer, also known as a holding chamber, is a device that makes using an inhaler easier and more effective. A mouthpiece or mask at one end of the device is attached to the patient, and the other end of the device is attached to the mouthpiece of the inhaler. Spacers are recommended for patients who have difficulty coordinating the action of pressing down on the inhaler and breathing in at the same time. Spacers are only used with MDIs because this type of inhaler requires the patient to press down on the metal canister to activate the release of a dose. DPIs are primed prior to use, then the dose can be inhaled without pressing a button. Most inhalers are used to treat asthma or COPD.

Spacers are commonly prescribed for children but are also used for elderly patients or those with arthritis who have difficulty pressing on the inhaler to activate it. Spacer devices can be purchased OTC without a prescription, but most patients obtain a prescription in order to bill the device to their insurance plan.

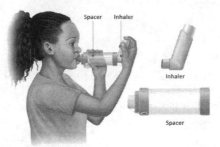

SUPPLIES FOR BLOOD GLUCOSE TESTING

Diabetics prick their fingers every day to test their blood sugar. In order to do this, they need the following supplies: lancets, test strips, blood glucose monitor, alcohol swabs, and a sharps container. A lancet is a small, sharp needle used to prick the finger. Test strips are thin strips of paper that react with the glucose in blood. Blood glucose monitors, also known as glucometers, read the response of the test strips and determine the blood glucose level. There are many different types of glucose monitors available on the market. Each meter is compatible with different test strips, so you must ensure that you are dispensing the correct type of test strips.

1. Swab the finger that will be used for testing with an alcohol swab to disinfect the area.
2. Insert a new test strip into the glucose monitor.
3. Prick the side of the finger with a lancet.
4. Gently squeeze or massage the finger until a drop of blood forms.
5. Touch and hold the drop of blood to the edge of the test strip.
6. The meter will display the blood glucose level after a few seconds.
7. Dispose of the used lancet in a sharps container.

PEN NEEDLES AND SYRINGES

Syringes are used to administer injectable medications from a vial. With syringes, the patients or their caregiver must draw up the dose of medication from the vial using the syringe. The markings on the syringe are used to determine how much fluid or what amount of medication is in the syringe. Any insulin that is packaged in a multiuse vial requires syringes for administration. Examples include Lantus, Novolog, Humalog, Humulin R, and Novolin N. Many other medications require syringes to administer. In general, any injectable medication that is not packaged in an IV bag or pen device must be drawn up using syringes.

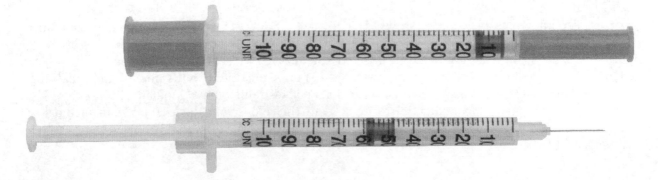

Pen needles are very short, thin needles that attach to injectable pen devices prior to administration. Pen needles are used for prefilled or refillable pen devices or cartridges. Examples of diabetic treatments that require pen needles for administration include Lantus SoloStar, Levemir FlexTouch, NovoLog FlexPen, Humalog KwikPen, Toujeo SoloStar, Byetta, and Victoza. Although pen devices are commonly used to administer insulin, there are some nondiabetic medications that use this technology as well, such as Forteo and Tymlos.

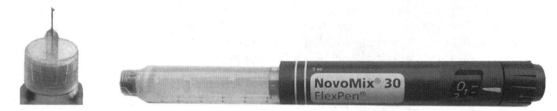

EQUIPMENT TO MEASURE VOLUME

Graduated cylinders are tall, narrow measuring tubes that have volumetric markings on them. They are commonly used for measuring volumes of liquid between 10 mL and 1000 mL. They are used to measure the amount of water needed for reconstituting a powder and measuring volumes of liquid ingredients to be used in compounding. There are various sizes of graduated cylinders available. The smallest possible size should be used to measure the volume of liquid required.

Volumetric flasks are pear-shaped glass measuring cups. They have markings on the side that indicate the fill volume. These are usually used in compounding to measure volumes of liquids. Volumetric flasks range in size from 10 ml to 2000 mL (2 L).

Syringes are used to measure small volumes of liquids. Syringes are used by patients and other healthcare professionals to measure out a volume of drug solution intended for injection into the body. They are also used in sterile compounding to transfer small volumes of solutions from one vial or container to another. Oral syringes are used to measure liquid doses between 5 mL and 10 mL for oral administration.

SELECTION OF MEDICAL SYRINGES

Medical syringes are selected based on three different categories: volume, length, and gauge.

The **volume** of a syringe is simply the amount of volume that it holds. Syringes are available in many volumes, including 1 mL, 3 mL, 5 mL, 10 mL, 20 mL, and 50 mL. The abbreviation cc is often used instead of mL. The 1 mL syringes are the most common type dispensed in retail pharmacies because they are used to inject insulin. Each 1 mL insulin syringe holds 100 units of insulin and has markings that indicate the fill volume in units.

The **length** indicates the length of the needle. Subcutaneous medications, including insulin and some vaccinations, generally use a shorter syringe between 5/8 and 1/2 inch in length. Intramuscular injections, including many vaccines, require longer syringes between 1 inch and 1.5 inches.

The **gauge** refers to the diameter or thickness of the needle. Needles vary in size from 16 to 30 gauge. Needles with a larger gauge have a smaller diameter and are preferred in patients who are smaller or frail. Needles with smaller gauges are preferred for larger patient with more body fat. Certain types of injections may also require a specific gauge needle.

UNIT DOSE PACKAGING

Unit dose packaging refers to tablets or capsules that are packaged in blister packs or individual dose packets that contain a single dose or an individual tablet/capsule. They are often used in hospital pharmacies to package and store individual doses for inpatients. Pharmacies can repackage larger containers into individual unit dose packages so long as the drug name, strength, manufacturer, lot number, and expiration date are listed on each unit dose packet. Some products are available from wholesalers already packaged in unit dose blister packs. Blister packaging is seldom used in retail pharmacies because it is inconvenient for patients. However, hospital pharmacies prefer blister packages because they do not require repackaging into unit dose packaging for administration to patients. Some medications are only available in unit dose blister packs due to stability issues or complex administration regimens. For example, orally disintegrating tablets are only available in blister packs because they would quickly disintegrate from the moisture in the air if packaged in multidose containers. Birth control pills, hormone replacement therapies, prednisone dosing packs, medication starter packs, and some DPI capsules are also packaged in unit dose blister packs.

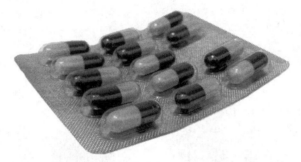

Lot Numbers, Expiration Dates, and NDC Numbers

BEYOND-USE DATES VS. EXPIRATION DATES

An **expiration date** is preassigned by the drug manufacturer and is the date after which a product can no longer be used. This date is required to be printed on the product container along with a lot number. The product can be used up to the expiration date, but not after. For example, you have short-dated amoxicillin tablets sitting on the pharmacy shelf that expire in September 2020. These tablets can be used by patients until September 30, 2020, but they expire starting on October 1, 2020. Some manufacturer expiration dates will include a date and month, but if only a month and year are listed, the expiration date is assumed to be at the end of the month.

A **beyond-use date** is assigned by the pharmacy or compounding facility; it is the date after which a compounded preparation can no longer be used. Beyond-use dates are assigned during compounding and are calculated from the date and time of preparation. For example, amoxicillin suspension is reconstituted for a patient on 4/1/2020 and has a beyond-use date of 14 days after reconstitution. Therefore, the beyond-use date that you should write on the label is 4/15/2020.

ASSIGNING BEYOND-USE DATES TO NONSTERILE COMPOUNDED PREPARATIONS

Beyond-use dates are expiration dates assigned to compounded or prepared products. They are defined as the date after which the product should not be used and are calculated or based on the date of preparation. If a compound has an official USP-NF monograph, the beyond-use date listed in the monograph should be used instead. If the compound is not listed in the USP-NF, but the beyond-use date of the compounded product is listed in the manufacturer's leaflet, use the manufacturer's beyond-use date. If the beyond-use date is not listed in either of these references, use the general USP-NF guidelines listed in the table below:

Type of Product	Maximum Beyond-Use Date
Oral solutions and water-based preparations	14 days
Topical and semisolid preparations	30 days
Nonaqueous (oil-based) preparations	6 months or the earliest expiration date of any of the ingredients, whichever is earlier

NDC NUMBER

A **National Drug Code (NDC) number** is a unique product identifier that is assigned to each product by the FDA. An NDC number is a 10-digit number divided into three parts. The first 4 digits identify the manufacturer. The second 4 digits identify the product strength, dosage form, and formulation. The last 2 digits identify the package size. The FDA is currently transitioning to 11-digit NDC numbers, so you will notice that some medications have 5 digits in the first part of their NDC number. For NDC numbers with only 10 digits, some computer systems will require the addition of a zero at the beginning of the number.

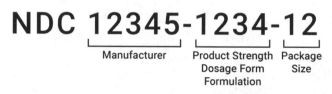

Because each drug product has a unique NDC number, it is useful for verifying that the correct product was dispensed when filling a prescription. NDC bar codes are also used to identify products in computer systems, Pyxis machines, dispensing robots, and barcode scanners.

LOT NUMBER

A lot number is a unique identification number assigned to a product by the manufacturer. By law, the lot number of a product must be listed on the product package. The lot number is usually stamped on the medication package next to the expiration date. Lot numbers signify a lot, batch, or particular group of products. In other words, products that are produced during the same time frame will have the same lot number. Most of the time, products with the same lot number also have the same expiration date.

Lot numbers are useful for identifying products during a product recall. The recall information will usually list the lot numbers of the products that are affected by the recall. This assists with identifying which products must be removed from the shelf and which products are safe to dispense. Without lot numbers, all products with the recalled NDC number would have to be discarded.

Procedures for Identifying and Returning Medications and Supplies

DISTRIBUTING AND TRANSPORTING MEDICATIONS IN HOSPITALS

Hospitals are big places, and each pharmacy must usually service a large area. One of the important roles of pharmacy personnel is to transport medications to the different areas of the hospital that need them. Many hospitals have tube systems that are used to transport medications from one department to another. These tubes systems are similar to the one that you use at the bank drive-through. Each hospital will have a list of medications near the tube station that cannot be tubed.

Controlled substances, expensive medications, patient's personal medications from home, and medications that should not be shaken are all on this list. Therefore, pharmacy technicians will always have to hand-deliver certain medications. Pharmacy technicians that are responsible for delivering medications throughout the hospital are known as drug runners. Runners are also responsible for preloading medications into robots and Pyxis machines that are located in most hospital departments. These machines allow nurses and other healthcare providers to access medications immediately without having to wait for the pharmacy to deliver them.

INDICATIONS OF A FORGED PRESCRIPTION

The following are characteristics of a prescription that may indicate that it is a forged prescription:

- The handwriting is too legible.
- The prescription is written for an unusually high quantity or dose.
- The prescription is written for a product that is rarely prescribed by local doctors.
- Nonstandard medical abbreviations are used.
- Unusual medical language is used.
- The prescription contains spelling errors.
- The prescription appears to be photocopied or has a watermark.
- The directions are written in full with no abbreviations.
- Parts of the prescription are written with a different color of ink or in different handwriting.
- The patient has never used your pharmacy before.
- There are no noncontrolled medications written for the same patient.
- The prescriptions are written for an unusual combination of drugs (e.g., stimulants and depressants).
- The prescription is written for a different person other than the customer presenting the prescription.
- The patient requests to pay out of pocket for the medication or denies having insurance.
- The prescription is written by a prescriber that you have never heard of.

CREDIT RETURN

When a medication is dispensed in a retail or outpatient pharmacy, the prescription is also billed through the computer system and a price is generated. Because billing is done during label production, this means that the insurance company has paid for the prescription before the patient picks it up. If the prescription needs to be returned for any reason, it must be **credit returned** in the computer system. This means that the prescription fill is reversed, the insurance claim is reversed, and the inventory is updated to accommodate the returned medication.

The most common reason for credit returns is the failure of the patient to pick up the prescription. A patient may refuse the medication, determine that it is too expensive, or forget to pick it up. Most insurance companies require pharmacies to return medications that have not been picked up by the patient within 10 to 14 days of the date of dispensing/billing. In some instances, you may need to credit return a prescription so that you can bill it through a different insurance plan or correct a billing issue (e.g., incorrect days' supply or incorrect quantity dispensed).

SCENARIOS IN WHICH A MEDICATION CAN AND CANNOT BE RETURNED TO STOCK

Returning a medication to stock means that you are returning it to the pharmacy shelf to be dispensed to another patient at another time. The most common reason for returning a medication to stock is because the patient failed to pick up the medication and it was credit returned. A patient may also request that a medication be returned to stock because it is too expensive, or they are no longer taking the medication. Stock bottles that were pulled for dispensing should also be returned if there is still medication remaining in the bottle.

Medications CANNOT be returned to stock if they have left the pharmacy. Once a patient picks up a medication and leaves the pharmacy with it, it cannot be returned to stock and dispensed to another patient. This is the law and is nonnegotiable. If a patient does not want a medication, it must be credit returned at the pharmacy counter before pickup. Products that are expired, damaged, or recalled cannot be returned to stock either.

RETURNING A MEDICATION TO STOCK

Before a medication can be returned to stock, the prescription must first be credit returned in the computer system. This reverses the payment from the insurance company, returns the refill to the patient's drug profile, and adjusts the inventory to reflect the returned quantity.

Medication information leaflets and packaging associated with the prescription that does not contain patient information can be disposed of in the regular trash. Documents that contain patient information must be disposed of with other PHI or HIPAA documents.

For products in their original packaging (e.g., a full box/bottle), attempt to remove the entire prescription label while preserving the lot number and expiration date printed on the container. If the label cannot be removed or for products that are not in their original packaging (e.g., amber prescription vials), mark out the patient's name and date of birth on the label using a thick black marker. Do NOT remove prescription labels from a vial because they contain important expiration date information. Do NOT combine the contents of a vial with an open container of the same product on the shelf because potentially serious errors may result. Additionally, the lot numbers for the products may not match.

CLEANING AND DISINFECTING STERILE COMPOUNDING AREAS OR CLEANROOMS

Guidelines for sterile compounding and cleaning sterile compounding areas are outlined in USP 797. Always follow the protocols and procedures in place at your facility first, and consult USP 797 if needed. General guidelines for cleaning include cleaning from the cleanest to the dirtiest area and from top to bottom, using single-use cleanroom wipes, replacing used wipes often, and using overlapping unidirectional strokes rather than circular motions. It is best to dedicate separate cleaning tools for use in each room or area. Cleaning should not occur while compounding is taking place, and only USP 797-approved cleaning products should be used. Approved cleaning products include sterile 70% isopropyl alcohol and PeridoxRTU.

Laminar flow hoods and biological safety cabinets should be cleaned at the beginning of each shift, before each batch, after a spill, and every 30 minutes while compounding. Countertops, work surfaces, and floors should be cleaned daily. Walls, ceilings, and shelves should be cleaned monthly. A cleaning log should be used to document the dates and times that cleaning has been completed.

DISPOSING OF EXPIRED, DAMAGED, RETURNED, OR RECALLED MEDICATIONS

For environmental and public safety reasons, medications must be disposed of properly. Damaged medications can usually be returned to the wholesaler or distributor. Check with your pharmacy's wholesaler for the specific return process, which usually includes filling out return authorization paperwork that includes the original purchase order information, item number, quantity, and reason for the return. A return authorization request can be made by telephone or through the online portal. Recalled medications should be returned to manufacturer. The recall notification will provide you with instructions on which medications should be returned and how to return them. Expired medications and patient-returned medications must be destroyed or sent to an authorized reverse distributor. Reverse distributors will usually give the pharmacy a return credit for medications returned minus a fee for their services. Returning medications to a reverse distributor usually involves filling out a paper or online form that lists the name, strength, dosage form, NDC number, and quantity of each medication being returned.

ENTERAL PRODUCTS

Enteral products provide nutrients or food in liquid form to patients through a feeding tube. Enteral nutrition differs from parenteral nutrition in that enteral nutrition is provided through a feeding tube into the enteral (digestive) system, whereas parenteral nutrition is infused into the venous system (veins). Different types of feeding tubes enter the digestive system at different locations: nasogastric (NG), orogastric (OG), gastrostomy (G-tube), and jejunostomy (J-tube).

Elemental enteral products contain all the nutrients that a patient requires, including sugars, proteins, and fats. The food components are broken down into their smallest components (predigested) to make it easier for patients to digest the product. Elemental formula examples include Vivonex T.E.N. and Vivonex PLUS.

Semielemental (peptide) products also contain sugars, proteins, and fats. However, the components are only partially predigested and require the patient to have some digestive tract function. An example is Peptamen AF.

Polymeric (standard) enteral formulas contain whole proteins, complex sugars (carbohydrates), and fats that have not been predigested. These are used for patients who have a fully working digestive tract. Polymeric products include Boost, Ensure, Nutren, and Replete. These products are commonly dispensed in retail pharmacies and are available over the counter.

Chapter Quiz

Ready to see how well you retained what you just read? Scan the QR code to go directly to the chapter quiz interface for this study guide. If you're using a computer, simply visit the bonus page at **mometrix.com/bonus948/ptcb** and click the Chapter Quizzes link.

Supplemental Content – Not Tested

Transform passive reading into active learning! After immersing yourself in this chapter, put your comprehension to the test by taking a quiz. The insights you gained will stay with you longer this way. Scan the QR code to go directly to the chapter quiz interface for this study guide. If you're using a computer, simply visit the bonus page at **mometrix.com/bonus948/ptcb** and click the Chapter Quizzes link.

State Requirements and Practice Standards

LICENSURE, REGISTRATION, AND/OR CERTIFICATION OF PHARMACY TECHNICIANS
LICENSURE OF PHARMACY TECHNICIANS

Just over a decade ago, pharmacy technicians were not required to be qualified or licensed at all. As the career has started to become more advanced, state laws have started requiring more and more training for pharmacy technicians. Initially, the only qualification required was to obtain licensure by examination through the Pharmacy Technician Certification Board (PTCB), a nationwide certification program. Today, most states also require pharmacy technicians to complete additional training and licensure requirements with the state board of pharmacy.

Laws governing the licensure of pharmacy technicians vary greatly from state to state. Only 20 of the 50 US states require PTCB certification in order to become a licensed pharmacy technician: Arizona, Idaho, Illinois, Iowa, Kansas, Louisiana, Mississippi, Montana, Nevada, New Mexico, North Carolina, North Dakota, Oregon, South Dakota, Texas, Utah, Vermont, Virginia, Washington, and Wyoming. In addition to or instead of PTCB licensure, most states require pharmacy technicians to become registered or licensed by the state board of pharmacy. New York, Pennsylvania, and Wisconsin are the only exceptions. Some states accept PTCB certification as qualifications for licensure, other states require completion of an additional training program or work experience, and a few states require hardly any qualifications at all.

PHARMACY TECHNICIAN CERTIFICATION WITH THE PTCB

The Pharmacy Technician Certification Board (PTCB) is a nationwide program that trains and certifies pharmacy technicians. Originally, PTCB certification was the only recognized certification program for pharmacy technicians. Then, individual states started requiring pharmacy technicians to also become licensed with their state board of pharmacy.

Initially, PTCB certification merely involved taking and passing the Pharmacy Technician Certification Exam, completing a criminal background check, and obtaining a high school diploma. As of 2020, the PTCB program is now requiring candidates to complete a PTCB-recognized training program or at least 500 hours of equivalent work experience in place of the high school diploma requirement.

Once PTCB certification is obtained, candidates must maintain their certification by completing at least 20 hours of continuing education (CE) during each 2-year renewal cycle. At least 1 CE credit must be in the subject of pharmacy law, and at least 1 CE credit must be in the subject of patient safety.

ROLES AND RESPONSIBILITIES OF PHARMACY EMPLOYEES

ACTIVITIES AND ROLES OF PHARMACY TECHNICIAN

Pharmacy technicians are legally allowed to perform the following roles in the pharmacy:

- Receive and enter paper or faxed prescription orders
- Receive refill requests from patients
- Receive a refill authorization from a prescriber or their agent
  - Any changes or new information to add to the existing prescription order other than refills must be made or added by a pharmacist
- Enter prescription orders and insurance information into the pharmacy software system
- View and enter patient data
- Check patients out at the cash register
- Count or measure out drug products in order to prepare a prescription order
- Manage pharmacy inventory
- Load drug-dispensing devices (e.g., Pyxis machines) in a hospital setting
- Distribute medications in a hospital setting
- Prepare sterile IV admixtures and nonsterile compounds under the supervision of a pharmacist

These roles are based on federal regulations. Some states have specific regulations in place to allow technicians to perform other roles, such as administering flu vaccines or performing accuracy checks in hospitals (tech-check-tech programs).

ACTIVITIES AND ROLES OF UNLICENSED PERSONNEL

Unlicensed pharmacy staff members are also referred to as supportive personnel. By law, unlicensed pharmacy personnel cannot be involved in dispensing medications, counseling patients, or entering information into a patient's profile. Pharmacy employees must always be supervised by a licensed pharmacist. Although state laws vary, unlicensed pharmacy staff members are generally allowed to perform the following tasks:

- Bookkeeping, prescription filing, and documenting third-party reimbursements
- Sending pharmacy orders and updating drug prices in the computer system
- Receiving the pharmacy order, unpacking medications, and putting stock away on the shelf
- Delivering medications to a patient's home
- Answering phone calls and transferring calls to licensed pharmacy staff members
  - Unlicensed personnel cannot receive prescription refill requests, refill authorizations, receive new prescriptions, or answer pharmacy questions over the phone
- Receiving a new prescription from a patient
  - Unlicensed personnel cannot enter new prescriptions into the computer system, so they must hand the prescription to a licensed pharmacist or pharmacy technician
- Helping customers find products in the pharmacy
  - If patients have questions about pharmacy products, they must be referred to a pharmacist
- Acting as a cashier for the sale of prescription and OTC medications

FACILITIES, EQUIPMENT, AND SUPPLY

CLEANLINESS, EQUIPMENT, AND FACILITY STANDARDS

State laws dictate the general requirements that must be met for pharmacy facilities. State boards of pharmacy are responsible for inspecting pharmacies to ensure that facility standards are met. An initial inspection is required when a pharmacy first opens or relocates. The frequency of inspection thereafter varies by state. Most states have similar requirements for pharmacy facilities:

- Adequate lighting, ventilation, and sanitation.
- A sink with hot and cold running water that is separate from any restroom.
- Cleanrooms should not have sinks or floor drains.
- All entrances to drug storage must be equipped with a lock.
- If controlled substances are dispensed, the pharmacy must have a security/alarm system that detects and provides notice of unauthorized entry when the facility is closed.
- The pharmacy should be maintained at controlled room temperature.
- If medications are stored in refrigerators, the pharmacy must keep daily written or electronic logs of the refrigerator temperatures on the days of operation.
- Retail pharmacies must have a private counseling area.
- If engaged in compounding, a working class III balance is often required.

STATE INSPECTION REQUIREMENTS AND REFERENCE MATERIALS REQUIRED IN THE PHARMACY

State boards of pharmacy reserve the right to inspect pharmacy facilities at any time. Inspections occur during the initial pharmacy opening, after a relocation, and periodically as determined by the state board of pharmacy. The general requirements for pharmacy staff and reference sources in pharmacies are as follows:

- The licenses of all pharmacy staff members should be displayed or readily retrievable for inspection.
- The pharmacy should maintain a list of all licensed pharmacy employees that includes their name, license classification, license number, and expiration date.
- All pharmacy personnel should wear a clearly visible and readable badge that identifies their name and position.
- Current editions of relevant reference sources must be kept in the pharmacy. This requirement varies by state, but many states require a current copy of the state law book, federal law book, and at least one clinical reference source.

STATE AND FEDERAL REQUIREMENTS FOR FILING AND STORING PRESCRIPTIONS

Federal law requires prescriptions to be kept on file at the pharmacy for a minimum of 2 years from the date of last dispensing. State laws usually require prescriptions to be kept on file for longer than 2 years, but the length of time varies from state to state. Additionally, insurance contracts and company policies often have even stricter requirements for the length of time that prescriptions must be kept.

There are three different ways that prescription records can be filed. The easiest and most common way to file prescription records is to have three separate files for schedule II controlled substances, schedules III–V controlled substances, and noncontrolled substances. Pharmacies are also allowed to maintain two separate files with schedule II controlled substances in one file and all schedules III–V controlled substances and noncontrolled substances together in another file. If only two prescription files are used, each prescription for schedules III–V controlled substances must be stamped with a red letter C in the lower right corner so that they can be readily identified.

Inventory Management

Transform passive reading into active learning! After immersing yourself in this chapter, put your comprehension to the test by taking a quiz. The insights you gained will stay with you longer this way. Scan the QR code to go directly to the chapter quiz interface for this study guide. If you're using a computer, simply visit the bonus page at **mometrix.com/bonus948/ptcb** and click the Chapter Quizzes link.

PROCEDURES TO ADDRESS IMPROPERLY STORED INVENTORY

Once a medication becomes expired or its beyond-use date has passed, it must be quarantined or separated from the rest of the pharmacy stock until it is disposed of. Products that become damaged or adulterated must also be disposed of, for example: a refrigerated product that is left out of the refrigerator for too long, a cough syrup bottle that is cracked and leaking, or a product that was compounded incorrectly and is not usable. Medications that have been dispensed to a patient and left the pharmacy and are then returned by the patient are also considered to be adulterated and cannot legally be re-dispensed. These medications should be quarantined and labeled as patient returns. If a drug recall is issued and the pharmacy determines that some of their stock is affected, these recalled medications must also be quarantined and disposed of.

AUTOMATED EQUIPMENT INVENTORY MANAGEMENT

Inventory management is the process of maintaining an adequate supply of drugs in the pharmacy. In order to achieve this, a perpetual or continuous inventory of the medications in stock must be maintained so that medications can be reordered in a timely manner. Medication orders are usually placed by a pharmacy buyer/purchaser in hospitals and large pharmacies, whereas most retail pharmacies have a computer system that automatically places orders based on par levels and current inventory. Pharmacy technicians should periodically correct on-hand inventory quantities. In hospital pharmacies, technicians may also be responsible for loading or reconfiguring Pyxis drawers and adjusting par levels.

Although technicians are responsible for maintaining schedules III–V and noncontrolled medication inventories, pharmacists are responsible for maintaining schedule II inventories and ordering schedule II drugs. By law, a perpetual inventory must be kept and monitored constantly. Every time a schedule II drug is received in the order or dispensed to a patient, the pharmacist must make a record in the controlled substance logbook. Every 10 days, all schedule II drugs must be counted and reconciled with the controlled substance logbook. Pharmacy technicians can assist with this inventory process under the direction of a pharmacist.

FORMULARY OR APPROVED/PREFERRED PRODUCT LIST

A formulary is a list of medications that are approved for use in the pharmacy. Formularies are used in hospital and facility settings to identify drugs that are safe and cost-effective. Formularies are also useful for identifying products that are normally kept in stock in the pharmacy. When submitting medication orders, the facility computer system will let the prescriber know which medications are on the formulary list and are readily available in the pharmacy. Some hospitals have protocols in place that allow pharmacists to substitute certain nonformulary drugs for a therapeutically equivalent drug that is on the formulary list. The pharmacy may be able to order and dispense nonformulary medications with prior approval from the management.

Insurance companies also use formularies to keep costs to a minimum. A preferred product list is a list of products or medications that are preferred by the insurance plan. Preferred products have a less expensive copay than nonpreferred products. Some nonpreferred products require prior authorization before the insurance company will pay for them.

SUITABLE ALTERNATIVES FOR ORDERING

TRANSFERRING OR BORROWING MEDICATION FROM ANOTHER PHARMACY

You may run into a scenario in which a patient needs a medication urgently, but you do not have the medication in stock at your pharmacy. Sometimes, you can assist the patient in finding the medication at a different pharmacy. The patient can either take a new prescription to that pharmacy, or you can have the pharmacist at your location transfer the prescription to the other pharmacy. Perhaps the patient is unable to go to the other pharmacy location or they are an inpatient at your hospital or facility. You could also come across a scenario in which the patient's insurance plan is not accepted at the other pharmacy, or the patient lives in a state that the other pharmacy is not licensed to ship medications into. In these scenarios, you may have to borrow or transfer the medication from another pharmacy closer to your location.

PROCEDURE

Federal law allows pharmacies to transfer, sell, or give away prescription drugs to licensed pharmacies, hospitals, or prescribers' offices. To prevent drug diversion and exploitation, most states place restrictions on the amount of drugs that pharmacies can sell, usually up to 5% of total annual drug sales. If pharmacies are under common ownership, an unlimited amount of prescription drugs can be transferred between facilities. If the pharmacies are not under common ownership, the receiving facility should use a purchase order to request the medication and the distributing pharmacy should issue an invoice. Documentation is especially important when transferring controlled substances. For the transfer or sale of schedule II controlled substances, a DEA Form 222 is required. The receiving facility must complete a DEA Form 222, keep copy 3, and send copies 1 and 2 to the distributing pharmacy. The distributing pharmacy should keep copy 1 and send copy 2 to the DEA. Once the transfer is complete, the receiving facility must record the amount of medication received on copy 3 of the DEA Form 222 and keep this form on file at the pharmacy for at least 2 years.

MEDICATION QUALITY CONTROL SYSTEM REQUIREMENTS

AUTOMATED DISPENSING SYSTEMS

Many retail pharmacies used automated counting systems, such as Parata Max, to assist with dispensing, error reduction, and inventory control. Pharmacy technicians will load the machine by scanning the stock bottle and entering the quantity that is being added to the system. When the system receives a prescription, it will count, fill, cap, and label the prescription. It will automatically deduct the amount dispensed from the running inventory.

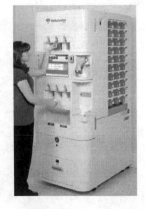

146

Hospital pharmacies use automated dispensing cabinets, such as Pyxis or Omnicell, to store medications and keep track of inventory. Pharmacy technicians deliver medications to Pyxis machines located in different areas throughout the hospital. Technicians will scan the medications into the correct pocket of the machine and update the on-hand inventory as they add medications to the system. Healthcare providers each have their own login to access the system and remove medications. When a medication is removed, the running inventory is automatically updated. The central pharmacy can access the running inventory in real time, and the system can send alerts to the pharmacy when medications are running low and need to be refilled.

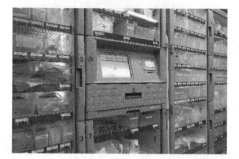

EMERGENCY DRUG KIT

An emergency drug kit, also referred to as a code tray or crash cart, is a kit containing drugs that are necessary to treat patients during emergency situations. Medications that are commonly contained within an emergency drug kit include epinephrine, atropine, dextrose, glucagon, naloxone, amiodarone, EpiPen, adenosine, diphenhydramine, sodium bicarbonate, dobutamine, and phenytoin. The contents of these kits vary depending upon the needs of the facility and the types of patients that are being treated. For example, pediatric code trays contain different medications and different dosages of medications than adult code trays.

Emergency drug kits should be labeled with the list of contents and their expiration date. The outside of the kit should show the earliest expiration date of drugs in the kit as well as the verifying pharmacist's initials and a statement that the kit is for emergency use only. The kit should be secured with a tamper-evident seal and kept in a secure area. Drugs in the kit should only be used by authorized personnel upon written or verbal orders from a provider. Once a kit has been opened or contents have expired, it should be returned to the pharmacy to be restocked.

FLOOR STOCK

Floor stock refers to prescription or OTC medications that are stored in a department of a hospital or facility other than the pharmacy. Floor stock medications are usually stored in a nurses' station or medical supply room. All prescription and floor stock medications are required to be stored in a secured environment that is only accessible by authorized personnel. Floor stock medications should only be dispensed with verbal or written orders from a provider. Some hospital departments may also have a Pyxis storage cabinet that is maintained and restocked by the pharmacy department. Medications contained within automated dispensing cabinets are not considered to be floor stock.

The pharmacy department does not usually maintain an inventory of floor stock medications. Therefore, any controlled medications cannot be kept as floor stock. The types of medications allowed to be kept as floor stock generally include sterile water, saline solutions, irrigation fluids, certain IV fluids (e.g., lactated Ringer's solution), heparin flushes, medical gases (e.g., oxygen), and prescription devices.

BAR-CODE SCANNING TECHNOLOGY

Barcode scanning is used in the dispensing process to verify that the correct medication was dispensed. In retail or outpatient settings, the bar code of each stock bottle is scanned during the dispensing process to ensure that the NDC number matches the NDC number dispensed on the label or in the computer system. In hospital pharmacies, barcode scanning is also used when delivering medication to automated dispensing cabinets (e.g., Pyxis machines). When the pharmacy technician restocks the machine, they first scan the medication. This triggers the machine to open the pocket or drawer assigned to that medication. This reduces the likelihood of stocking the drug in the wrong location. It also reduces the likelihood that nurses or providers will dispense and administer the wrong medication. Additionally, nurses use barcode scanning technology to ensure that they are administering the right drug to the right patient. First, they scan the drug, and then they scan the patient identifier code on the patient's wristband before drug administration.

INVENTORY CONTROL PRACTICES AND RECORD KEEPING

COMPUTERIZED INVENTORY CONTROL SYSTEMS

Inventory control is an important part of the pharmacy technician role. Inventory is not just about counting pills. Maintaining appropriate stock levels of medications is an important need that balances patient safety and satisfaction with efficiency and profitability.

Most pharmacies have computerized inventory control systems that continuously update on-hand medication quantities as prescriptions are dispensed. Additionally, computer systems will automatically reorder medications whose on-hand quantities have fallen below a set **par level**. A par level is the minimum amount of inventory that is required to be on hand for the pharmacy to function efficiently. Par levels are determined from drug usage patterns and turnover rates and can usually only be overridden by pharmacy management.

Because medication orders are placed based on current inventory levels, it is important to maintain an accurate perpetual or continuous inventory of all dispensable medications. Shelves should be periodically inventoried and searched for expired medications. Expired drugs should be quarantined and removed from the computerized inventory.

DOCUMENTATION REQUIREMENTS FOR PHARMACY INVENTORIES

A full inventory of all pharmacy products must be performed at least every 2 years. Records of the inventory should include the date of the inventory and the results of the inventory. The completed inventory record should be signed and dated by the person taking the inventory as well as the pharmacist in charge within 3 business days of the inventory taking place. Inventory records should be kept on file for a minimum of 2 years according to federal law, but some states require records to be kept for longer periods of time. Each registered pharmacy location should have separate inventory records kept on file at each facility.

Inventory records for schedule II controlled substances should be kept separate from inventory records of other medications. Additionally, a perpetual inventory must be kept in the controlled substance logbook. A record must be made every time a schedule II substance is received, sold, delivered, or dispensed to a patient.

PROCEDURES TO PERFORM PHYSICAL INVENTORY

PERFORMING A PHARMACY INVENTORY

An inventory should be performed either before the pharmacy opens or after the pharmacy closes for the day. A separate inventory should be done for each registered pharmacy location. All pharmacy stock must be inventoried, including expired drugs and medications contained within robotic dispensing systems or automated dispensing cabinets (e.g., Pyxis).

For noncontrolled drugs, the number of full bottles of each product should be counted. For partially empty containers, the exact count of the contents can be estimated.

For schedules III–V controlled medications, follow the same procedures as for noncontrolled medications. For partially empty containers, an estimated count or measure of the container contents is sufficient for inventory purposes unless the container holds more than 1000 tablets or capsules. For containers holding more than 1000 units, an exact count of the contents should be made.

For schedule II controlled substances, an exact count or measure of the container contents must be performed and documented in the inventory record. There are no exceptions for partially empty containers. Inventory records for schedule II substances should be kept separate.

Once the inventory is complete, the person performing the inventory and the pharmacist in charge should sign and date the inventory record.

SCENARIOS IN WHICH PHARMACY INVENTORY IS REQUIRED

All pharmacies must complete an initial inventory prior to opening for business and engaging in the distribution or dispensing of medications. An inventory is also required when the pharmacy changes ownership or closes for business.

According to federal law, all pharmacies must also complete a full inventory every 2 years. However, many state laws, company policies, and accreditation bodies require annual inventories. The inventory may be completed any day within 2 years of the last inventory. Inventories should be completed before the pharmacy opens or after the pharmacy closes for the day.

Occasionally, medications can change schedules. If a controlled substance was formerly in a different schedule and becomes a schedule II controlled drug, an inventory of that drug must be completed. The inventory must be done before opening or after closing of the pharmacy date that the change in schedule becomes effective.

DAILY DISPENSING LOG, INVENTORY REPORT, AND DISCREPANCY REPORT

A **daily dispensing log** summarizes the amount and type of prescriptions filled by the pharmacy each day. This report is useful for analyzing workflow and pharmacy staffing levels.

An **inventory report** can generally be run for any drug, group of drugs, or schedule of drugs. These are very useful to pharmacy technicians because they allow us to cycle count medications. Cycle counting is like spot checking inventory levels for a group of drugs. Most pharmacies have established guidelines that state which medications should be inventoried for each period or quarter. The on-hand inventory levels of medication must be counted, and computer inventory levels should be updated if the quantities do not match. Inventory reports are also helpful for assisting pharmacists in investigating a schedule II controlled drug inventory discrepancy. Inventory reports for a specific drug allow pharmacists to track inventory changes and determine when the discrepancy occurred. Some dispensing systems will automatically generate a **discrepancy report** for controlled medications if a discrepancy is found between the quantity in the dispensing systems and the computer inventory.

Health and Wellness

FACTORS THAT CAN INFLUENCE EFFECTS OF MEDICATIONS

Patients respond differently to drugs depending upon their age, race, genetics, height, weight, gender, and diet. Most drugs have different recommended doses for pediatric patients because children metabolize medications at a different rate. Many medications have a greater or longer lasting effect in elderly patients because those patients break down drugs more slowly. Some medications require dosage adjustment in the elderly. Height and weight may also influence drug effects. Some drugs are dosed based on weight or body surface area. Gender, race, and genetics can also play roles in drug dosing. Patients of a certain race or gender and those with certain genetic conditions may require dosage adjustments for certain medications. Diet can also affect the metabolism of certain medications. For example, patients who take warfarin should be cautious of their vitamin K intake because it can affect the actions of warfarin. Some other medications (e.g., tetracyclines) can be affected by ions, such as calcium, and should not be taken with milk.

DEVICES COMMONLY DISPENSED BY PHARMACIES

Medical devices are a broad category that includes anything from diabetic test strips to implantable pacemaker devices. Many medical devices are used by surgical departments and are billed medically. However, some devices are dispensed by pharmacies. For example, diabetic test strips, lancets, and syringes may be considered medical devices. For most insurance companies, these devices are billed under the normal pharmacy plan. Medicare requires these devices to be billed under the medical side, Medicare Part B. Blood glucose monitors and nebulizer machines are also billed under Medicare Part B. Many commercial insurance plans do not cover glucose monitors, so patients must purchase them out of pocket or through a manufacturer coupon program. Blood pressure monitors and spacer devices that are used in conjunction with inhalers are medical devices that are commonly sold by pharmacies. Most insurance companies will not reimburse for these devices, so patients generally must purchase them out of pocket.

COMPLIANCE AND THE MEDICATION ADHERENCE RATIO

Compliance occurs when the patient adheres to the prescribed drug regimen. It can sometimes be difficult to determine whether a patient is taking their medication according to the prescribed directions and getting the full benefit from their treatment. The best way for pharmacy technicians to assess patient compliance is to pay attention to computer alerts for early or late refills. Refilling early means that the patient is running out of medication quicker than they should. This is of concern for medications with a high potential for abuse, such as opioids and benzodiazepines. Late refills mean that patients are missing doses or not taking the medication as often as prescribed.

The **medication possession ratio (MPR)** is the ratio of the days' supply dispensed to the number of days between refills. This ratio can be multiplied by 100 to get a percentage. Ideally, the MPR should be 1:1 or 100%. The lower the MPR, the less adherent the patient is.

Billing and Reimbursement

CHARACTERISTICS OF REIMBURSEMENT POLICIES AND PLANS
GOVERNMENT-SPONSORED HEALTH INSURANCE PLANS

Medicare is a federally funded program that provides health insurance coverage for patients older than 65 years old, disabled people, and patients with kidney failure or amyotrophic lateral sclerosis.

- **Part A** (standard) — covers hospital inpatient services, nursing facilities, and hospice care
- **Part B** (optional, additional premium) — covers outpatient services, doctor visits, medical supplies, and certain pharmacy medications (e.g., vaccinations, nebulizer solutions, diabetic test strips)
- **Part C** (Medicare Advantage Plans) — Part A and B benefits offered by private insurers
- **Part D** (optional, additional premium) — Medicare Prescription Drug Plan. Patients are subject to different deductibles and copays depending upon their chosen plan.

Medicaid provides medical coverage to individuals or families with low incomes or with a disability. Medicaid is jointly funded by federal and state governments. Medicare and Medicaid are governed by the Centers for Medicare & Medicaid Services (CMS). However, individual states decide on eligibility, coverage, and copays.

> **Review Video: Medicare & Medicaid**
> Visit mometrix.com/academy and enter code: 507454

Tricare is a federal program that provides health coverage to military members, retirees, and their families. A third party (e.g., Express Scripts) provides the actual billing services, and patients can use any in-network pharmacy. The Veterans Health Administration (VHA) provides healthcare benefits to veterans, but it only covers services provided by VHA doctors or VHA pharmacies.

PRIVATE INSURANCE PLANS

Private insurance coverage is when a health insurance plan is being paid for by an individual person or their employer rather than by the government or another third party (e.g., worker's compensation, patient assistance programs, copay card). There are two main categories of private insurance plans: HMOs and PPOs.

Health maintenance organizations (HMOs) are a network of pharmacies and providers that work with an insurer or are contracted to work with them. With HMO insurance plans, patients are usually required to use an in-network pharmacy. Additionally, HMO plans often require patients to use a generic medication or a medication that is on their preferred product list.

Preferred provider organizations (PPOs) are a network of pharmacies and providers that work with an insurer but will partially reimburse patients for services from an out-of-network provider or pharmacy. Like HMOs, PPO plans will usually require patients to use a generic medication or a medication that is on their preferred product list. However, with PPO plans, patients can use an out-of-network provider or pharmacy if they are willing to pay a higher copay or cost.

DAW CODE

A **dispense-as-written (DAW) code** is a system used by prescribers, pharmacies, and insurance companies to signify the intention of the prescriber or patient regarding generic substitution of the prescribed medication. Insurance companies require generic substitution for most medications unless special circumstances are indicated using a DAW billing code. If no DAW code is noted on the prescription, it is assumed that generic substitution is permitted by the prescriber.

DAW Codes			
0	No product selection is indicated.	5	The branded product is dispensed at the generic price.
1	Substitution is NOT allowed by the prescriber; use the branded product.	6	Override.
2	Substitution is allowed, but the patient requested branded product.	7	Substitution is NOT allowed; the branded product is required by law.
3	Substitution is allowed, but the pharmacist selected a branded product.	8	Substitution is allowed, but the branded product is not available.
4	Substitution is allowed, but the generic equivalent is not in stock.	9	Other.

IMPACT OF THE AFFORDABLE CARE ACT ON PHARMACY SERVICES

The Affordable Care Act (ACA), commonly referred to as Obamacare, was signed into law in 2010. The ACA was enacted mainly to offer all Americans essential health coverage, including emergency, preventative, and mental health services. For patients who were unable to enroll in affordable health coverage through their employer but weren't eligible for Medicaid, the ACA offered several government-subsidized health coverage options. The cost of the insurance coverage was subsidized based on the patient's income. The ACA also required all Americans to have essential insurance coverage. Without proof of health coverage, patients would be charged a tax penalty. This tax penalty is no longer in effect.

The ACA also created accountable care organizations, which are groups of providers that work together to provide health care to different populations. The main impact of this concept on pharmacies is that Medicare and other insurance companies started requiring and paying pharmacies to provide medication therapy management services, which are provided by pharmacists to help improve patient care in addition to providing extra income.

STRATEGIES TO RESOLVE THIRD-PARTY REJECTED CLAIMS

BILLING PHARMACY CLAIMS AND PROCESSING AN INSURANCE CLAIM

Most pharmacy computer systems will bill the patient's insurance benefit in real time as their prescription is processed. Once the pharmacy technician gathers the necessary information from the patient and enters it into the computer system, the computer transmits that information to the insurer and the results will be displayed in the claim response screen. This screen will tell you whether the claim was approved or denied, what copay (out-of-pocket cost to the patient) will be owed, whether the patient is required to pay a deductible (the amount the patient must pay before coverage begins), and what the insurer reimbursed for the services.

Information Required to Bill/Process an Insurance Claim

- Insurance Plan Information
  - BIN number — Pharmacy benefit international identification number
  - Cardholder ID number
  - Group number
  - DAW code (if applicable)

- Prescription Information
  - Medication information and NDC number
  - Quantity dispensed
  - Days' supply
  - Date the prescription was written
  - Date the prescription is dispensed
  - Prescriber's identification number (DEA number or National Provider Identifier)
- Patient Information
  - Patient name
  - Patient's gender/sex
  - Patient's date of birth (DOB)
  - Patient's relationship to cardholder
- Pricing/Cost Information
  - Ingredient cost
  - Dispensing fee
  - Total amount billed to the insurance plan

REJECTION OF PHARMACY INSURANCE CLAIM

The following are examples of reasons for a pharmacy insurance claim rejection and ways to resolve the issues:

1. Nonmatch of insurance information and patient information
   a. Verify insurance information and obtain a copy of the card if possible. Check that the information given matches the information in the computer.
   b. Verify patient information, including DOB and name. Some insurance plans require that the patient name in the computer matches the name on the insurance card exactly (e.g., Medicare).
2. Refill too soon
   a. Check that the days' supply was calculated correctly from the previous fill. If not, call the insurance company to rebill the old claim.
   b. Verify that the patient is taking the medication as prescribed.
   c. If special circumstances require early refill (e.g., lost medication, vacation), contact the insurance company for an early refill override.
3. Prior authorization required
   a. Insurance companies require prior authorizations for expensive or nonformulary medications. This requires paperwork to be sent to the patient's prescriber, who will call or fax the insurance company to complete the authorization. Approval is usually granted within 1 week, but insurance companies sometimes deny coverage of the medication.
4. Pharmacy is not in the network
   a. Contact the insurance company to check if a one-time override is available. In most cases, the prescription must be transferred to an in-network pharmacy.

REIMBURSEMENT MODELS

The **wholesale acquisition cost (WAC)**, also known as the **average sale price (ASP)**, is the average cost of a particular medication in the USA. Insurance companies use this price as their basis for reimbursement of brand-name medications.

The **maximum allowable cost (MAC)** is a set cost that an insurance company will reimburse for a particular product or medication. Insurance companies use a set MAC price to reimburse pharmacies for generic medications. MAC prices are updated more frequently than WAC prices and are a better indicator of current market price. The insurance company will reimburse the same amount regardless of how much the pharmacy paid for the product. Therefore, this reimbursement system encourages pharmacies to purchase drugs at the lowest possible price in order to make a greater profit.

For inpatient and facility services, many insurance plans use a fee-for-service reimbursement system. The facility is reimbursed a set price to provide a specific service to a patient, regardless of the cost incurred. The average manufacturer's price of products is used to calculate this cost. Because facilities are reimbursed by service rather than by treatment, this reimbursement method discourages facilities from providing unnecessary or excessive treatments/services and encourages them to purchase drug at the lowest possible price.

PROCEDURES TO COORDINATE BENEFITS

Coordination of benefits is the process of determining in which order to bill insurance plans when a patient has multiple active insurance plans.

The first step in coordinating benefits is determining which plan is the primary one, the plan that should be billed first. If you ask the patient, they usually know which plan is their primary plan. Alternatively, insurance companies usually have access to this information. In fact, if you attempt to bill a secondary insurance first, the claim will likely be rejected stating that the patient has another primary insurance that must be billed first.

If the patient has a private insurance plan as well as a government insurance plan (e.g., Medicare, Medicaid, Tricare), the private insurance must always be billed first. If that isn't tricky enough, consider what to do if a patient has two government insurance plans: Medicaid should be billed second after any Medicare or Tricare plan.

Manufacturer coupon cards should be billed last. For instance, if the patient only has one insurance plan, the coupon card should be billed second. If the patient has two insurance plans, the coupon card should be billed third. Manufacturer coupons cannot be used if a patient has any government insurance plan.

LEVEL-OF-SERVICE BILLING
MEDICAL AND PHARMACY INSURANCE COVERAGE

Medical insurance is used to cover hospital visits, outpatient clinic visits, and primary care visits. Medical services are billed to a patient's medical insurance after their appointment or visit is complete. Medical facilities usually have a dedicated medical billing team that submits claims to medical insurers. Pharmacy insurance is used to cover medications and devices. Insurance claims for medications are billed at the point of sale (at the time of dispensing). Once the patient's insurance information is added into their profile, the computer system will automatically bill the patient insurance during dispensing. Generally, pharmacy technicians only deal with pharmacy insurance, but there are some instances in which medication insurance should be used in a pharmacy. Some insurance plans require vaccinations, medical equipment, medical devices, home infusions, and certain medications to be billed to the medical plan. For example, when Medicare patients receive a flu vaccine at the pharmacy, their Medicare Part B medical insurance coverage must be billed. Nebulizer solutions, diabetic testing strips, and some types of medical equipment must also be billed to Medicare Part B. Some insurance plans also require IV solutions, such as hemophilia blood factors, to be billed to their medical plan.

MINIMIZING PATIENT'S OUT-OF-POCKET COSTS

It's not a secret that medications can be very expensive. For patients without insurance, there are free discount plans available to help with insurance costs. The most popular one is GoodR. The patient can go online and print a coupon for a medication in order to reduce their out-of-pocket cost. Not all pharmacies accept GoodR coupons, but there are other programs available depending upon your location. In some cases, a medication may be so expensive that no discount will reduce the cost to a reasonable price. The pharmacist may need to get involved to suggest a cheaper generic alternative. If the cheaper alternative is not therapeutically equivalent with the prescribed drug, the pharmacist will need to contact the prescriber to approve the medication change. Suggesting a cheaper alternative is an option for patients with insurance as well. Dispensing a generic equivalent generally leaves the patient with a less expensive copay than with brand-name products. If a product is only available as a branded product, many manufacturers offer coupons to patients with commercial insurance to reduce their copay. These coupons are generally available on the manufacturer's website. However, they cannot be used for patients with government insurance.

FORMULARY TIERS

A **formulary tier** is a list of medications that are grouped together by insurance companies for pricing purposes. Tier 1 medications are the least expensive and are the insurance plan's preferred products. Tier 1 drugs are generic medications that are inexpensive and are associated with low copays. Tier 2 drugs are generic medications that are more expensive or nonpreferred. Patient copays are usually still low, but they may be higher than for tier 1 drugs. Tiers 3 and 4 drugs are more expensive brand-name medications that impose a higher copay upon the patient compared to tiers 1 and 2 drugs. Tier 3 brand-name drugs are preferred over other branded drugs and are associated with a lower copay than nonpreferred tier 4 branded drugs. Tier 5 medications are very expensive specialty medications. These drugs are associated with high copays. Some insurance companies require patients to fill tier 5 medications at a specialty or preferred pharmacy.

Tier	Drug Type
1	Preferred generic
2	Generic
3	Preferred brand
4	Nonpreferred brand
5	Specialty

CHAPTER QUIZ

Ready to see how well you retained what you just read? Scan the QR code to go directly to the chapter quiz interface for this study guide. If you're using a computer, simply visit the bonus page at **mometrix.com/bonus948/ptcb** and click the Chapter Quizzes link.

PTCB Practice Test #1

Want to take this practice test in an online interactive format?
Check out the bonus page, which includes interactive practice questions and much more: **mometrix.com/bonus948/ptcb**

1. Which of the following is an example of a brand name of a medication?
   a. Amlodipine
   b. Bisoprolol
   c. Lasix
   d. Fluticasone

2. Which of the following products is the brand-name equivalent for clopidogrel?
   a. Coumadin
   b. Lovenox
   c. Plavix
   d. Lotrel

3. Which of the following products would be considered therapeutically equivalent to sumatriptan 50 mg tablets?
   a. Sumatriptan 6 mg/0.5 mL solution for injection
   b. Imitrex 50 mg tablets
   c. Sumatriptan 20 mg nasal spray
   d. Effexor 50 mg capsules

4. Which of the following would be an example of a drug-disease interaction?
   a. A patient who takes warfarin and aspirin is at an increased risk for bleeding.
   b. Beta-blockers can cause airway constriction, so they are contraindicated in patients who have asthma or chronic obstructive pulmonary disease.
   c. Patients who take simvastatin should not drink grapefruit juice because it can increase their risk of side effects.
   d. A patient taking rifampicin has orange-colored urine.

5. Tetracycline capsules should be taken on an empty stomach, at least 1 hour before or 2 hours after food. This is because certain foods, particularly dairy products, reduce its absorption. This is an example of a:
   a. Drug-drug interaction
   b. Drug-disease interaction
   c. Drug-food interaction
   d. Drug-laboratory interaction

6. Which of the following would be a common side effect of anticoagulants?

    a. Skin rash
    b. Excessive bruising or bleeding
    c. Hair loss
    d. Hypertension

7. All of the following medications are indicated for epilepsy EXCEPT:

    a. Keppra
    b. Risperdal
    c. Dilantin
    d. Depakote

8. All of the following medication classes should be avoided in elderly patients EXCEPT:

    a. Antihistamines
    b. Tricyclic antidepressants
    c. Benzodiazepines
    d. Proton pump inhibitors

9. Thalidomide (Thalomid) is known to be harmful when taken during pregnancy. It has a high risk of causing significant birth defects in babies. The term used to describe this type of side effect is:

    a. Myelosuppression
    b. Teratogenicity
    c. Ototoxicity
    d. Nephrotoxicity

10. Which of the following would be an appropriate temperature to store a medication that is required to be kept at room temperature?

    a. 85 °F
    b. 15 °C
    c. 22 °C
    d. 45 °F

11. What is the appropriate temperature range for storing a refrigerated medication?

    a. 20-40 °F
    b. 36-46 °F
    c. 25-35 °F
    d. 26-36 °F

12. Which of the following antihypertensive drugs is a beta-blocker?

    a. Verapamil
    b. Bisoprolol
    c. Losartan
    d. Ramipril

13. All of the following are common side effects of anticancer chemotherapy agents EXCEPT:

a. Immunosuppression
b. Vomiting
c. Hair loss
d. Tremors

14. All of the following are common side effects of opioids EXCEPT:

a. Nausea
b. Diarrhea
c. Respiratory depression
d. Dependence

15. Which of the following statements is TRUE regarding dietary supplements?

a. A list of ingredients is not required by law.
b. The packaging may state that the product can be used to prevent or treat a disease.
c. The products must be proven to be safe and effective.
d. The packaging may claim that the product improves the general function of the body.

16. Which of the following medications has a narrow therapeutic index?

a. Xarelto
b. Phenytoin
c. Fluoxetine
d. Lisinopril

17. Most insulin products require refrigeration prior to dispensing. Once dispensed, insulin can be stored at a controlled room temperature for how long?

a. up to 6 months
b. up to 28 days
c. until the expiration date listed on the vial
d. up to 14 days

18. Which of the following pieces of information is the pharmacy NOT required to include on the dispensing label?

a. Prescriber's phone number
b. Date of filling
c. Prescription number
d. Name of prescriber

19. Which of the following products has been adulterated?

a. A bottle of valsartan that is not labeled with the phrase "℞ Only"
b. A vial of insulin that has been stored in a patient's car during a hot summer day
c. A bottle of over-the-counter (OTC) sleep aid tablets that does not have a child-resistant cap
d. A bottle of Crestor that does not contain the generic name on the label

20. Which of the following products is misbranded?

    a. A tube of triamcinolone cream that has been stored at a warehouse that was shut down by the FDA for unsanitary conditions

    b. A vial of insulin that has been stored in a patient's car during a hot summer day

    c. A bag of IV vancomycin that was compounded using a diluent that is not compatible with vancomycin

    d. A bottle of tablets that is labeled as valsartan 40 mg, but the contents of the bottle contain valsartan 80 mg tablets

21. Which of the following forms is used to order schedule II controlled substances?

    a. DEA Form 106

    b. DEA Form 222

    c. The same form used to order noncontrolled medications

    d. DEA Form 224

22. What is the maximum amount of pseudoephedrine that can be sold to a customer in a 24-hour period?

    a. 9 g

    b. 4 g

    c. 3.6 g

    d. 1.8 g

23. Which of the following medications is required to participate in a REMS program due to its potential to cause serious adverse effects in pregnant women?

    a. Digoxin (Lanoxin)

    b. Isotretinoin (Accutane)

    c. Lithium (Lithobid)

    d. Gabapentin (Neurontin)

24. All of the following are appropriate methods for filing prescriptions EXCEPT:

    a. Schedule II prescriptions, schedules III–V prescriptions, and noncontrolled prescriptions are stored in three separate files.

    b. Schedule II prescriptions are stored in their own separate file, but schedules III–V and noncontrolled prescriptions are filed together.

    c. All controlled substance prescriptions may be stored in the same file as noncontrolled prescriptions if controlled substance prescriptions are stamped with a red letter "C."

    d. Electronic prescription records retained for 2 years with controlled substances easily retrievable from all other records.

25. Prescriptions must be kept on file at the pharmacy for a minimum of __ years according to federal law.

    a. 1

    b. 2

    c. 3

    d. 4

26. Federal law requires a full inventory of all pharmacy items to be performed how frequently?

a. Every 6 months
b. Yearly
c. Every 2 years
d. Every 3 years

27. Which of the following Medicare programs covers prescription drugs?

a. Medicare Part A
b. Medicare Part B
c. Medicare Part C
d. Medicare Part D

28. Which of the following insurance plans provides coverage to active-duty military personnel?

a. Medicaid
b. Tricare
c. AARP
d. Medicare

29. A patient drops off a prescription for Coumadin at your pharmacy. You notice that the prescriber has written "DAW 1" under the directions. You should:

a. Dispense the generic product warfarin if you do not have the brand-name product Coumadin in stock.
b. Dispense the generic equivalent, warfarin.
c. Do not dispense the prescription because handwritten prescriptions are not valid.
d. Dispense only the brand-name product Coumadin.

30. Which of the following insurance information is NOT needed to submit a point-of-sale prescription claim?

a. Lot number
b. BIN number
c. Cardholder ID number
d. Patient's gender

31. Which of the following insurance plans should be billed first?

a. Tricare
b. Private insurance plan
c. Medicaid
d. A manufacturer coupon card

32. Which of the following medications may be required to be billed to a patient's medical plan rather than their pharmacy plan?

a. Ramipril tablets
b. ProAir HFA metered-dose inhaler
c. Influenza vaccine
d. Cosopt ophthalmic solution

33. An unlicensed pharmacy staff member may perform all of the following tasks EXCEPT:

a. Receive the pharmacy order, unpack medications, and put stock away on shelves
b. Enter new prescription information into the pharmacy's computer system
c. Act as a cashier
d. Send pharmacy orders and update drug quantities and prices in the pharmacy's computer system

34. A patient turns in a prescription for Xalatan 0.005% ophthalmic solution. The directions are 1 gtt ou nightly. How many days will a 2.5 mL bottle last the patient? (Conversion factor: 20 drops/mL)

a. 50 days
b. 28 days
c. 25 days
d. 18 days

35. All of the following medications must be stored in a refrigerator EXCEPT:

a. NovoLog
b. EpiPen
c. NuvaRing
d. Pneumovax 23

36. Most vaccinations must be stored in a refrigerator. However, there are a few vaccine products that must be kept in a freezer. Which of the following vaccine products must be stored in a freezer?

a. Flulaval (influenza vaccine)
b. Varivax (varicella vaccine)
c. Measles, mumps, and rubella vaccine
d. Adacel (tetanus, diphtheria, and pertussis vaccine)

37. Which of the following medications is classified as a schedule III controlled substance?

a. Klonopin (clonazepam)
b. Lomotil (diphenoxylate/atropine)
c. Qdolo (tramadol)
d. Depo-Testosterone (testosterone)

38. Hydromorphone is a controlled substance belonging to which schedule?

a. II
b. III
c. IV
d. V

39. Which of the following is a requirement of the iPledge program that must be adhered to when dispensing a prescription for isotretinoin (Accutane)?

a. The prescription must be sent to the pharmacy electronically.
b. Female patients must be using at least one contraceptive method.
c. The quantity dispensed must not exceed a 30-day supply.
d. The prescription must be dispensed within 24 hours of receipt.

40. Which of the following statements regarding emergency drug kits is NOT true?

    a. They contain critical care drugs, such as epinephrine, naloxone, amiodarone, and glucagon.

    b. They should be labeled with an expiration date that is 6 months from the date of dispensing.

    c. They should only be used by authorized personnel in response to an order from a provider.

    d. The contents of the kit may vary depending upon the unit or hospital where the kit is located.

41. Which of the following prescription issues would prompt you to become suspicious that the prescription was forged or altered?

    a. The prescription is written for an unusually high quantity of tablets.

    b. The prescription is handwritten and difficult to read.

    c. The directions on the prescription contain abbreviations.

    d. The prescription is written for one of your regular patients.

42. Pharmaceutical products are each assigned a unique National Drug Code (NDC) number. What do the last two digits of this number signify?

    a. The manufacturer of the product

    b. The product strength, dosage form, and formulation

    c. The product's package size

    d. The product's batch number

43. A patient drops off a prescription for levothyroxine 0.125 mg tablets, dispense #30 tablets, take 1 am. You notice that the bottles of levothyroxine in your pharmacy are labeled in micrograms (mcg). What strength of levothyroxine tablets would be equivalent to the 0.125 mg tablets prescribed?

    a. 1.25 mcg

    b. 12.5 mcg

    c. 125 mcg

    d. 1,250 mcg

44. Which of the following classes of medication recalls is voluntary and unlikely to cause adverse effects if administered by the patient?

    a. Class I

    b. Class II

    c. Class III

    d. Class IV

45. In which of the following scenarios can a product be placed in the normal pharmacy stock for future dispensing?

    a. A drug product that has become expired

    b. A medication that is returned from will call because the patient did not collect it within 10 days

    c. A medication that is returned by the patient after picking it up because their doctor recently changed their medication

    d. A drug product that arrives from the distributor damaged and missing a product label

46. This category of medications decreases the amount of fluid that a person has in their body compartments by promoting water loss in the urine:

a. Expectorants
b. Diuretics
c. Vasodilators
d. Corticosteroids

47. A patient is currently taking oral prednisolone, a corticosteroid, for a severe asthma flare-up. Which of the following would be a side effect of prednisolone?

a. Hypoglycemia (low blood sugar)
b. Weight loss
c. Increased risk of infection
d. Fluid loss

48. When a patient fails to complete their full course of antibiotics, this can lead to:

a. Allergy
b. Increased side effects
c. Arrhythmias
d. Bacterial resistance

49. Which of the following OTC creams is used to treat athlete's foot?

a. Lamisil
b. Fleet
c. Aloe vera
d. Cortizone-10

50. Which of the following medications is given orally to treat diabetes mellitus by lowering blood glucose levels?

a. Insulin glargine
b. Metformin
c. Exenatide
d. Glucagon

51. Progesterone-only contraceptives (POCs) are used by many women because there are fewer side effects and they can be used while breastfeeding. Which of the following is an example of a POC?

a. Ethinyl estradiol/drospirenone (Yaz)
b. Ethinyl estradiol/etonogestrel (NuvaRing)
c. Levonorgestrel (Mirena)
d. Ethinyl estradiol/norgestimate (Estarylla)

52. Which of the following antibiotic suspensions can be stored at room temperature and does not require reconstitution prior to dispensing?

a. Bactrim
b. Amoxicillin
c. Augmentin
d. Cephalexin

53. Nitroglycerin tablets are stored in brown bottles, and nitroglycerin IV solutions are stored in either brown or foil bags. The reason for this is that nitroglycerin is:

    a. Sensitive to moisture in the air

    b. Sensitive to changes in temperature

    c. Incompatible with certain plastics

    d. Sensitive to light

54. Which of the following is true regarding a prescription transfer request for oxycodone tablets?

    a. The pharmacist must obtain the DEA number of the pharmacy upon transferring the prescription.

    b. The prescription can only be transferred between pharmacies one time because oxycodone is a controlled medication.

    c. The prescription cannot be transferred between pharmacies because oxycodone is a schedule II controlled substance.

    d. The prescription can be transferred between pharmacies within the same chain an unlimited number of times until it expires.

55. Which of the following is an antihyperlipidemic drug used to treat high cholesterol?

    a. Bisoprolol

    b. Simvastatin

    c. Nifedipine

    d. Methylcellulose

56. Which of the following pieces of information is required on a controlled drug prescription but is NOT required to be on a prescription for a noncontrolled drug?

    a. The prescriber's DEA number

    b. The prescriber's written or electronic signature

    c. The date the prescription was issued or written

    d. The total quantity of medication prescribed

57. A patient hands you a prescription for zolpidem 5 mg tablets, dispense #30 with eight refills. How should you proceed?

    a. Enter the prescription into the computer system as written, and give the patient eight refills as instructed by the prescriber.

    b. Enter the prescription into the computer system, and give the patient five refills because this is the maximum allowed by law.

    c. Allow the patient to refill the prescription as many times as desired until the expiration date of 12 months from the date it was written.

    d. Contact the prescriber to get a new prescription because zolpidem is not available in 5 mg tablets.

58. Which of the following legislative acts established a tracing system for medications and requires drug distributors to supply pharmacies with a drug pedigree that tracks and records the movement of drugs?

    a. The Omnibus Reconciliation Act of 1990 (OBRA '90)

    b. The Health Insurance Portability and Accountability Act of 1996

    c. The Drug Supply Chain Security Act

    d. The Poison Prevention Packaging Act

59. Which of the following DEA numbers is valid?

    a. AW2976452
    b. BF8976134
    c. AS8524616
    d. XD7491655

60. Which of the following abbreviations should NOT be used due to a high potential for confusion and error?

    a. qod
    b. po
    c. hs
    d. sol

61. What quantity of clobetasol propionate is contained within a 30 g tube of clobetasol propionate 0.05% cream?

    a. 1.5 g
    b. 1.5 mg
    c. 15 mg
    d. 15 g

62. You are compounding topiramate 20 mg/mL oral suspension. This product is being compounded specifically for this patient because there is no equivalent product available on the market. What beyond-use date should you use for this product?

    a. 7 days
    b. 10 days
    c. 14 days
    d. 30 days

63. How many continuing education (CE) credits are required to renew a pharmacy technician's PTCB certifications?

    a. 10
    b. 15
    c. 20
    d. 30

64. Which of the following is classified as a schedule IV controlled substance?

    a. Phenergan with codeine (Phenergan)
    b. Testosterone (Depo-Testosterone)
    c. Pentobarbital (Nembutal)
    d. Tramadol (Qdolo)

65. All of the following codeine solutions would be classified as a schedule V controlled substance EXCEPT:

    a. A solution containing 6.25 mg promethazine and 10 mg codeine per 5 mL of syrup
    b. A solution containing 20 mg dextromethorphan and 50 mg codeine per 20 mL of syrup
    c. A solution containing 100 mg guaifenesin and 10 mg codeine per 5 mL of syrup
    d. A solution containing 24 mg chlorpheniramine and 30 mg codeine per 15 mL of syrup

66. All of the following actions may be performed by a licensed pharmacy technician EXCEPT:

   a. Receive a prescription refill authorization from a prescriber
   b. Load automated dispensing systems with drug stock
   c. Prepare sterile IV admixture compounds
   d. Receive a new prescription order via telephone from a prescriber

67. Which of the following is considered a high-alert medication?

   a. Methotrexate
   b. Esomeprazole
   c. Polyethylene glycol
   d. Docusate

68. In which of the following scenarios may a fax be accepted as a hard copy prescription for a schedule II controlled substance?

   a. Schedule II substance prescriptions may always be accepted via fax.
   b. The prescription specifically states that the drug is for a hospice patient.
   c. The prescriber calls ahead to notify you that they will be faxing the prescription.
   d. The hard copy prescription is mailed to the pharmacy within 7 days.

69. A DEA Form 222 is required in all of the following scenarios EXCEPT:

   a. Ordering schedule II controlled substances
   b. Selling controlled substances to a prescriber for office use
   c. Reporting a theft or loss of controlled substances
   d. Returning a schedule II controlled substance to a reverse distributor

70. Which of the following legislative acts requires pharmacists to offer medication counseling to all Medicaid patients?

   a. The Omnibus Reconciliation Act of 1990 (OBRA '90)
   b. The Health Insurance Portability and Accountability Act of 1996
   c. The Drug Supply Chain Security Act
   d. The Poison Prevention Packaging Act

71. For which of the following adverse reactions events is it MOST important for the pharmacy to report to the FDA's MedWatch program?

   a. A patient experiences a rash after taking oral penicillin.
   b. A patient fails to rinse their mouth after using their inhaler, resulting in oral thrush.
   c. A patient taking ticagrelor (Brilinta) has a severe epidural hemorrhage that causes him to be hospitalized.
   d. A patient on a daily aspirin regimen receives a mild bruise after hitting their hand on a corner of their desk.

72. The wrong strength of a medications is dispensed to a patient. Before the patient realizes that the pharmacy has made an error, they have already ingested two doses of the incorrect strength. This is an example of:

   a. A near miss
   b. A prescription error
   c. Adulteration
   d. Misbranding

73. Which of the following describes an unlawful disclosure of protected health information (PHI)?

a. Prescription records are stored in a locked closet outside of the pharmacy area.
b. A copy of a prescription is thrown in the regular store trash bin.
c. Patient information is electronically shared between pharmacies within the same store chain.
d. A copy of a prescription is shredded by pharmacy personnel, and then it is thrown in the regular trash bin.

74. A terminally ill patient in a long-term-care facility has an ongoing prescription for oxycodone. The prescriber has noted on the prescription that the patient is terminally ill. Which of the following is true regarding this prescription?

a. Because oxycodone is a schedule II controlled drug, the full quantity must be dispensed at one time.
b. The prescription can be partially filled an unlimited number of times until the prescription expires 6 months after the written date.
c. Because schedule II prescriptions cannot be refilled, any partial fill will result in the remaining balance of the prescription being voided.
d. Because the patient is terminally ill and living in a long-term-care facility, the prescription can be partially filled an unlimited number of times within a 60-day period.

75. You are preparing an IV solution of vancomycin 500 mg in 500 mL of sodium chloride. The compounding guide suggests using a 500 mg/5 mL vial. However, this vial size is out of stock, and all you have available is a 5 g/20 mL vial. What quantity (in mL) of the 5 g/20 mL stock solution is needed to prepare the 500 mg/500 mL IV solution?

a. 0.2 mL
b. 1 mL
c. 2 mL
d. 5 mL

76. Which of the following vitamins should be avoided in patients who take warfarin?

a. Vitamin A
b. Vitamin D
c. Folic acid
d. Vitamin K

77. Orally disintegrating/dissolving tablet dosage forms should be:

a. Placed on the gums under the upper lip or under the cheek and allowed to disintegrate/dissolve
b. Placed under the tongue and allowed to disintegrate/dissolve
c. Placed on the tongue and allowed to disintegrate/dissolve
d. Swished around in the mouth, then spit out after 30 seconds

78. Which of the following medications is EXEMPT from the Poison Prevention Packaging Act child-proof packaging requirements?

a. Phenergan with codeine oral suspension
b. Nitroglycerin sublingual tablets
c. Methotrexate oral tablets
d. Lidocaine viscous solution

79. All of the following pieces of information are legally required to be on the package or label of an OTC medication EXCEPT:

    a. Name and address of the manufacturer
    b. Lot number
    c. NDC number
    d. Name of each active and inactive ingredient

80. Pharmacies are permitted to compound medications, but they are not allowed to manufacture medications without becoming licensed and approved as a manufacturer by the FDA. Which of the following compounding activities is NOT permitted by pharmacies who are licensed as manufacturers?

    a. Preparing a small quantity of cream for a patient specific to a prescription
    b. Preparing an oral solution without using commercial-grade equipment
    c. Reconstituting a vancomycin suspension from a manufactured kit
    d. Preparing a small quantity of cream for a prescriber's office without a patient-specific prescription

81. A patient is receiving total parenteral nutrition. The prescription order is for 1500 mL to be administered over 12 hours. What rate, in mL/min, should the nurse set the infusion at?

    a. 1.25 mL/min
    b. 2.08 mL/min
    c. 25 mL/min
    d. 125 mL/min

82. Which of the following is true regarding pharmacy inventories?

    a. An exact count of all medications in stock should be measured.
    b. Inventory records for all drug schedules can be kept together.
    c. An exact count should be measured for all containers holding more than 1,000 units.
    d. Drug inventory in automated dispensing cabinets or Pyxis machines should not be counted as pharmacy stock.

83. Which of the following medications is used to treat hyperlipidemia (high cholesterol)?

    a. Amlodipine
    b. Enoxaparin
    c. Zocor
    d. Losartan

84. Advair is commonly used to treat which of the following conditions?

    a. Cystic fibrosis
    b. Asthma
    c. Psoriasis
    d. Pulmonary hypertension

85. Which of the following antihistamines is considered to be non-drowsy or cause less drowsiness than other antihistamines?

    a. Phenergan
    b. Hydroxyzine
    c. Meclizine
    d. Loratadine

86. Which of the following is a common side effect of most antibiotics?

a. Immunosuppression
b. Diarrhea
c. Cough
d. Muscle pain

87. Which of the following insulin products is long-acting and usually given once a day in the evening?

a. Insulin detemir
b. Insulin aspart
c. Insulin NPH
d. Insulin glulisine

88. A patient's prescription instructs them to administer one ounce of solution per dose. How many milliliters should the patient be instructed to measure out for each dose?

a. 5 mL
b. 10 mL
c. 30 mL
d. 65 mL

89. You are preparing to compound 100 g of triamcinolone 0.1% cream. The only triamcinolone cream preparation that you have in stock is 3%. What quantity of 3% cream should be mixed with white petroleum ointment to product 100 g of 0.1% triamcinolone cream?

a. 0.3 g
b. 3.3 g
c. 33 mg
d. 33 g

90. Which of the following is an antipsychotic medication that is commonly used to treat schizophrenia?

a. Risperidone
b. Prozac
c. Levetiracetam
d. Duloxetine

Answer Key and Explanations for Test #1

1. C: Lasix is the brand name for furosemide. The other three medications listed are generic names. Amlodipine is the generic name for Norvasc, bisoprolol is the generic for SANDOZ, and fluticasone is the generic name for Flovent.

2. C: The brand-name product for clopidogrel is Plavix. Coumadin is the brand name for warfarin, Lovenox is the brand name for enoxaparin, and Lotrel is the brand name for tablets containing amlodipine and benazepril.

3. B: Therapeutically equivalent medications have the same active ingredients, the same efficacy, and the same safety profile. They must also be equivalent in their dosage form (e.g., tablet, capsule, cream, patch, injection) and the way in which the body is able to absorb it (bioavailability). Answer A is an injection, and answer C is a nasal spray, so they are not equivalent. Answer D is Effexor, which is the brand name of venlafaxine. The correct answer is B. Imitrex is the brand name for sumatriptan, and the strength and dosage form (tablets) are equivalent.

4. B: Drug-disease interactions occur when a drug interacts with or interferes with an existing medical condition. Another example would be that pseudoephedrine increases blood pressure and is not recommended in patients who have hypertension (high blood pressure). If the scenario had discussed how beta-blockers, such as propranolol, reduce the effectiveness of albuterol, an inhaled medication used to treat asthma, then this would be a drug-drug interaction.

5. C: Drug-food interactions occur when the effects of a drug are changed when taken in combination with a particular food. Another example is how grapefruit juice decreases the ability of statin drugs to be metabolized (broken down). If the patient was taking a calcium supplement that reduced the absorption of tetracycline, then this would have been a drug-dietary supplement interaction. If the question said that tetracycline affected the way that calcium is absorbed or used in the body, resulting in reduced blood calcium levels, then this would have been a drug-nutrient interaction. This is not a true statement; it is merely being used as an example.

6. B: Anticoagulants are also known as blood thinners because they prevent the blood from forming clots. The most common complaint with anticoagulant use is bruising or bleeding easily. Patients should watch for stomach pain or black, tarry stool, which indicates gastrointestinal bleeding. Signs and symptoms of a head bleed would be sudden headache, nausea, vomiting, blurred vision, weakness or numbness on one side of the body, or difficulty speaking.

7. B: Epilepsy is a medical diagnosis assigned to patients who have a seizure disorder. An indication is a diagnosis or disease state for which a medication is used. There are many antiepileptic drugs, and there are 8 in the top 200 drugs: gabapentin (Neurontin), lamotrigine (Lamictal), topiramate (Topamax), pregabalin (Lyrica), levetiracetam (Keppra), phenytoin (Dilantin), oxcarbazepine (Trileptal), and divalproex sodium (Depakote). Risperidone (Risperdal) is an antipsychotic drug that is used to treat schizophrenia and other psychoses. It is not indicated for epilepsy.

8. D: Elderly patients have a reduced ability to metabolize (break down) and excrete medications, and they are generally more susceptible to adverse effects. Sedating drugs can lead to delirium and confusion in elderly patients as well as increase their risk of falling. Classes of medications that should be used with caution in elderly patients include antihistamines, tricyclic antidepressants, muscle relaxers, benzodiazepines, hypnotics (sleeping pills), antipsychotics, antihypertensives, cardiac glycosides (digoxin), and nonsteroidal anti-inflammatory drugs.

9. B: Teratogenicity is the ability of a drug to be toxic to a fetus/embryo and lead to birth defects. Teratogenicity is an adverse effect of medications that are contraindicated in pregnancy. Some examples of medications that are teratogenic include isotretinoin (Accutane), thalidomide, angiotensin-converting enzyme inhibitors, anticoagulants, chemotherapy drugs, testosterone, antiepileptics, lithium, nonsteroidal anti-inflammatory drugs, and some antibiotics (e.g., tetracycline, sulfamethoxazole).

10. C: The correct answer is C. Most medications can be stored at room temperature, which is defined as 20-25 °C (59-77 °F). This includes most tablets, capsules, liquid solutions, creams, inhalers, and patches.

11. B: The correct answer is B. Some medications require refrigeration at 2-8 °C (36-46 °F). Medications that usually require refrigeration include injectables, vaccines, and antibiotic suspensions.

12. B: Beta-blockers end with the suffix *-olol*. They are commonly prescribed to treat high blood pressure, arrhythmias, and heart failure. Verapamil is a calcium channel blocker, losartan is an angiotensin receptor blocker, and ramipril is an angiotensin-converting enzyme inhibitor.

13. D: Most antineoplastic agents have the same classic chemotherapy side effects. These include hair loss, increased risk of infection (immunosuppression), low red blood cell count (anemia), bruising or bleeding easily, skin rashes (especially at the site of injection), fatigue, nausea, vomiting, diarrhea, constipation, gastrointestinal ulcers, mouth sores, and weight loss. Tremors are not a common side effect of chemotherapy.

14. B: Opioids are central nervous system depressants used to treat pain. Common side effects of opioids include dependence, addiction, nausea, vomiting, respiratory depression (slow respiratory rate), and slowing of the digestive system. Opioids slow down the movement of the digestive tract and can lead to reduced bowel movements. Therefore, they commonly cause constipation, NOT diarrhea.

15. D: Although dietary supplements such as vitamins, minerals, and medical foods are still regulated by the Food and Drug Administration (FDA), the regulations are not as strict as they are for drugs. The FDA ensures that dietary supplements are manufactured using good manufacturing practices, but no proof of safety or efficacy is required. The packaging must state the name and quantity of each ingredient, but no other information is required. Dietary supplements cannot advertise that the product can cure, diagnose, or prevent any disease. However, dietary supplements can claim that they improve general structures or functions in the body. If a dietary supplement wants to claim that it can be used to treat or prevent a disease or condition, this claim must first be preapproved by the FDA.

16. B: The following medications have a narrow therapeutic index: lithium (Lithobid), warfarin (Coumadin), digoxin (Lanoxin), phenytoin (Dilantin), theophylline (Theo-24), cyclosporine (Sandimmune), tacrolimus (Prograf), and many chemotherapy agents. This means that there is a narrow range of safe dosages and even minor changes in the dose can cause serious side effects in the patient. Rivaroxaban (Xarelto), fluoxetine (Prozac), and lisinopril (Zestril) do not have a narrow therapeutic index.

17. B: Insulin products should be stored in a refrigerator at 2-8 °C (36-46 °F). However, they can be stored at controlled room temperature for up to 28 days. Patients should be counseled on these storage requirements.

18. A: The following information is required to be on a pharmacy dispensing label: date of fill, name and address of the filling pharmacy, name of prescriber, prescription number, name of patient, name and strength of the drug, directions for use, generic name of the drug, and drug expiration date. The prescriber's phone number is NOT a requirement for a dispensing label. For controlled substances, the phrase "Caution: Federal law prohibits transfer of this drug to any person other than the patient to whom it was prescribed" must also be on the dispensing label.

19. B: Adulteration occurs when a drug product or device is contaminated, impure, or is not of the advertised strength. Adulteration can occur if the product is prepared, packaged, or stored under unsanitary conditions. Products that require refrigeration, such as insulin, become adulterated if they are stored outside of a refrigerator. Products can also be adulterated if they are manufactured, processed, packaged, or stored in a warehouse that is unsanitary or not following FDA standards. Adulterated products also include banned devices and the use of unapproved color additives. Products can become adulterated if stored inappropriately or if mixed or packaged so as to reduce their quality or purity, for example, intravenous (IV) products that have been mixed with an incompatible diluent (e.g., dextrose 5% instead of normal saline) or that have been packaged in an IV bag that the drug is not compatible with are considered adulterated.

20. D: Misbranding occurs when a drug product's labeling is false, misleading, or contains incorrect information. For example, the drug strength may differ from the bottle contents. Misbranding also occurs if information required by law to be on the label is missing such as the generic drug name, quantity or proportion of active ingredients, directions for use, address and phone number for reporting adverse drug reactions, manufacturer's name and address, storage requirements, or "R-Only" phrase. Misbranding also occurs when a product is the exact imitation of another product (i.e., counterfeit medication). Intentional falsification of a prescription, false or misleading advertising, or promotion of a drug for off-label use is also considered misbranding. Misbranding at the pharmacy level includes dispensing an "R-Only" drug without a prescription, improper labeling or dispensing (i.e., dispensing error), failure to comply with the Risk Evaluation and Mitigation Strategy (REMS), selling at item labeled "Not for resale," or failure to provide child-resistant packaging in accordance with the law.

21. B: A Drug Enforcement Agency (DEA) Form 222 is required for ordering schedule II controlled substances. A DEA Form 106 is used to report a loss or theft of controlled substances. DEA Form 224 is used to initially register with the FDA to dispense controlled substances. Schedule II medications cannot be ordered using the same form or online order as noncontrolled substances. Some pharmacies are able to use an online DEA Form 222 to submit schedule II orders. These orders still remain separate from noncontrolled substances and schedules III–V controlled substances.

22. C: The Combat Methamphetamine Epidemic Act of 2005 began restricting OTC sales of pseudoephedrine, ephedrine, and phenylpropanolamine. This law requires these medications to be kept behind a counter or in a locked cabinet and places restrictions on the OTC sale of these products. Customers must be ≥18 years old and must show a valid photo ID to purchase pseudoephedrine products. The maximum amount of pseudoephedrine that the customer can purchase in a 24-hour period is 3.6 g. Up to 9 g can be sold to that same customer in a 1-month period. Records of pseudoephedrine sales must be kept on file for at least 2 years. The following information must be recorded: photo ID number; date and time of transaction; product name; quantity sold; purchaser's name, address, and date of birth; and purchaser's signature.

23. B: The FDA does not usually approve medications that pose serious safety risks, but sometimes the benefits outweigh the risks. The FDA can approve these medications conditional of participation in a postmarketing safety program or a Risk Evaluation and Mitigation Strategy (REMS) program. REMS programs are specific to the medication, but they usually involve supplemental patient counseling, patient education, and laboratory monitoring (e.g., pregnancy testing). There may even be extra training or continuing education required for the prescriber and dispensing pharmacist. The following medications require REMS: isotretinoin (Accutane), clozapine (Clozaril), pomalidomide (Pomalyst), lenalidomide (Revlimid), and thalidomide (Thalomid).

24. C: There are three different ways that prescription records can be filed. The easiest and most common way to file prescription records is to have three separate files for schedule II controlled substances, schedules III–V controlled substances, and noncontrolled substances. Pharmacies are also allowed to maintain two separate files with schedule II controlled substances in one file and schedules III–V controlled substances and noncontrolled substances together in another file. If only two prescription files are used, each prescription for a schedule III–V controlled substance must be stamped with a red letter "C" in the lower right corner so they can be readily identified. Electronic prescription filing is allowed if all records are easily read and controlled substance records are easily retrievable from all other records. Using only one file for all controlled substances and noncontrolled substances is NOT allowed.

25. B: Federal law requires prescriptions to be kept on file at the pharmacy for a minimum of 2 years from the date of last dispensing. State laws usually require prescriptions to be kept on file for longer than 2 years, but the length of time varies from state to state. Additionally, insurance contracts and company policies often have even stricter requirements for the length of time that prescriptions must be kept.

26. C: According to federal law, all pharmacies must complete a full inventory every 2 years. However, many state laws, company policies, and accreditation bodies require annual inventories. The inventory may be completed any day within 2 years of the last inventory. Inventories should be completed before the pharmacy opens or after the pharmacy closes for the day. Pharmacies must also complete an initial inventory prior to opening for business and when the pharmacy changes ownership or closes for business.

27. D: Medicare is a federally funded program that provides health insurance coverage for patients over 65 years old, disabled people, and patients with kidney failure or amyotrophic lateral sclerosis.

- Part A (standard): covers hospital inpatient services, nursing facilities, and hospice care.
- Part B (optional, additional premium): covers outpatient services, doctor visits, medical supplies, and certain pharmacy medications (e.g., vaccinations, nebulizer solutions, diabetic test strips).
- Part C (Medicare Advantage Plans): parts A and B benefits offered by private insurers.
- Part D (optional, additional premium): Medicare prescription drug plan. Patients are subject to different deductibles and copays depending upon their chosen plan.

28. B: Tricare is a federal program that provides health coverage to military members, military retirees, and their families. A third party (e.g., Express Scripts) provides the actual billing services, and patients can use any in-network pharmacy. The Veterans Health Administration (VHA) provides healthcare benefits to veterans, but it generally only covers services provided by Department of Veterans Affairs (VA) doctors or VA pharmacies.

Medicare is a federally funded program that provides health insurance coverage for patients over 65 years old, disabled people, and patients with kidney failure or amyotrophic lateral sclerosis.

Medicaid provides medical coverage to individuals or families with low incomes or with a disability. Medicaid is jointly funded by federal and state governments. Medicare and Medicaid are governed by the Centers for Medicare and Medicaid Services (CMS).

29. D: A dispense-as-written (DAW) code is a system used by prescribers, pharmacies, and insurance companies to signify the intention of the prescriber or patient regarding generic substitution of the prescribed medication. Insurance companies require generic substitution for most medications unless special circumstances are indicated using a DAW billing code. If no DAW code is noted on the prescription, it is assumed that generic substitution is permitted by the prescriber.

DAW Codes			
0	No product selection is indicated.	5	The branded product is dispensed at the generic price.
1	Substitution is NOT allowed by the prescriber; use the branded product.	6	Override.
2	Substitution is allowed, but the patient requested the branded product.	7	Substitution is NOT allowed; the branded product is required by law.
3	Substitution is allowed, but the pharmacist selected the branded product.	8	Substitution is allowed, but the branded product is not available.
4	Substitution is allowed, but the generic equivalent is not in stock.	9	Other.

30. A: Most pharmacy computer systems will bill the patient's insurance benefit in real time (point-of-sale claims) as their prescription is processed. Once the pharmacy technician gathers the necessary information from the patient and enters it into the computer system, the computer transmits that information to the insurer and the results will be displayed in the claim response screen. The following information is required for insurance billing and processing:

Information Required to Bill and Process an Insurance Claim

- Insurance Plan Information
  - BIN number: Pharmacy benefit international identification number
  - Cardholder ID number
  - Group number
  - DAW code (if applicable)
- Prescription Information
  - Medication information and NDC number
  - Quantity dispensed
  - Days' supply
  - Date the prescription was written
  - Date the prescription is dispensed
  - Prescriber's identification number (DEA number or National Provider Identifier)
- Patient Information
  - Patient name
  - Patient's gender/sex
  - Patient's date of birth (DOB)
  - Patient's relationship to cardholder

- Pricing and Cost Information
  - Ingredient cost
  - Dispensing fee
  - Total amount billed to the insurance plan

31. B: If the patient has a private insurance plan as well as a government insurance plan (e.g., Medicare, Medicaid, Tricare), the private insurance must always be billed first. Manufacturer coupon cards should always be billed last. For instance, if the patient only has one insurance plan, the coupon card should be billed second. If the patient has two insurance plans, the coupon card should be billed third. Manufacturer coupons cannot be used if a patient has any government insurance plan.

32. C: Pharmacy insurance is used to cover prescription medications, whereas medical insurance is used to cover hospital visits, outpatient clinic visits, and primary care visits. Pharmacies generally only deal with pharmacy insurance, but there are some instances when medical insurance must be used in a pharmacy. Some insurance plans require vaccinations, medical equipment, medical devices, home infusions, and certain medications to be billed to the medical plan. For example, when Medicare patients receive an influenza vaccine at the pharmacy, their Medicare Part B medical insurance coverage must be billed. Nebulizer solutions, diabetic test strips, and some types of medical equipment must also be billed to Medicare Part B.

33. B: Unlicensed pharmacy staff members, also referred to as supportive personnel, cannot be involved in dispensing medications, counseling patients, or entering information into a patient's profile. Although state laws vary, unlicensed pharmacy staff members are generally allowed to perform the following tasks: bookkeeping, prescription filing, documenting third-party reimbursements, sending pharmacy orders, updating drug quantities and prices in the computer system, receiving pharmacy orders, unpacking medications, putting stock away on the shelves, delivering medications to a patient's home, answering phone calls, helping customers find products in the pharmacy, acting as a cashier for the sale of prescription and OTC medications, and taking in new prescriptions from patients. Unlicensed personnel CANNOT answer questions about medications, enter new prescription information into the computer system, receive prescription refill requests over the phone, or be involved in the dispensing process.

34. C: 1 gtt ou nightly means that the patient is to administer 1 drop into each eye every night. Therefore, the patient will be using 2 drops daily. There are 2.5 mL in each bottle. Multiply 2.5 mL by the conversion factor of 20 drops/mL to find out how many total drops are in the stock bottle. 2.5 mL × 20 drops/mL = 50 drops. Divide the total number of drops in the stock bottle (50 drops) by the number of drops that the patient is using daily (2 drops) to get the days' supply. Therefore, the correct answer is 25 days.

General formula to calculate days' supply:

Total # of units prescribed ÷ # of units per dose ÷ # of doses per day

35. B: NovoLog is a type of insulin. All insulin products must be stored in a refrigerator. NuvaRing is a contraceptive formulated as a vaginal ring. It must be stored in a refrigerator. Pneumovax 23 is a pneumococcal vaccine. Most vaccines must be stored in a refrigerator. EpiPen is an injection used to treat severe, emergent allergic reactions that involve anaphylaxis. EpiPens should be stored at room temperature. The injection is sensitive to and should not be exposed to cold temperatures or heat.

36. B: There are two vaccines that must be stored in a freezer: Varivax (varicella vaccine), which protects against chicken pox, and Zostavax (herpes zoster vaccine), which protects against shingles but is no longer available in the US. All other vaccines available on the market require refrigeration. This includes a newer version of the vaccine used to protect against shingles called Shingrix. Other commonly used vaccines that require refrigeration are influenza vaccines (Fluad, Flulaval, Fluzone), tetanus, diphtheria, and pertussis vaccines (Daptacel, Adacel, Boostrix), hepatitis B vaccines (Engerix-B, Recombivax HB), hepatitis A vaccines (Havrix, Vaqta), *Haemophilus influenzae* type B vaccine (ActHIB, PedvaxHIB), meningococcal vaccines (Menactra, Menveo), measles, mumps, and rubella vaccination, human papillomavirus vaccination (Gardasil), and pneumococcal vaccines (Pneumovax 23, Prevnar 13).

37. D: Schedule III controlled substances include synthetic cannabinoids (marijuana derivatives) such as dronabinol (Marinol); anabolic steroids, including testosterone (Depo-Testosterone); barbiturates, including pentobarbital and secobarbital formulated as a suppository or in combination with another noncontrolled substance; ketamine (Ketalar); and some opioid pain medications, including buprenorphine. Codeine and dihydrocodeine are considered schedule III substances when the product contains ≤90 mg per dosage unit or ≤1.8 g per 100 mL of solution when used in combination with another noncontrolled substance. Morphine is a schedule III substance if it is used in combination with a noncontrolled substance and the product contains ≤50 mg per 100 mL or 100 g.

38. A: Hydromorphone (Dilaudid) is a schedule II controlled substance, meaning that it has a high potential for abuse and prescribers must adhere to stricter prescription and storage requirements. Opioids, attention-deficit/hyperactivity disorder stimulants, and barbiturates are classified as schedule II substances. Other commonly prescribed schedule II substances are codeine, dihydrocodeine, hydrocodone, morphine (MS Contin), oxycodone (Oxycontin, Percocet), oxymorphone, fentanyl, methadone, meperidine (Demerol), amphetamine (Adderall), methylphenidate (Ritalin, Concerta), and pentobarbital.

39. C: The use of isotretinoin (Accutane) is restricted because it can cause serious fetal abnormalities or fetal death in women who are pregnant. All prescribers, pharmacies, and patients who deal with isotretinoin are required to adhere to the iPledge program. Permitted prescriptions for isotretinoin may be via telephone, fax, or email, and dispensed to the patient within 7 days of a negative pregnancy test. A maximum of 30 days' supply can be dispensed at a time. Female patients must agree to monthly pregnancy testing and comply with using two methods of contraception throughout the duration of treatment and for 30 days after treatment.

40. B: An emergency drug kit, also referred to as a code tray or crash cart, contains drugs that are necessary to treat patients during emergency situations. Medications that are commonly contained within an emergency drug kit include epinephrine, atropine, dextrose, glucagon, naloxone, amiodarone, EpiPen, adenosine, diphenhydramine, sodium bicarbonate, dobutamine, and phenytoin. The contents of these kits vary depending upon the needs of the facility and the types of patients that are being treated. Emergency drug kits should be labeled with the list of contents and pharmacist's initials. The earliest expiration date of all of the drug contents should be noted on the outside of the kit. The kit should be secured with a tamper-evident seal and kept in a secure area. Drugs in the kit should only be used by authorized personnel upon written or verbal orders from a provider. Once a kit has been opened or contents have expired, it should be returned to the pharmacy to be restocked.

41. A: There are certain characteristics that may indicate that a prescription was forged: The handwriting is too legible, the prescription is written for an unusually high quantity or dose, the prescription is written for a product that is rarely prescribed by local doctors, nonstandard medical abbreviations are used, unusual medical language is used, the prescription contains spelling errors, the prescription appears to be photocopied or has a watermark, the directions are written in full with no abbreviations, parts of the prescription are written with a different color of ink or in different handwriting, the patient has never used your pharmacy before, there are no noncontrolled medications written for the same patient, the prescriptions are written for an unusual combination of drugs (e.g., stimulants and depressants), the prescription is written for a different person other than the customer presenting the prescription, the patient requests to pay out-of-pocket for the medication or denies having insurance, or the prescription is written by a prescriber that you have never heard of previously. You should bring these types of prescriptions to the attention of a pharmacist for further inspection.

42. C: A National Drug Code (NDC) number is a unique product identifier that is assigned to each product by the FDA. These are useful for identifying products and using barcode scanning technology to ensure that the correct product was dispensed. An NDC number is a 10- or 11-digit (newer products) number divided into three parts. The first 4 or 5 digits identify the manufacturer. The second 4 digits identify the product strength, dosage form, and formulation. The last 2 digits identify the package size. For NDC numbers with only 10 digits, some computer systems will require the addition of a zero at the beginning of the number.

43. C: A gram (g) is the basic metric unit of mass or weight. All other metric units of mass are centered around the gram. Metric units of measure can easily be converted from one form to another by moving the decimal place. A kilogram (kg) is 10^3 or 1,000 times larger than a gram. Therefore, to convert grams to kilograms, the decimal place must be moved to the left three places. Milligrams (mg) and micrograms (mcg) are smaller than a gram. A milligram is 10^{-3} or 1,000 times smaller than a gram, whereas a microgram is 10^{-6} or 1,000,000 times smaller than a gram. To convert grams to milligrams, the decimal place must be moved to the right three places. To convert grams to micrograms, the decimal place must be moved to the right six places.

Unit of Measure	Kilogram	Gram	Milligram	Microgram
Conversion Factor	10^3	1	10^{-3}	10^{-6}
Sample conversion	0.008	8	8,000	8,000,000

44. C: If a medication causes adverse effects, is contaminated, damaged, or mislabeled, the FDA may require the manufacturer to recall the medication. The manufacturer will then have to supply distributors and pharmacies with information about the product that is being recalled (product name, lot number, package size, and reason for the recall). **Class I recalls** occur when the drug or device could cause serious adverse health consequences or death if administered. All of the affected medication in stock at the pharmacy must be isolated. A notice must also be issued to all patients to whom the drug has been dispensed asking the patients to return the medication to the pharmacy. **Class II recalls** occur when drugs or devices could cause temporary, reversible effects or have a small chance of causing serious adverse effects if administered. All affected drug stocks at the pharmacy must be isolated, but a notice to patients is not usually required. **Class III recalls** occur when the affected drugs or devices are unlikely to cause any adverse health effects if administered. They usually result from a packaging or labeling violation. These recalls are usually voluntary (not required). Class IV is not a type of drug recall.

45. B: The most common reason for returning a medication to stock is because the patient failed to pick up the medication, and it was credit returned. A patient may also request that a medication be returned to stock because it is too expensive or because they are no longer taking the medication. Stock bottles that were pulled for dispensing should also be returned if there is still medication remaining in the bottle. Medications CANNOT be returned to stock once they have left the pharmacy. Once a patient picks up a medication and leaves the pharmacy with it, it cannot be returned to stock and redispensed to another patient. This is the law and is nonnegotiable. If a patient does not want a medication, it must be credit returned at the pharmacy counter before pickup. Products that are expired, damaged, or recalled cannot be returned to stock either.

46. B: Diuretics, such as furosemide and hydrochlorothiazide, treat edema (swelling) and high blood pressure (hypertension) by promoting the excretion of water in the urine. Expectorants, such as guaifenesin, help thin the mucus that builds up during a cold or respiratory illness so that it can be expelled more easily. Vasodilators increase the diameter of blood vessels in order to lower blood pressure or treat chest pains (angina). Corticosteroids are anti-inflammatory medications that are used to treat a wide variety of diseases. They promote fluid retention, NOT fluid excretion.

47. C: Corticosteroids, such as prednisolone, have a lot of side effects. They are used to reduce inflammation, but they also reduce the body's immune response. Therefore, they increase the risk of infection. They also cause fluid retention, weight gain, hyperglycemia (high blood glucose), and hypokalemia (low potassium).

48. D: When patients do not complete their full course of antibiotics, bacteria can develop resistance to the antibiotic so that it will be less effective in the future. Up to 10% of patients are allergic to penicillin antibiotics, but failing to finish the course will not increase the likelihood of allergy. Failing to finish the course will not lead to side effects of arrhythmias either. In fact, many patients stop taking their antibiotic due to side effects. It is common to get nausea, vomiting, diarrhea, and abdominal pain with antibiotics.

49. A: OTC antifungal creams include clotrimazole (Lotrimin), ketoconazole (Ketodan), miconazole (Monistat), and terbinafine (Lamisil). Fleet is a glycerin enema that is available OTC as a laxative. Aloe vera is an herbal cream or gel used to treat burns, scrapes, and psoriasis. Hydrocortisone is a corticosteroid cream (that comes in various strengths) used to treat skin irritation (rashes, swelling, itching), poison oak, poison ivy, and eczema.

50. B: Metformin (Glumetza, Riomet) is a first-line treatment for diabetes mellitus type 2. Insulin glargine (Lantus) is a long-acting insulin. It cannot be administered orally and must be injected. Exenatide (Byetta) is a newer antidiabetic medication called an incretin mimetic. It cannot be administered orally and must be injected. Glucagon (GlucaGen) is an injectable medication used to increase blood glucose levels during a hypoglycemic emergency. A hypoglycemic emergency occurs when a patient's blood sugar falls too low due to a high dose of insulin or antidiabetic medications.

51. C: Progesterone-only contraceptives (POCs) do not contain an estrogen; they only contain a progesterone. Combined oral contraceptives (COCs) contain an estrogen and a progesterone. Estrogens are responsible for many side effects, such as breast tenderness, weight gain, high blood pressure, breakthrough vaginal bleeding, increased breast cancer risk, and increased risk of blood clotting. The estrogen typically used in COCs is ethinyl estradiol. There are many types of progesterones that are used: norethindrone, levonorgestrel, drospirenone, norgestrel, desogestrel, norgestimate, norelgestromin, etonogestrel, and medroxyprogesterone.

52. A: Most antibiotics are unstable in water, so they are formulated as a powder for reconstitution. This means that water must be added prior to dispensing to prepare the oral suspension. Most formulations that require reconstitution must be refrigerated after mixing and have a shortened beyond-use date of 7–14 days, depending upon the product. Bactrim (trimethoprim/sulfamethoxazole) is unique in that it does NOT require reconstitution. It is already prepared as a suspension and is stable at room temperature. It can be kept on the pharmacy shelf with the rest of the room-temperature liquids.

53. D: Medications that are stored in brown bottles or bags or in foil are often required to be protected from light in order to preserve their shelf life. Although nitroglycerin must also be protected from moisture, high temperatures, and certain plastics, the brown packaging will not help with this. The reason for the brown or foil packaging is because nitroglycerin is particularly sensitive to light.

54. C: Oxycodone is a schedule II medication. Schedule II controlled substance prescriptions cannot be transferred between pharmacies, and they are not refillable. A new prescription must be obtained for each fill. Schedules III and IV substances can only be transferred between pharmacies one time. Schedule V and noncontrolled substances can be transferred between pharmacies an unlimited number of times so long as the total fill quantity is not exceeded and no refills are issued after the prescription expiration date (12 months for noncontrolled substances or 6 months for schedule V substances). Schedules III and IV substances can also be transferred an unlimited number of times between pharmacies if the pharmacies share a common database.

55. B: The most common antihyperlipidemic medications used to treat high cholesterol (hypercholesterolemia) are the HMG-CoA reductase inhibitors, known as *statins* because they end with the suffix *-statin*. Some antihyperlipidemic medications, such as ezetimibe and cholestyramine, prevent the absorption of cholesterol in the gastrointestinal tract. Below is a list of the commonly prescribed antihyperlipidemic medications.

Generic Name	Brand Name
Ezetimibe	Zetia
Simvastatin	Zocor
Atorvastatin	Lipitor
Rosuvastatin	Crestor
Cholestyramine	Questran
Colestipol	Colestid

56. A: The following information is required to be on ALL prescription orders: date issued/written, name of the patient, drug name, drug strength, drug dosage form, total quantity of drug prescribed, directions for use, name and address of the prescriber, prescriber's signature (digital or electronic signatures are acceptable).

In addition, prescriptions for controlled drugs must contain the following information: the patient's address and the prescriber's DEA number. Most states allow controlled substance prescription to be sent electronically, but some states may require special software or special prescription paper. Some states also require controlled substance prescriptions to be written on their own separate form.

The number of refills allowed is not a required element of a prescription. If no refill number is listed, it can be assumed that the prescription is not refillable.

57. B: Zolpidem is a schedule IV medication. Schedules III–IV controlled substances can be refilled up to five times (a total of six fills). Answer A is not correct because eight refills exceed the maximum amount allowed by law. Schedules III and IV medications expire 6 months from their

179

written date (NOT 12 months as suggested in answer C). All fills, partial fills, and refills must be issued within 6 months of the date the prescription is written. If refills remain after the 6-month period, they are no longer valid because the prescription has expired. Schedules III–IV prescriptions may be transferred between pharmacies only ONE time. Chain pharmacies that share a common database can transfer prescriptions an unlimited amount of times.

58. C: The Drug Supply Chain Security Act was enacted in 2013 as an effort to reduce the prevalence of counterfeit drugs. This act established a national tracing system for medications, known as a drug pedigree. These pedigrees track and record drug movement. Tracking begins at the manufacturing facility where the drug is produced. Any time a drug is moved to a new location, such as a distribution facility or pharmacy, this is documented in the drug pedigree. The types of tracking information contained in the drug pedigree include the name, strength, and dosage of the product; the NDC number; the container size; the number of containers; the product lot numbers; the transaction date; the shipment date; the name and address of the seller and purchaser; and the transaction history. Pharmacies are required to obtain drug pedigree information and maintain drug pedigrees for 6 years.

59. C: A DEA number is an identifier assigned to any health care provider that prescribes or dispenses controlled substances. This number helps identify and authenticate prescribers. A DEA number consists of two letters and seven numbers.

The first letter indicates the type of practitioner or facility.

- Medical doctors, doctors of osteopathic medicine, veterinarians (doctors of veterinary medicine), dentists, and podiatrists = A, B, or F
- Midlevel practitioners (e.g., physician assistants and certified registered nurse practitioners) = M
- Prescribers authorized to prescribe under a narcotic treatment program = X

The second letter is the first letter of the prescriber's last name.

The numerical digits provide a mechanism for verifying the authenticity of a DEA number.

1. Add digits 1 + 3 + 5.
2. Add digits 2 + 4 + 6, and multiply this number by 2.
3. Calculate the total sum from steps 1 and 2.
4. The last digit of the total sum should equal the 7th digit of the DEA number.

DEA numbers can also be electronically verified on the DEA's website.

60. A: The following abbreviations should NOT be used: U (unit), IU (international unit), qd (daily), qod (every other day), chemical abbreviations of drugs (e.g., $MgSO_4$, NaCl, KCl), and drug name abbreviations (e.g., MS, HCTZ, NS). Trailing zeros (e.g., 5.0 mg) and leading decimal points (e.g., .5mg) should be avoided for numbers. Therefore, answer A is the correct answer. The other three answer choices are approved abbreviations: po (by mouth), hs (at bedtime), and sol (solution).

61. C: Percentages can be converted into a fraction by placing the number in the numerator and 100 in the denominator. For creams and other solids, the units are g/100 g. For solutions or suspensions, the fraction should be expressed in g/100 mL. For liquid in liquid formulations, such as emulsions, percentages can be expressed as mL/100 mL.

$$0.05\% = 0.05 \text{ g per } 100 \text{ g}$$

180

To solve using dimensional analysis:

$$\frac{0.05\ \text{g}}{100\ \text{g}} = \frac{50\ \text{mg}}{100\ \text{g}} = \frac{5\ \text{mg} \times 3}{10\ \text{mg} \times 3} = \frac{15\ \text{mg}}{30\ \text{g}}$$

To solve using cross-multiplication:

$$\frac{0.05\ \text{g}}{100\ \text{g}} = \frac{(x)\ \text{g}}{30\ \text{g}}$$

$$(0.05\ \text{g})(30\ \text{g}) = (100\ \text{g})(x)$$

$$1.5\ \text{g} = (x)100\ \text{g}$$

$$x = 0.015\ \text{g} = 15\ \text{mg}$$

62. C: Beyond-use dates are expiration dates assigned to compounded or prepared products. They are defined as the date after which the product should not be used and are calculated based on the date of preparation. If possible, a manufactured product should be used. The directions and beyond-use date on the packaging should be adhered to in these cases. However, occasionally a product is not available on the market, so a product must be specifically compounded. The following beyond-use date guidelines should be used for such compounded products:

Type of Product	Maximum Beyond-Use Date
Oral solutions and water-based preparations	14 days
Topical and semisolid preparations	30 days
Nonaqueous (oil-based) preparations	6 months or the earliest expiration date of any of the ingredients, whichever is earlier

63. C: The Pharmacy Technician Certification Board (PTCB) is a nationwide program that trains and certifies pharmacy technicians. Some states accept PTCB for their licensing requirements, whereas other states have separate training programs. Once PTCB certification is obtained, candidates must maintain their certification by completing at least 20 hours of continuing education (CE) during each 2-year renewal cycle. At least 1 CE credit must be in the subject of pharmacy law, and at least 1 CE credit must be in the subject of patient safety. Most states also require pharmacy technicians to register with the state board of pharmacy and maintain a separate license. Your state license may have different CE requirements and a different timeline for license renewal.

64. D: Most drugs in the schedule IV classification are benzodiazepines: alprazolam (Xanax), chlordiazepoxide, clobazam, clonazepam (Klonopin), diazepam (Valium), flurazepam, loprazolam, lorazepam (Ativan), nitrazepam, oxazepam, temazepam, and triazolam. Z drugs used to treat insomnia are similar to benzodiazepines and are also schedule IV substances: zaleplon, zolpidem (Ambien), zopiclone (Imovane), and eszopiclone (Lunesta). Central nervous system stimulants used to aid in weight loss are schedule IV substances: phentermine (Adipex-P), diethylpropion, and mazindol. Modafinil (Provigil), a stimulant used to treat sleep disorders, is also a schedule IV substance. Some muscle relaxers are schedule IV controlled substances, including dextropropoxyphene and carisoprodol (Soma). The opioid pain medication tramadol (Qdolo) is also a schedule IV substance. The central nervous system depressant phenobarbital, which is used to treat seizure disorders, is also a schedule IV medication.

Phenergan with codeine (Phenergan) is a schedule V drug, and testosterone is a schedule III drug. Pentobarbital is similar in nature to phenobarbital, but it is more potent and is classified as a schedule II controlled substance.

65. B: Schedule V substances are generally combination products that contain a schedule II, III, or IV controlled substance in another noncontrolled substance. This includes the opiates dihydrocodeine and codeine. In order to be classified as a schedule V substance, codeine products must contain no more than 200 mg per 100 mL or 100 g of another noncontrolled ingredient.

Answer A contains 10 mg codeine per 5 mL of syrup. Therefore, it contains 200 mg (the legal maximum) of codeine per 100 mL. These are the active ingredients in Phenergan with codeine syrup.

Answer B contains 50 mg of codeine per 20 mL. Therefore, it contains 250 mg of codeine per 100 mL. This is above the legal maximum for the schedule V classification.

Answer C contains 10 mg codeine per 5 mL of syrup. Therefore, it contains 200 mg (the legal maximum) of codeine per 100 mL. These are the active ingredients in Coditussin AC and Maxi-Tuss AC.

Answer D contains 30 mg codeine per 15 mL of syrup. Therefore, each 5 mL contains 10 mg of codeine. If we multiply these numbers by 20, we can determine that each 100 mL contains 200 mg of codeine (the legal maximum).

Other schedule V controlled substances:

Products that contain ≤100 mg of dihydrocodeine per 100 mL of 100 grams of a noncontrolled substance. Pregabalin (Lyrica) is also schedule V.

Diphenoxylate (a schedule II controlled substance on its own) is a schedule V substance when no more than 2.5 mg is combined with at least 25 mcg of atropine per dosage unit. Therefore, the medication Lomotil (2.5 mg diphenoxylate/0.025 mg atropine) used to treat diarrhea is a schedule V substance.

66. D: The following actions CAN legally be performed by a pharmacy technician: receive and enter paper or faxed prescription orders, receive refill requests from patients, receive a refill authorization from a prescriber or their agent (given that there are no changes to the prescription), enter prescription orders and insurance information into the pharmacy software system, view and enter patient data, act as a cashier, count or measure out drug products in order to prepare a prescription order, manage pharmacy inventory, load drug-dispensing devices (e.g., Pyxis machines) or automated dispensing robots, distribute or deliver medications, and prepare sterile IV admixtures and nonsterile compounds under the supervision of a pharmacist.

The following actions must be performed by a licensed pharmacist: provide medication counseling or give medical advice to patients, receive new verbal or telephone prescription orders, perform a clinical review of prescription orders, perform clinical interventions (e.g., drug interaction, prescription alteration), perform a drug utilization review. In most cases, only pharmacists are allowed to transfer prescriptions from one pharmacy to another. Most states also require immunizations to be performed by pharmacists, although some states are allowing specially trained technicians to immunize patients.

67. A: High-alert medications have the potential to cause significant harm if an error is made. These include:

- IV adrenergic agonists (e.g., epinephrine)
- IV adrenergic antagonists (e.g., propranolol)
- Anesthetics (e.g., propofol)
- IV antiarrhythmics (e.g., amiodarone)
- Antithrombotic agents (e.g., warfarin, alteplase, apixaban)
- Chemotherapy agents (e.g., methotrexate)
- Dextrose solutions ≥20% (hypertonic dextrose)
- Dialysis solutions
- Epidural administration of any medication
- Oral hypoglycemic agents (e.g., glyburide, glimepiride, metformin)
- IV inotropic agents (e.g., digoxin)
- Insulin
- Intrathecal administration of any medication
- Liposomal formulations (e.g., liposomal amphotericin B)
- Narcotics/opioids (e.g., oxycodone, hydrocodone, hydromorphone)
- Neuromuscular blocking agents (e.g., succinylcholine, rocuronium, vecuronium)
- IV nitroprusside sodium
- Parenteral nutrition
- IV potassium chloride or potassium phosphate
- IV radiocontrast agents
- Sedation agents (e.g., chloral hydrate, midazolam, dexmedetomidine)
- Sterile water for injection, inhalation, and irrigation in containers of ≥100 mL
- IV sodium chloride >0.9% (hypertonic saline)
- IV vasopressin

68. B: Schedule II controlled medications are generally NOT allowed to be accepted by facsimile transmission.

Faxed schedule II prescriptions are permitted ONLY in the following circumstances: The patient is a resident of a long-term-care facility; the patient is enrolled in a hospice care program licensed by the state or certified by Medicare and the prescription specifically states that it is for a hospice patient; a narcotic pain therapy drug is prescribed for a terminally ill patient (e.g., home infusion/IV pain therapy); or the medication is a parenteral, intravenous, intramuscular, subcutaneous, or intraspinal infusion that is going to be compounded for direct administration to a patient. Valid, signed schedule II prescriptions may also be faxed to the pharmacy by the prescriber, patient, or patient's agent in order to expedite predispensing preparations, but the original prescription must be received by the pharmacy prior to actual dispensing.

Schedules III–V controlled medications can always be accepted via fax.

69. C: A DEA Form 222 is required to order, sell, or transfer schedule I or II controlled substances between distributors, pharmacies, or practitioner's offices. Each form has three carbon copies: copy 1 (brown) is kept by the supplier/distributor/wholesaler, copy 2 (green) is sent to the DEA by the supplier at the end of each month, and copy 3 (blue) is kept by the purchaser/pharmacy. The form must be written in indelible ink or typewritten with no changes or erasures permitted. Electronic DEA Form 222 submission is also available. Only the registrant and those authorized by power of attorney on behalf of the registrant can complete this form. Orders may be partially filled by the supplier, but the remaining quantity must be shipped within 60 days.

DEA Form 224: controlled substance registration for manufacturers, distributors, or dispensers that wish to handle controlled substances

DEA Form 41: controlled substance destruction/disposal

DEA Form 106: to report theft or loss of controlled substances

All controlled substance records, including DEA forms, must be kept on file at the pharmacy for a minimum of 2 years according to federal law.

70. A: The OBRA '90 Act elevated the standards for drug therapy reviews and patient counseling in the pharmacy setting. Although OBRA '90 standards only apply to Medicaid patients, most states have passed similar regulations that apply to all pharmacy patients.

Under OBRA '90, a pharmacist must conduct a review of drug therapy prior to dispensing each prescription, which involves screening for therapeutic duplications, drug interactions, allergies, and contraindications. The pharmacist must also make a reasonable effort to obtain the following information for the patient's profile: name, address, telephone number, date of birth, gender, allergies, list of current medications, relevant medical history.

OBRA '90 also requires pharmacists to offer each Medicaid patient counseling on their prescriptions. The law requires the pharmacist to counsel on information deemed significant by the pharmacist, such as the name and description of the medication, route of administration, directions for use, common side effects, proper storage, duration of treatment, and special precautions.

71. C: The FDA's MedWatch program can be used to report adverse effects associated with any human drug (whether it is OTC or prescription-only), biologic (blood components, tissue-based products), medical device, vaccine, dietary supplement, infant formula, cosmetic, food, or beverage. MedWatch can even be used to report medication errors. Anyone can submit adverse drug reaction information to MedWatch, including pharmacists, pharmacy technicians, prescribers, or even patients. Although it is time-consuming, the FDA encourages use of the MedWatch reporting system, even if you are not certain of all the details of the event. Adverse event reporting through MedWatch is particularly encouraged for serious adverse reactions that involve hospitalization, a life-threatening reaction, result in disability or permanent damage, or result in death. The FDA also encourages the reporting of quality or safety concerns with a product, such as suspected contamination, suspected counterfeit products, defective products, inadequate packaging or labeling, or stability issues.

72. B: A prescription error occurs when a mistake has been made in the prescribing, dispensing, or administration process. Near misses are prescription errors that are caught before the medication reaches the patient. In this scenario, the patient has picked up the medication and ingested the incorrect tablets. Therefore, it is a prescription error NOT a near miss. Other examples of prescription error events include dispensing the wrong drug, the wrong strength of drug, or the wrong formulation of the drug (e.g., tablets instead of liquid); dispensing a drug to the incorrect patient (patient name mix-ups); dispensing the incorrect quantity of medication; refilling a prescription too early (which can lead to medication abuse or overdose); incorrect labeling or directions; incorrect infusion rate information; compounding a medication incorrectly (e.g., adding too much or too little water); preparing an IV admixture in an incompatible solution or an incompatible bag; dispensing a drug to a patient with a known allergy or contraindication;

dispensing a drug that interacts with another medication that the patient is taking; failure to provide adequate counseling or information to the patient; or shipping a medication order to the incorrect address.

73. B: The Health Insurance Portability and Accountability Act of 1996 placed restrictions on the storage, access, and transfer of electronic, paper, or oral patient health information. Protected health information (PHI) includes any document that contains a patient's name, address, date of birth, medical history, insurance information, or other identifying information. PHI that is stored or transmitted must have safeguards in place to prevent unauthorized access. Computer systems must be password-protected and backed up daily to prevent data loss. Paper documents must be stored in a locked area.

PHI must be disposed of in a secure manner. Some smaller pharmacies shred all of their PHI. Most pharmacies accumulate too much PHI for this to be feasible. Retail pharmacies usually have a large trash bin into which PHI is dumped. At regular intervals, a document shredding company will pick up the bin's contents and dispose of them properly. Smaller PHI trash bins are usually scattered around the pharmacy, and then the contents are combined into the large PHI bin at the end of the day. Hospitals and facilities have PHI information receptables scattered around the facility. They usually look like gray boxes that have an opening for paper. A shredding or disposal service will collect these at regular intervals.

74. D: Schedules III–V controlled substances CAN be partially filled so long as the maximum quantity prescribed is never exceeded and any fills are not dispensed beyond 6 months after the date that the prescription was written.

The law allows schedule II medications to be partially filled so long as the remaining balance is supplied within 72 hours. This means that the patient must pick up the partial balance within 72 hours; most retail pharmacies find this service too risky to offer. If the partial fill is not supplied within 72 hours, the remaining balance on the prescription must be voided and the prescriber must be notified.

There are certain exceptions to this rule that allow prescriptions to be partially filled for up to 60 days from the date of issuance of the prescription. These exceptions include patients in long-term-care facilities and patients who are terminally ill. In these cases, the prescription must indicate either "LTCF" or "Terminally ill," respectively. The prescription can be partially filled an unlimited number of times within the 60-day period so long as the pharmacist records the date, quantity dispensed, remaining quantity authorized, and dispensing pharmacist's name for each fill.

75. C: 2 mL

$$500 \text{ mg} = 0.5 \text{ g}$$

We have 5 g/20 mL, and we want to find out what quantity contains 0.5 g, so we need to use cross-multiplication:

$$\frac{0.5 \text{ g}}{x} = \frac{5 \text{ g}}{20 \text{ mL}}$$

$$(0.5 \text{ g})(20 \text{ mL}) = (5 \text{ g})(x)$$

$$x = 2 \text{ mL}$$

Or, we can solve it by reducing the fraction:

$$\frac{5 \text{ g}}{20 \text{ mL}} \rightarrow \frac{0.5 \text{ g}}{2 \text{ mL}}$$

76. D: Vitamin K is a warfarin K antagonist that interferes with blood clotting. Therefore, vitamin K should be avoided because it reduces the effectiveness of warfarin. Patients should be instructed to avoid vitamin K supplements and vitamin K-rich foods, such as spinach and green, leafy vegetables. In fact, vitamin K (menadiol, phytomenadione) is an antidote or reversal agent used to treat warfarin overdoses. Vitamin D (ergocalciferol) is used to promote bone health and treat osteoporosis and renal failure. Vitamin B_{12} (hydroxocobalamin) is used to prevent or treat deficiencies in patients with gastrointestinal disorders. Folic acid (folate) is used to prevent neural tube defects in pregnant women; it is also used alongside methotrexate therapy in order to reduce side effects.

77. B: Orally disintegrating/dissolving tablets or sublingual tablets should be placed under the tongue and allowed to disintegrate or dissolve. Buccal tablets should be placed on the gums under the upper lip or under the cheek and allowed to disintegrate. Some OTC medications use a dissolving film or oral drug strip that can be placed on the tongue and allowed to dissolve. Lidocaine viscous solution is unique in that it is intended to be swished around in the mouth until the patient's pain has resolved, and then it should be spit out. Orally disintegrating/dissolving tablets, buccal tablets, and dissolving films are not intended to be swallowed like typical tablets and capsules are.

78. B: The Poison Prevention Packaging Act of 1970 requires that medications be packaged in a childproof container. Patients can request (orally or in writing) that non-safety caps be used for all of their medications, and prescribers can only request non-safety caps for each specific prescription. Certain products are exempt from this childproof cap requirement:

- Topical creams/lotions/ointments (except lidocaine, dibucaine, and minoxidil)
- Sublingual nitroglycerin
- Isosorbide dinitrate ≤10 mg
- Cholestyramine/colestipol powder
- Oral contraceptives and medroxyprogesterone
- Unit dose potassium <50 mEq
- Erythromycin tablets ≤16 mg/package or suspension ≤8 g/package
- Effervescent tablets of aspirin or acetaminophen
- Drugs administered on site at a hospital or nursing home
- Lozenges
- Inhalers
- Pancrelipase
- Sucrose
- Mebendazole ≤600 mg/package
- Dental products (except products with >264 mg sodium fluoride)
- Steroid dose packs: methylprednisolone <84 mg, betamethasone <12.6 mg
- One package size of an OTC product if the label states "this package is for households without young children" (the same product must also be available in child-proof packaging)

79. C: The following information is required on the packaging of an OTC product:

- For each active ingredient, the name and general pharmacological category (e.g., antihistamine) of the drug must be listed
- List of inactive ingredients in alphabetical order
- Name and address of the manufacturer, packager, or distributor
- Net quantity in the package
- Drug facts panel, which includes the following: directions for use, indications, side effects, dosages, administration route(s), contraindications, and other warning or precautions
- Any required preparation for use (e.g., shake well)
- Lot number and expiration date
- Phone number for questions and comments
- Cautions and warnings, including: "For external use only"; "For rectal/vaginal use only"; "Do not use in..."; "Ask a doctor or pharmacist before use if you have certain conditions"
- Special storage instructions (e.g., "Keep in a refrigerator")
- Note: The NDC number is NOT mandatory on OTC medication labels

80. D: Compounding is when a pharmacy makes or prepares small, reasonable quantities of a product in anticipation of receiving a prescription. Pharmacies are only allowed to compound a product if they have or expect to have a prescription for a specific patient. Compounds cannot be sold to another pharmacy, prescriber, or hospital unless that pharmacy, prescriber, or hospital has obtained a special outsourcing facility license. In order to compound a product, the pharmacy must only use FDA-approved ingredients. Compounding that occurs in pharmacies is only intended to be small in scale, and the use of commercial-grade equipment is not allowed. The final product cannot duplicate a product that is commercially available for purchase, and the compound must not be a product that was withdrawn from the market for safety reasons.

Manufacturing is when a facility that has been licensed, inspected, and approved by the FDA produces, repackages, or relabels drug products. Manufacturing facilities have a different license than a pharmacy does, which allows them to prepare products that are approved by the FDA. Unlike pharmacies, they must follow strict quality control measures and must follow current good manufacturing practices.

81. B: One way to solve this problem is by using dimensional analysis:

$$\frac{1500 \text{ mL}}{12 \text{ hrs}} \times \frac{1 \text{ hr}}{60 \text{ min}} = \frac{1500 \text{ mL}}{720 \text{ min}} = \frac{2.08 \text{ mL}}{\text{min}}$$

Another way to solve this problem is by using the flow rate equation:

$$\text{Flow rate} = \frac{\text{mL of solution}}{\text{hours or minutes}}$$

First, we must figure out how many minutes are in 12 hours. Therefore, we need to multiply 12 hours by 60 minutes, which equals 720 minutes. Then we can plug this information into the equation.

$$\text{Flow rate} = \frac{1500 \text{ mL}}{720 \text{ min}} = \frac{2.08 \text{ mL}}{\text{min}}$$

82. C: An inventory should be performed either before the pharmacy opens or after the pharmacy closes for the day. A separate inventory should be done for each registered pharmacy location. All pharmacy stock must be inventoried, including expired drugs and medications contained within robotic dispensing systems or automated dispensing cabinets (e.g., Pyxis).

For noncontrolled drugs, the number of full bottles of each product should be counted. For partially empty containers, the exact count of the contents can be estimated.

For schedules III, IV, and V controlled medications, follow the same procedures as for noncontrolled medications. For partially empty containers, an estimated count or measure of the container contents is sufficient for inventory purposes unless the container holds more than 1,000 tablets or capsules. For containers holding more than 1,000 units, an exact count of the contents should be made.

For schedule II controlled substances, an exact count or measure of the container contents must be performed and documented in the inventory record. There are no exceptions for partially empty containers. Inventory records for schedule II substances should be kept separate.

Once the inventory is complete, the person performing the inventory and the pharmacist in charge should sign and date the inventory record.

83. C: Amlodipine (Norvasc) is a calcium channel blocker used to treat hypertension (high blood pressure). Enoxaparin (Lovenox) is a blood thinner. Losartan (Cozaar) is an angiotensin receptor blocker used to treat hypertension. Zocor (simvastatin) belongs to a category of drugs used to treat high cholesterol (antihyperlipidemics). They are commonly referred to as *statins* and include atorvastatin (Lipitor), pravastatin, rosuvastatin (Crestor), and lovastatin (Altoprev). Other common medications used to treat hyperlipidemia includes fenofibrate (Tricor), ezetimibe (Zetia), gemfibrozil (Lopid), and omega-3 acid (Lovaza).

84. B: Advair is an inhaler that contains a combination of two medications, salmeterol (a bronchodilator) and fluticasone (a corticosteroid). Bronchodilators dilate, or open, the airways to make it easier for patients to breathe. They are used to treat respiratory diseases, such as asthma and chronic obstructive pulmonary disease, but they can also be used short term during a respiratory illness to help relieve shortness of breath. Corticosteroids are anti-inflammatory medications that are used to treat a wide range of diseases, including respiratory illnesses such as asthma. Other similar medications that are commonly prescribed include Symbicort (budesonide, formoterol), another combination of a bronchodilator and a corticosteroid used to treat asthma. Albuterol (Ventolin, ProAir, Proventil) is a quick-acting bronchodilator used to treat acute asthma attacks. Tiotropium (Spiriva) is a long-acting bronchodilator used to treat chronic obstructive pulmonary disease.

85. D: Promethazine (Phenergan), hydroxyzine (Vistaril), and meclizine (Bonine) are drowsy antihistamines that usually cause significant sedation or fatigue in patients. Loratadine (Claritin) and cetirizine (Zyrtec) are non-drowsy antihistamines that cause less sedation in most patients. Antihistamines are used to treat seasonal allergies, allergic reactions, flu symptoms, and cold symptoms.

86. B: Antibiotics are used to treat bacterial or microbial infections. All antibiotics have the potential to cause nausea, vomiting, diarrhea, stomach upset, and abdominal pain. Antibiotics can also kill the normal flora (good bacteria) in the body and lead to secondary infections, such as thrush or intestinal infection (colitis, *Clostridium difficile*). This is more common with broad-spectrum (less-specific) antibiotics and longer courses of treatment. Patients can take a probiotic to help prevent this side effect. Penicillin (e.g., amoxicillin, penicillin) allergies occur in 1–10% of patients, with about 10% of those patients also being allergic to cephalosporins (e.g., cephalexin).

Tetracyclines (e.g., tetracycline, doxycycline) cause sensitivity to sunlight and staining of the teeth, so they should be avoided in children. Quinolones (e.g., ciprofloxacin, levofloxacin) can cause tendon rupture and increase the risk of seizures in at-risk patients.

87. A: The following are types of insulin used to treat diabetes mellitus:

Insulin Type/Generic Name	Brand Name	Duration of Action
Rapid-Acting Insulins		
Insulin glulisine	Apidra	1–3 hours
Insulin aspart	NovoLog, NovoPen	3–5 hours
Insulin lispro	Humalog, HumaPen	3–4 hours
Short-Acting Insulins		
Insulin regular	Novolin R, Humulin R	4–6 hours
Intermediate-Acting Insulins		
Insulin NPH	Novolin N, Humulin N	10–18 hours
Long-Acting Insulins		
Insulin glargine	Lantus	24 hours
Insulin detemir	Levemir	18–24 hours

88. C: A fluid ounce is equivalent to 30 mL of fluid. A teaspoon is equivalent to 5 mL of fluid. A tablespoon is equivalent to 15 mL of fluid. Answer D may have been confused with the conversion for grains; there are approximately 65 mg in one grain.

89. B: The following equation should be used to solve this problem:

$$C_1 \times V_1 = C_2 \times V_2$$

where C_1 is the concentration of stock cream, V_1 is the volume or quantity of stock cream that will be required for the preparation, C_2 is the desired concentration of the cream to be prepared, and V_2 is the volume or quantity of cream to be prepared. Therefore, the numbers that should be plugged into the equation are as follows:

$$(3\%)\, V_1 = (0.1\%)(100 \text{ g})$$

$$(3\%)\, V_1 = 0.1 \text{ g}$$

$$V_1 = 3.33 \text{ g}$$

Therefore, 3.3 g of 3% cream should be mixed with 96.7 g of white petroleum ointment to make 100 g of 0.1% triamcinolone cream.

90. A: Risperidone (Risperdal), quetiapine (Seroquel), and aripiprazole (Abilify) are antipsychotic medications used to treat schizophrenia. Fluoxetine (Prozac), sertraline (Zoloft), citalopram (Celexa), escitalopram (Lexapro), duloxetine (Cymbalta), venlafaxine (Effexor), paroxetine (Paxil), and mirtazapine (Remeron) are antidepressants. Levetiracetam (Keppra), lamotrigine (Lamictal), topiramate (Topamax), phenytoin (Dilantin), and oxcarbazepine (Trileptal) are commonly used to treat epilepsy or seizure disorders.

PTCB Practice Test #2

1. Which of the following medications belongs to the same drug class as pantoprazole (Protonix)?

    a. Esomeprazole (Nexium)
    b. Cimetidine (Tagamet)
    c. Famotidine (Pepcid)
    d. Nizatidine (Axid)

2. Which of the following is a fluoroquinolone?

    a. Cefadroxil
    b. Ciprofloxacin
    c. Cefazolin
    d. Cephalexin

3. Which of the following drug classes is NOT used to treat hypertension?

    a. Beta-blockers
    b. Thiazolidinediones
    c. Diuretics
    d. ACE inhibitors

4. In order for a drug to be considered a generic or therapeutic equivalent to a brand-name drug, the drug must meet which of the following conditions?

    a. It must have the same shape, color, and scoring as the brand-name drug.
    b. It must have the same inert ingredients as the brand-name drug.
    c. It must be bioequivalent to the brand-name drug.
    d. It must be priced comparably according to the average wholesale price and federal upper limit price listed in the Micromedex Red Book.

5. Which drug reference is published annually by the FDA and provides a list of all prescriptions approved as safe and effective, along with therapeutic equivalence determinations using a two-letter therapeutic evaluation code?

    a. Red Book database
    b. *Orange Book*
    c. *Physicians' Desk Reference*
    d. *Drug Facts and Comparisons*

6. When selecting a therapeutically equivalent drug product, which of the following TE codes represent drug products for which there are no known or suspected bioequivalence problems?

    a. AA
    b. AB
    c. BC
    d. BD

7. A patient presents to the pharmacy with a prescription for citalopram (Celexa). However, his patient profile shows that he has already been prescribed sertraline (Zoloft). Which of the following possible life-threatening drug interactions can occur with this combination?

    a. Stein-Leventhal syndrome
    b. Stevens-Johnson syndrome
    c. Sjögren's syndrome
    d. Serotonin syndrome

8. Which of the following foods would affect the way warfarin (Coumadin) might work in the body?

    a. Kale
    b. Eggplant
    c. Bananas
    d. Cucumbers

9. Which of the following drug classes should be avoided in patients with hypertension?

    a. Beta-blockers
    b. Decongestants
    c. ACE inhibitors
    d. Calcium channel blockers

10. What is the dosage form for nitroglycerin (Nitrostat)?

    a. Intravenous (IV)
    b. Extended-release capsule
    c. Sublingual tablet
    d. Oral suspension

11. Through which route of administration is insulin glulisine (Apidra) commonly administered?

    a. Oral
    b. Subcutaneous
    c. Topical
    d. Inhalation

12. A prescription for Augmentin 45 mg/kg/day PO divided BID for 10 days is sent to the pharmacy for a pediatric patient (20 months old) weighing 20 pounds. The prescription is for the treatment of acute bacterial otitis media. Which of the following dosage forms would you use to fill this prescription?

    a. Augmentin 200 mg/5 mL oral suspension
    b. Augmentin 200 mg chewable tablet
    c. Augmentin ES 600 mg/5 mL oral suspension
    d. Augmentin XR 1,000 mg tablet

13. Which of the following black box label warnings are associated with ALL antidepressants?

    a. Serious adverse reactions, including tendinitis and tendon rupture.

    b. Increased risk of serious gastrointestinal (GI) adverse events, including bleeding, ulcer, and perforation.

    c. May cause tardive dyskinesia, a serious and often irreversible movement disorder.

    d. Increased suicidality risk in children, adolescents, and young adults.

14. Which of the following side effects is commonly associated with the use of antibiotics?

    a. Dizziness

    b. GI upset

    c. Insomnia

    d. Hyperhidrosis

15. Which of the following adverse effects is associated with the use of lisinopril?

    a. Headache

    b. Constipation

    c. Dry cough

    d. Hypertension

16. A 75-year-old female patient presents to the pharmacy complaining about muscle pain and cramps in her legs. The pharmacist reviews her patient profile in the computer and determines which of the following drugs to be the possible cause?

    a. Gabapentin

    b. Sucralfate

    c. Rosuvastatin

    d. Atomoxetine

17. Which of the following drugs is commonly used to treat diabetes?

    a. Metformin

    b. Risperidone

    c. Aripiprazole

    d. Ziprasidone

18. Which of the following OTC supplements is commonly used by patients to help lower triglyceride levels?

    a. Fenofibrate

    b. Glucosamine

    c. St. John's wort

    d. Fish oil

19. Which of the following OTC supplements is commonly used by patients to help improve insomnia?

    a. Elderberry

    b. Saw palmetto

    c. Melatonin

    d. Echinacea

20. Which of the following drugs is commonly used to treat depression?

    a. Levothyroxine
    b. Metoprolol
    c. Alprazolam
    d. Citalopram

21. Unlike their dry powder counterpart, nonpreserved compounded oral preparations reconstituted using water must be marked with a beyond-use date of

    a. 7 days
    b. 14 days
    c. 28 days
    d. 45 days

22. At what temperature should unopened insulin vials, pens, and cartridges be stored in the pharmacy?

    a. Controlled room temperature
    b. Controlled cold temperature
    c. Cool temperature
    d. Freezing temperature

23. Factors affecting the compatibility and stability of a compounded sterile preparation include all of the following EXCEPT

    a. Temperature sensitivity
    b. Light sensitivity
    c. Plastic containers
    d. IV bag size

24. A prescription for oral clarithromycin suspension 15 mg/kg/day divided BID × 7 days is faxed to the pharmacy for a female pediatric patient weighing 44 pounds. The maximum single dose is 500 mg. Which bottle size should be selected to fill this prescription?

    a. Clarithromycin 125 mg/5 mL (50 mL)
    b. Clarithromycin 125 mg/5 mL (75 mL)
    c. Clarithromycin 125 mg/5 mL (100 mL)
    d. Clarithromycin 125 mg/5 mL (150 mL)

25. Which of the following drugs is considered a narrow-therapeutic-index (NTI) medication?

    a. Metformin
    b. Lithium
    c. Eszopiclone
    d. Dextromethorphan

26. Which of the following oral anticoagulant agents is considered an NTI drug?

    a. Dabigatran
    b. Warfarin
    c. Rivaroxaban
    d. Apixaban

27. Which of the following drugs is NOT an NTI drug?

    a. Theophylline
    b. Phenytoin
    c. Digoxin
    d. Phenelzine

28. Which of the following is a sign of physical instability in a nonsterile compounded medication?

    a. Creams that exhibit crystallization and emulsion breakage.
    b. Suppositories with the absence of excessive softening or shriveling.
    c. Gels with a uniform appearance, without discoloration or inappropriate odor.
    d. Ointments lacking grittiness or granularization.

29. Which of the following is NOT a sign of chemical instability in a compounded solution?

    a. Precipitation
    b. Haziness
    c. Difficulty resuspending
    d. Discoloration

30. Which of the following is NOT a factor that affects the stability of nonsterile compounded medications?

    a. Tightly closed containers
    b. Humidity
    c. Light
    d. Adverse temperatures

31. Which of the following antibiotic suspensions needs to be refrigerated after reconstitution?

    a. Cefdinir (Omnicef)
    b. Clarithromycin (Biaxin)
    c. Amoxicillin-clavulanate (Augmentin)
    d. Nitrofurantoin (Macrobid)

32. An opened vial of insulin detemir (Levemir) can be stored at room temperature for how many days?

    a. 10 days
    b. 14 days
    c. 30 days
    d. 42 days

33. Which of the following drugs is NOT sensitive to light exposure?

    a. Daunorubicin
    b. Doxorubicin
    c. Didanosine
    d. Dacarbazine

34. Where should syringes and glass vials be disposed?

   a. Trash can
   b. Sharps container
   c. Biohazard container
   d. Autoclave bag

35. Once a pharmacy technician has finished compounding a chemotherapeutic agent, where should the waste be disposed?

   a. Yellow nonhazardous waste bin
   b. Black hazardous waste bin
   c. Red biohazard bag
   d. Sharps container

36. How often must a pharmacy technician change gloves when compounding chemotherapy and other hazardous drugs?

   a. Every 30 minutes
   b. Every 45 minutes
   c. Every 60 minutes
   d. Every 2 to 3 hours

37. How many times can a prescription for Lortab be refilled?

   a. None
   b. Once
   c. Three times
   d. Five times

38. How many times can a prescription for zolpidem (Ambien) be transferred between different pharmacies?

   a. None
   b. Once
   c. Three times
   d. Five times

39. A prescription for the combination medication butalbital-aspirin-caffeine must include the following information, EXCEPT

   a. Date of issue
   b. Drug name, strength, and dosage form
   c. Patient's name and address
   d. Date of filling

40. Which controlled substance schedule does tramadol (Qdolo) belong to?

   a. Schedule I
   b. Schedule II
   c. Schedule III
   d. Schedule IV

41. A patient presents to the pharmacy with a prescription for oxycodone (OxyContin) 15 mg tab #100. The prescription is from Dr. Boice Howard, and the DEA number listed on the prescription is BH8253285. Which of the following statements regarding the DEA number is correct?
   a. The first letter of the DEA registration number is the first initial of the prescriber's first name.
   b. The second letter of the DEA registration number is the first initial of the prescriber's last name.
   c. The last two numbers of the DEA registration number are called the check digits.
   d. The DEA registration number provided on this prescription is valid.

42. What form is used to order schedule II medications?
   a. DEA Form 41
   b. DEA Form 106
   c. DEA Form 222
   d. DEA Form 224

43. Besides being kept in a locked cabinet, how else can schedule II drugs be stored in a pharmacy?
   a. Schedule II drugs can be stored in the original delivery box behind the counter.
   b. Schedule II drugs can be dispersed throughout the stock of noncontrolled substances.
   c. Schedule II drugs can be stored together with all other schedule drugs under the pharmacy counter.
   d. Schedule II drugs can be stored in the narcotic safe with a turn dial.

44. While filling a medication order for morphine 0.2 mg/kg of body weight for a patient weighing 165 pounds using a 15 mg/mL vial, the pharmacy technician accidentally drops the vial, causing it to break. Which of the following steps must occur after cleanup?
   a. Report the spill to the supervising pharmacist and try filling the order again.
   b. Report the spill to the supervising pharmacist, and allow someone else to fill the medication order.
   c. Report the spill to the supervising pharmacist, and fill out a DEA Form 41.
   d. Report the spill to the supervising pharmacist, and fill out a DEA Form 106.

45. Which of the following is NOT a REMS program established to mitigate the potential risk for harm with the use of prescription drugs?
   a. Naprosyn REMS
   b. iPLEDGE Program
   c. Clozapine REMS
   d. THALOMID REMS

46. What is the maximum daily limit of pseudoephedrine (PSE) base that a patient can purchase, regardless of the number of transactions?
   a. 3.6 grams
   b. 7.5 grams
   c. 9 grams
   d. 10.8 grams

47. A patient presents to the pharmacy asking to buy two boxes of Sudafed Sinus Congestion, which contain 30 mg tablets of PSE and 24 tablets per box. After taking down their information and entering it into the electronic logbook, it's revealed that in the past 28 days, the patient has purchased the following through multiple transactions:

- two boxes of Wal-Phed D (120 mg PSE × 10 caplets per box)
- one box of Claritin-D 24-Hour (240 mg PSE × 10 tablets per box)
- one box of Sudafed 24-Hour (240 mg PSE × 10 tablets per box)

Which of the following statements regarding this potential transaction is correct?

a. The products can't be sold because the patient has purchased the maximum amount of PSE that is legally allowed.
b. The person is suspected of collecting PSE in large batches for illegal purposes; therefore, the state's DEA representative should be notified.
c. The pharmacist should be summoned to assist with this matter.
d. The transaction is valid, and the requested medicine can be sold to the patient.

48. A patient receives a recall notice from the pharmacy stating that their Keflex 250 mg (urinary tract infection treatment) was found to contain less of the active ingredients than what was labeled and that the FDA has issued a recall of the drug. Which of the following FDA drug recall classifications would this fall under?

a. Class I recall
b. Class II recall
c. Class III recall
d. Class IV recall

49. Once a pharmacy technician removes a recalled medication from the floor, where must it be stored in the pharmacy?

a. Controlled substance lockbox
b. Under the counter
c. Separate from the other medications
d. With other drug stock boxes

50. Which of the following products is NOT under strict FDA regulations?

a. Prescription medications
b. OTC medications
c. Dietary supplements
d. Medical devices

51. Which of the following drug classes is NOT listed on the ISMP list of high-alert medications in community/ambulatory health care?

a. Anticoagulants
b. Insulin
c. Opioids
d. Antidepressants

52. Which of the following pair of drugs would NOT likely be found on the ISMP's list of confused drug names?

    a. Zyrtec and Zovirax
    b. Mirapex and Miralax
    c. Ditropan and Diprivan
    d. Reminyl and Amaryl

53. Which organization provides guidelines and resources on medication safety, including a list of high-alert medications for different care facilities?

    a. FDA
    b. DEA
    c. TJC
    d. ISMP

54. Which of the following tall man lettering drug name pairs is NOT correct?

    a. CARBOplatin and CISplatin
    b. SANDOstatin and SANDimmune
    c. FLUoxetine and DULoxetine
    d. PHENobarbital and PENTobarbital

55. Which of the following is NOT an example of a medication that should not be crushed, split, or opened?

    a. Remeron
    b. Cardizem CD
    c. Theo-24
    d. Ambien CR

56. Which of the following prescription inscriptions has a higher probability of resulting in a medication error?

    a. Synthroid 25 mcg
    b. Lipitor 20 mg
    c. Latanoprost 0.005%
    d. Humalog 14 U @ HS

57. A patient approaches the pharmacy counter asking for OTC suggestions for allergy medications. What should you do?

    a. Recommend that they try cetirizine (Zyrtec) because it has a quicker onset and longer duration of action.
    b. Recommend that they try desloratadine (Clarinex) because it is only once-daily dosing and has a lower incidence of daytime drowsiness.
    c. Contact the primary care doctor for further assistance.
    d. Refer the patient to the pharmacist for further assistance.

58. A patient brings in a new prescription from their cardiologist for Crestor. Upon entering the information into the computer, the new prescription is checked against all of the medications in the patient's profile and a therapeutic duplication warning appears on the screen. This reveals that the patient is also taking Lipitor, which was prescribed by their primary care physician. What should be done?

    a. Fill the prescription because the doctors know what is best for the patient.
    b. Inform the patient that the prescription cannot be filled and that they should contact their doctors for further assistance.
    c. Inform the pharmacist of the situation and wait for further instruction.
    d. Contact the cardiologist and primary care doctor to have them decide how to proceed.

59. Which of the following is NOT a medication error reporting system?

    a. MedWatch
    b. FAERS
    c. VAERS
    d. ISMP MERP

60. Which of the following scenarios would be best described as a near-miss error?

    a. Ampicillin was ordered for a patient allergic to penicillin. However, the pharmacist was alerted to the allergy during the computer order entry process and the physician was called to review other treatment options.
    b. A patient discovers that they were dispensed Seroquel 200 mg tablets instead of 300 mg tablets prior to taking a dose.
    c. A nurse administers potassium chloride 20 mEq instead of cefazolin 2 g due to the stark similarities between the two vials, resulting in a sentinel event.
    d. The pharmacy technician dispenses 10 mL Novolog vial in place of 10 mL Novolin vial, causing a patient to experience an adverse event.

61. Which of the following statements about MEDMARX is INCORRECT?

    a. MEDMARX is overseen by the *United States Pharmacopeia* (USP).
    b. MEDMARX is a voluntary reporting system that tracks adverse drug reactions and medication errors.
    c. Information gathered through MEDMARX is used to determine the individual(s) responsible for the errors.
    d. MEDMARX is designed for use by hospitals and health systems to collect, track, and analyze medication errors.

62. A patient presents to the outpatient clinic pharmacy for a refill of their lisinopril 10 mg. During the filling process, the pharmacy employee notices that this patient has not refilled this prescription in 48 days. Based on this information, what kind of medication error should the pharmacy employee suspect has occurred?

    a. Omission error
    b. Compliance error
    c. Prescribing error
    d. Monitoring error

63. A patient presents to the pharmacy with a prescription for amoxicillin 500 mg TID for seven days. After entering the information into the computer, the system alerts the pharmacy technician to a potential drug-allergy interaction. The technician notifies the pharmacist, who then confirms that the patient has a penicillin allergy. Based on this information, what kind of medication error has likely occurred?

   a. Prescribing error
   b. Dispensing error
   c. Administration error
   d. Unauthorized drug error

64. The hospital pharmacy receives a medication order for a fentanyl 25 mcg patch. However, the pharmacy technician dispenses a fentanyl 75 mcg patch instead. Based on this information, what kind of medication error do you believe has occurred?

   a. Prescribing error
   b. Dispensing error
   c. Administration error
   d. Deteriorated drug error

65. Which of the following procedures is NOT required when compounding sterile products?

   a. Gloves should be thoroughly sprayed and rubbed with isopropyl alcohol 70% and then allowed to air dry before proceeding with sterile compounding.
   b. When cleaning a horizontal laminar flow hood, it is best practice to spray the entire inside of the hood, including the high-efficiency particulate air (HEPA) filter, with isopropyl alcohol 70%.
   c. The compounding area must be saturated with isopropyl alcohol 70% and allowed to remain for at least 30 seconds prior to the beginning of each shift.
   d. Wipe the rubber top of the vial with an isopropyl alcohol 70% prep pad using firm strokes in a unidirectional sweeping motion at least three times and allow to air dry.

66. When donning personal protective equipment (PPE) just prior to entering the sterile compounding area, which of the following pieces of PPE should be put on first?

   a. Shoe covers
   b. Gloves
   c. Nonshedding gown
   d. Facial mask

67. A pharmacy technician is filling a prescription for Proscar 5 mg #30. It is essential that the technician immediately does which of the following after counting and packaging the tablets in the labeled prescription bottle?

   a. Apply the warning labels to the bottle.
   b. Clean the counting tray with isopropyl alcohol.
   c. Notify the pharmacist that the prescription is complete.
   d. Call the patient stating that the prescription is ready for pickup.

68. Which type of products must be sterile and isotonic?

   a. External medications
   b. Ophthalmic products
   c. Oral inhalation products
   d. Otic preparations

69. **A patient comes in with a prescription for 100 mg BID PO of cefdinir suspension for seven days. Upon reconstitution of the medication, which of the following auxiliary labels should be affixed to the bottle?**

   a. "For external use"
   b. "For otic use"
   c. "May cause dizziness"
   d. "Shake well"

70. **Which of the following may be used in a parenteral solution?**

   a. Purified water
   b. Water for injection
   c. Sterile water for injection USP
   d. Sterile water for irrigation USP

71. **A patient presents to the pharmacy with the following prescription:**

   Amoxicillin 500 mg cap
   Sig: tk i cap po TID × 7 days for bacterial rhinosinusitis
   Dispense QS

Using the information provided, how many capsules should be dispensed for an adult male patient weighing 75 kg?

   a. 3 capsules
   b. 14 capsules
   c. 21 capsules
   d. 30 capsules

72. **A patient presents to the pharmacy with a prescription for**

   Cefdinir 125 mg/5 mL
   Sig: 7 mg/kg BID × 7 days for acute bacterial otitis media.

Using the information provided, calculate the quantity to be dispensed for a pediatric patient weighing 46.5 pounds.

   a. Cefdinir 125 mg/5 mL (60 mL)
   b. Cefdinir 125 mg/5 mL (100 mL)
   c. Cefdinir 250 mg/5 mL (60 mL)
   d. Cefdinir 250 mg/5 mL (100 mL)

73. **A compounding pharmacy receives a prescription for 4.5 ounces of 4% hydrocortisone cream, but it only stocks 1% and 10% hydrocortisone cream. How many grams of each will be needed to prepare this order?**

   a. 3 g of the 1% hydrocortisone cream + 1.5 g of the 10% hydrocortisone cream
   b. 27 g of the 1% hydrocortisone cream + 13.5 g of the 10% hydrocortisone cream
   c. 90 g of the 1% hydrocortisone cream + 45 g of the 10% hydrocortisone cream
   d. 810 g of the 1% hydrocortisone cream + 405 g of the 10% hydrocortisone cream

74. The hospital pharmacy receives a STAT order of furosemide 150 mg IV in 250 mL lactated Ringer's solution to be infused over 60 minutes. There is 1% furosemide in stock. How many mL of this solution will be needed to fill this medication order?

   a. 2.5 mL
   b. 6.7 mL
   c. 9.2 mL
   d. 15 mL

75. A patient presents to the pharmacy with a prescription for

   Diclofenac 50 mg tab
   Sig: tk i tab po Q8–12h PRN
   #24

Using the information provided, calculate the day's supply.

   a. Two days
   b. Four days
   c. Six days
   d. Eight days

76. What is the percentage concentration of a solution that contains 250 mg/50 mL?

   a. 0.5%
   b. 1%
   c. 2.5%
   d. 5%

77. A prescription is electronically sent to the pharmacy for Proventil HFA. The patient is a 6-year-old male patient weighing 20 kg. Which of the following medical devices would be recommended to assist with proper usage?

   a. Tuberculin syringe
   b. Oral dose spoon
   c. Test strips
   d. Spacer

78. Which of the following medical devices is NOT commonly used in patients with diabetes?

   a. Oral syringe
   b. Alcohol swab
   c. Glucometer strips
   d. Lancet

79. Which needle gauge size has the largest lumen diameter?

   a. 13G
   b. 19G
   c. 22G
   d. 30G

80. Drug Bottle A has a National Drug Code (NDC) number of 0093-1723-01, and Drug Bottle B has an NDC number of 0093-7542-06. Based on this information, what can be said about these two drug products?

    a. Both drug bottles are for the same drug and dose.
    b. Both drugs are produced by the same manufacturer.
    c. Both drug bottles contain the same amount of medication.
    d. Both drugs have nothing in common.

81. When repackaging unit-dose drugs in a pharmacy, which of the following suggested FDA guidelines has been proposed for assigning an expiration date in the absence of stability studies?

    a. 12 months from the date of repackaging
    b. 9 months from the date of repackaging
    c. 6 months or 25% of the remaining manufacturer expiration date, whichever is earlier
    d. 9 months or 50% of the remaining manufacturer expiration date, whichever is earlier

82. A patient presents to the pharmacy with a prescription for Synthroid 112 mcg. The physician has handwritten "DAW" on the prescription. Which DAW code would be assigned to this prescription?

    a. DAW 0
    b. DAW 1
    c. DAW 2
    d. DAW 3

83. A patient drops off a prescription for cyclobenzaprine 5 mg TID #90. For 12 days, the pharmacy attempts to contact the patient to pick up the filled medication, but the patient remains out of reach. Company policy states that the order is canceled after 12 days and the prescription is stored on the patient's profile. What happens to the medication?

    a. The medication is disposed of by discarding it in a specialized pharmacy refuse container.
    b. The medication is removed from rotation, and the drug wholesaler is notified for pickup.
    c. The medication is returned to stock, and the charges are reversed.
    d. The prescription is canceled, and the patient will need to obtain a new prescription from the prescriber for future filling.

84. Which of the following is NOT a reason that a medication might be returned to a drug wholesaler or drug manufacturer?

    a. The medication was damaged in transit to the pharmacy.
    b. The medication is under FDA recall.
    c. The medication is close to expiration.
    d. The medication is no longer wanted by the patient.

85. Which of the following is the brand name for vilazodone?

    a. Wellbutrin
    b. Viibryd
    c. Remeron
    d. Trintellix

86. Which of the following is the generic name for Lipitor?

    a. Atorvastatin
    b. Lovastatin
    c. Rosuvastatin
    d. Simvastatin

87. Which of the following drugs would NOT likely be used in the treatment of asthma?

    a. Fluticasone
    b. Albuterol
    c. Nadolol
    d. Montelukast

88. How many 1-ounce jars can be filled with 476 grams of clotrimazole cream?

    a. 15 jars
    b. 16 jars
    c. 17 jars
    d. 18 jars

89. How many mcg are in 1/8 oz of erythromycin ophthalmic ointment 0.5%?

    a. 0.00000375 mcg
    b. 0.00375 mcg
    c. 3,750 mcg
    d. 3,750,000 mcg

90. Which USP guideline provides the standards and requirements for compounding nonsterile preparations?

    a. USP General Chapter <795>
    b. USP General Chapter <797>
    c. USP General Chapter <800>
    d. USP General Chapter <825>

Answer Key and Explanations for Test #2

1. A: Pantoprazole (Protonix) belongs to the proton pump inhibitor (PPI) drug class. Although all of the drugs listed are used to treat gastroesophageal reflux disease, only esomeprazole (Nexium) is a PPI. Other drugs in the PPI category include omeprazole (Prilosec), lansoprazole (Prevacid), dexlansoprazole (Dexilant), and rabeprazole (Aciphex). Cimetidine (Tagamet), famotidine (Pepcid), and nizatidine (Axid) are histamine-2 receptor antagonists.

2. B: Ciprofloxacin is a fluoroquinolone antibiotic, whereas the others are cephalosporins. (Hint: Most fluoroquinolone antibiotics end in *-floxacin*.) Cephalosporin antibiotics are a class of antibiotics widely used in patients who are allergic to penicillin. Within this class are cefadroxil, cefazolin, and cephalexin.)

3. B: Recall that "hypertension" means high blood pressure, which is commonly treated using angiotensin-converting enzyme (ACE) inhibitors, angiotensin II receptor blockers, alpha-blockers, beta-blockers, calcium channel blockers, and/or diuretics, to name a few. These medications work to reduce blood pressure. Thiazolidinediones are a class of oral hypoglycemic medications that may be used to treat type 2 diabetes.

4. C: In order for a generic drug to be therapeutically equivalent to the brand-name drug, the U.S. Food and Drug Administration (FDA) requires that generic drugs have the same active ingredient, strength (dose), dosage form, route of administration, and indications as the brand-name drug. In addition, generic drug manufacturers must submit bioequivalent studies to the FDA proving that the generic drug has the same clinical effect and safety profile as the brand-name drug. The appearance, inert ingredients (excipients), and pricing of the generic drug do not affect how the drug works and therefore are not required to be identical to the brand-name drug.

5. B: The *Orange Book*, also known as *Approved Drug Products with Therapeutic Equivalence Evaluations*, is used to determine whether a drug is therapeutically equivalent to another. The *Orange Book* serves as a guide for identifying suitable generic alternatives for branded products. This drug reference is nicknamed the *Orange Book* after its distinct bright-orange cover. The Red Book database provides information on drug pricing and product information on prescription and over-the-counter (OTC) drug products. The *Physicians' Desk Reference* and *Drug Facts and Comparisons* are the most commonly used drug reference books for clinical pharmacology information for more than 22,000 prescription and 6,000 OTC products.

6. A: Drug products that the FDA considers to be therapeutically equivalent to other products with no known or suspected bioequivalence problems are designated with the TE code AA. Products designated AB are also considered to be therapeutically equivalent, but only after actual or potential bioequivalence problems have been resolved with adequate in vivo and/or in vitro evidence supporting bioequivalence. Products designated with a TE code starting with a B (BA, BO, BP, BX, etc.) are considered NOT to be therapeutically equivalent to other pharmaceutically equivalent products. (Hint: "TE code" refers to therapeutic equivalence evaluation code.)

7. D: Recall that citalopram (Celexa) and sertraline (Zoloft) are antidepressants. Both drugs fall into the selective serotonin reuptake inhibitor (SSRI) category because they work by blocking the reuptake (reabsorption) of serotonin into the presynaptic neuron, thereby increasing the levels of serotonin available to bind to the receptor. However, when patients combine two serotonin-related medications or medications that increase serotonin levels, it can result in a rare but life-threatening interaction called serotonin syndrome. Symptoms of serotonin syndrome include elevated body temperature, agitation, confusion, overactive reflexes, tremors, profuse sweating, rapid heart rate, dilated pupils, vomiting, and diarrhea.

8. A: Recall that warfarin (Coumadin) is an anticoagulant drug used to prevent blood clots. It does this by inhibiting the synthesis of vitamin K-dependent clotting factors. Increasing vitamin K levels through diet or supplementation can promote clotting and reduce the effectiveness of warfarin. Foods that are high in vitamin K are typically leafy green vegetables such as kale, spinach, collard greens, turnip greens, mustard greens, broccoli, etc., but they can also include things such as asparagus, avocado, dill pickles, green tea, and margarine. Patients are suggested to limit their consumption of foods containing high amounts of vitamin K, or at least maintain the same level, while they are taking warfarin.

9. B: Patients with cardiovascular disease such as hypertension (high blood pressure) and heart disease should avoid the use of decongestants because they have been shown to cause adverse cardiovascular effects. Palpitations, tachycardia, arrhythmia, exacerbated hypertension, reflex bradycardia, coronary occlusion, cerebral vasculitis, myocardial infarction, cardiac arrest, and death have been reported. Patients with cerebrovascular insufficiency (stroke, transient ischemic attack, etc.) and hyperthyroidism are also warned to avoid or limit the use of decongestants. ACE inhibitors, beta-blockers, and calcium channel blockers are all drug classes that are used to treat hypertension.

10. C: Nitroglycerin (Nitrostat) is a vasodilator indicated for the acute relief of an attack or acute prophylaxis of angina due to coronary artery disease. Nitrostat is supplied as white, round, flat-faced sublingual tablets in three strengths (0.3, 0.4, and 0.6 mg). Nitroglycerin can evaporate from tablets if strict precautions are not taken. Nitroglycerin should be kept in its original glass container and must be tightly capped after each use to prevent loss of tablet potency. Heat, moisture, and light will damage the tablets and result in the loss of tablet potency. Nitrostat should be dissolved under the tongue (sublingually) or in the buccal pouch (between the gums and cheek) at the first sign of an acute angina attack. The dose may be repeated approximately every 5 minutes until relief is obtained. If the pain persists after a total of three tablets in a 15-minute period, or if the pain is different than is typically experienced, the patient should seek prompt medical attention. Furthermore, Nitrostat may be used prophylactically 5 to 10 minutes prior to engaging in activities that might precipitate an acute attack. Administer Nitrostat at rest, preferably in the sitting position.

11. B: Insulin glulisine (Apidra) is a rapid-acting insulin used in the treatment of type 1 or 2 diabetes in adults and type 1 diabetes in children older than the age of 4. All insulin products are commonly injected into subcutaneous (subcut) tissue at a 90-degree angle using a 4–5 mm needle. Common injection sites include the abdomen, thigh, and upper arm. Injection sites should be rotated within the same region (abdomen, thigh, or upper arm) from one injection to the next to reduce the risk of lipodystrophy. Apidra is used to improve blood glucose control in patients and should be administered at mealtime (within 15 minutes before a meal or within 20 minutes after starting a meal). Apidra should be used in a regimen with an intermediate- or long-acting insulin. All insulin products can possibly cause hypokalemia and should be used cautiously in patients who may be at risk for hypokalemia.

(Note: In the past, "subcutaneous" has been abbreviated "SC," "SQ," or "subQ." However, these abbreviations are on the Institute for Safe Medication Practices' (ISMP) list of error-prone abbreviations, symbols, and dose designations and should be avoided. For patient safety purposes, the subcutaneous route of administration can be safely abbreviated "subcut" or written out as "subcutaneously.")

12. A: Augmentin (amoxicillin and clavulanate potassium) is a combination antibiotic indicated in the treatment of certain bacterial infections. It is made of amoxicillin, which is a penicillin-class antibiotic; and clavulanic acid, which is beta-lactamase inhibitor. Dosing for Augmentin is based on the amoxicillin component. To answer this question, the required dose must first be calculated using the following steps:

1. Convert pounds into kilograms: $\frac{20 \text{ lb}}{2.2 \text{ kg/lb}} = 9$ kg.
2. Calculate the dose: $\frac{45 \text{ mg}}{\text{kg/day}} \times 9 \text{ kg} = 405 \frac{\text{mg}}{\text{day}} \div 2$ doses per day $= 202.5$ mg per dose.

Because this is a pediatric patient, it is best practice that the dosage be rounded down for safety purposes and ease of dosing. Therefore, the calculated dose would be 200 mg per dose.

Now the choices can be narrowed down by eliminating Augmentin XR tablets, which are not only the incorrect dose but also because tablets are not an appropriate dosage form option for pediatric patients. Augment ES comes in too high of a dose for what is necessary. Augmentin 200 mg chewable tablets are reserved for use by older patients and would be considered a choking hazard in a 20-month-old pediatric patient. The best option for this patient is Augmentin 200 mg/5 mL.

Hint:

- To convert pounds to kilograms, divide pounds by 2.2.
- To convert kilograms to pounds, multiply kilograms by 2.2.
- "BID" means twice a day; therefore, the total daily dose would be divided by 2.
- Allergy alert: Augmentin contains amoxicillin, which belongs to the penicillin drug class. Patients allergic to penicillin should not be given Augmentin.

13. D: The black box warning is the most stringent warning issued by the FDA about a medication's adverse drug events. These warnings must be added to drug labels and prescribing information. As a drug class, antidepressants all have a black box warning about the risk of increased suicidality in children, adolescents, and young adults with major depressive or other psychiatric disorders. Fluoroquinolone antibiotics carry a black box warning for the increased risk of tendinitis and tendon rupture, whereas nonsteroidal anti-inflammatory drugs carry a black box warning for the increased risk of serious GI adverse events. Metoclopramide (Reglan) is labeled with a black box warning that informs providers and patients about the risk of tardive dyskinesia.

14. B: Antibiotics commonly cause GI symptoms such as nausea, vomiting, abdominal pain, and diarrhea. These drugs are commonly prescribed to fight bacterial infections, and they work by reducing or killing certain bacteria, both the afflicting bacteria strain and the beneficial gut flora. This can disrupt the delicate balance among the various species in the intestines and can ultimately lead to GI upset.

15. C: Recall that lisinopril (Zestril) is an ACE inhibitor and is commonly used to treat hypertension. ACE inhibitors are associated with a dry, persistent cough in 5–35% of patients prescribed them and usually occurs within the first few months of treatment. Other common side effects include hypotension, dizziness, and increased serum creatinine. Patients experiencing an ACE inhibitor-induced cough often can be prescribed an angiotensin receptor blocker (ARB) for hypertension without the risk for cough. (Hint: The generic name of ACE inhibitors ends in *-pril*. The generic name of ARBs ends in *-sartan*.)

16. C: Rosuvastatin (Crestor) is a 3-hydroxy-3-methylglutaryl coenzyme A (HMG-CoA) reductase inhibitor drug (commonly known as "statins") and is used to treat hyperlipidemia (high cholesterol). In combination with diet, this drug class works to lower bad cholesterol (low-density lipoprotein [LDL]) and triglycerides and increase good cholesterol (high-density lipoprotein [HDL]) levels. One of the most common complaints of people taking statins is muscle pain, primarily involving large, proximal muscle groups such as the legs and/or back. Symptoms typically occur within four to six weeks after starting a statin, but they can occur at any time throughout the duration of treatment. Some risk factors for statin-associated muscle side effects include patients with the following characteristics: older than the age of 75, renal or hepatic insufficiency, history of musculoskeletal symptoms, Asian ancestry, female, low body mass index, frailty, and alcohol or drug abuse.

(Hint: The generic name of HMG CoA reductase inhibitors ends in *-statin*, which is why they are commonly referred to as "statins." Other drugs in this drug class include atorvastatin [Lipitor], fluvastatin [Lescol], lovastatin [Mevacor, Altocor], pravastatin [Pravachol], pitavastatin [Livalo], and simvastatin [Zocor].)

17. A: Metformin (Glumetza) is an oral antidiabetic agent (drug class: biguanide) used to treat type II diabetes mellitus. This drug is used to lower blood glucose levels by improving insulin sensitivity through peripheral glucose uptake and utilization. The most common side effect seen with this drug is GI upset (diarrhea, nausea, cramping) that tends to resolve or lessen with long-term use. Risperidone (Risperdal), aripiprazole (Abilify), and ziprasidone (Geodon) are all atypical antipsychotics.

18. D: Fish oil is a source of docosahexaenoic acid and eicosapentaenoic acid, commonly known as omega-3 fatty acids. Omega-3 fatty acids come solely from dietary sources, meaning they can't be manufactured in the body. Dietary sources of these omega-3 fatty acids include fatty fish (salmon, mackerel, etc.) and shellfish (mussels, oysters, crabs, shrimp). Patients commonly take fish oil to reduce the risk of heart attacks and strokes, as well as to treat high triglycerides. Although little evidence exists to support the use of fish oil to lower bad cholesterol (LDL), very high doses of purified fish oil can lower triglyceride levels and slightly increase good cholesterol (HDL). Fenofibrate (TriCor) is a prescription-only drug used to treat elevated cholesterol and triglycerides.

19. C: Melatonin is a natural hormone synthesized in the pineal gland in the brain. During the day, melatonin levels are low due to increased exposure to light. However, production peaks during the nighttime hours due to decreased light exposure, and this induces physiological changes that support sleep. Melatonin can also be synthetically made and is available as an OTC supplement. Evidence suggests that melatonin promotes sleep and is safe for short-term use. Zolpidem (Ambien), ramelteon (Rozerem), and doxepin (Silenor) are all prescription-only medications that are used to treat insomnia.

20. D: Citalopram (Celexa) is an SSRI antidepressant medication used to treat depression. Other agents in this drug class include escitalopram (Lexapro), fluoxetine (Prozac), fluvoxamine (Luvox), paroxetine (Paxil), and sertraline (Zoloft). Levothyroxine (Euthyrox, Levoxyl, Synthroid, Tirosint, and Unithroid) is used to treat hypothyroidism. Metoprolol (Lopressor and Toprol XL) is a beta-blocker and is used to treat angina, hypertension, and heart failure with reduced ejection fraction. Alprazolam (Xanax) is a benzodiazepine and is used to treat anxiety disorders, panic disorder, and preoperative anxiety.

21. B: According to the United States Pharmacopeia (USP) General Chapter <795>, the beyond-use date is the date after which a compounded preparation should not be used and is determined from the date that the preparation is compounded. Typically, in the absence of drug stability information, for water-containing formulations (prepared from solid form), the beyond-use date is no later than 14 days. This is because water is a viable growth medium for microorganisms to proliferate and it also has the potential to degrade the active ingredient.

22. B: Insulin is a temperature-sensitive protein in an aqueous medium. Because heat increases the rate of most chemical reactions, including protein denaturation, insulin is more stable when refrigerated at controlled cool temperatures between 36 °F and 46 °F (2°C and 8 °C). Because insulin is temperature sensitive, unopened insulin should not be frozen or stored at controlled room temperature (or higher).

23. D: Storing and maintaining intravenous (IV) solutions at the appropriate temperatures is an important consideration in preserving drug stability because temperature excursions can cause drug degradation. Exposure to light can also cause some drugs to break down, resulting in a loss of potency. Some drugs are incompatible with plastic containers and administration sets and can bind to the plastic material, thereby reducing their therapeutic efficacy. The size of an IV bag has no effect on a compounded preparation's compatibility and stability as long as the solution/diluent being used is compatible.

24. C: Clarithromycin is a macrolide antibiotic that works by binding to the 50S ribosomal subunit of susceptible bacteria, resulting in inhibition of protein synthesis. It is only available as a generic drug.

To answer this question, the required dose must first be calculated using the following steps:

1. Convert pounds into kilograms: $\frac{44 \text{ lb}}{2.2 \text{ kg/lb}} = 20$ kg.
2. Calculate the dose: $\frac{15 \text{ mg}}{\text{kg/day}} \times 20$ kg = 300 mg per day.
3. Calculate how many milliliters are required per day using the ratio-proportion method:

$$\frac{125 \text{ mg}}{5 \text{ mL}} = \frac{300 \text{ mg}}{x \text{ mL}}.$$

$$125 \text{ mg}(x) = 300 \text{ mg (5 mL)}.$$

$$x = \frac{300 \text{ mg (5 mL)}}{125 \text{ mg}} = 12 \text{ mL per day}.$$

4. Calculate how many milliliters are needed to fulfill this prescription:

$$12 \text{ mL per day} \times 7 \text{ days} = 84 \text{ mL total}.$$

The 50 mL and 75 mL bottles are too small, and the patient would run out of the medication before the end of their duration of therapy. The 150 mL bottle is too large and would result in too much waste. The most appropriate choice is the 100 mL bottle.

Clarithromycin oral suspension only comes in 125 mg/5 mL (50 mL, 100 mL) and 250 mg/5 mL (50 mL, 100 mL) doses and sizes.

25. B: The FDA defines narrow-therapeutic-index (NTI) drugs as those drugs in which small differences in the dose or blood concentration may lead to dose and blood concentration dependencies, serious therapeutic failures, or adverse drug reactions. Lithium carbonate is considered an NTI drug. It is used to treat bipolar disorder. Lithium blood levels must be closely monitored during the initiation of treatment (twice a week until the patient's status and blood levels are stable). Any deviation out of the narrow range of optimal therapy can result in either poor therapeutic efficacy (<0.5 mEq/L) or lithium toxicity (>1.5 mEq/L). Metformin (antidiabetic agent), eszopiclone (insomnia medication), and dextromethorphan (antitussive) do not require tight monitoring of drug levels.

26. B: Warfarin (Coumadin) is an oral anticoagulant used to reduce the risk of clots. Warfarin is considered an NTI drug because small fluctuations in dose can lead to subtherapeutic conditions (an increased risk for clots) or adverse reactions (an increased risk of bleeding and hemorrhage). International Normalized Ratio (INR) levels must be monitored in patients taking warfarin, and dosing must be adjusted so that the INR levels fall within the required range. Although dabigatran (Pradaxa), rivaroxaban (Xarelto), and apixaban (Eliquis) are oral anticoagulants, they are known as direct oral anticoagulants and do not require routine coagulation testing, unlike warfarin. Thus, these drugs do not fall into the NTI drug category.

27. D: Although the list of NTI drugs slightly varies between states as set forth by their boards of pharmacy, theophylline, phenytoin, and digoxin are all federally recognized NTI drugs. In addition to these, carbamazepine, levothyroxine, lithium, and warfarin are also on this list. Phenelzine (Nardil) is a monoamine oxidase inhibitor antidepressant.

28. A: Drug stability refers to the ability of an active pharmaceutical ingredient to maintain its physical and chemical properties and remain stable in a formulation. When ingredients are mixed for compounding purposes, there is the possibility for some instability to occur if the ingredients are not compatible. Other factors that influence drug stability include environmental factors (e.g., adverse temperature, humidity, light, etc.) and dosage form factors (pH, molecular binding, primary container, etc.). Drug instability and the resulting chemical degradation are difficult to detect without specific and costly analytical equipment, but excessive instability can result in observable physical changes. When compounded, creams should have a homogeneous appearance free of any grittiness, crystallization, microbial growth, or discoloration. Suppositories should not exhibit signs of excessive softening or hardening. Suppositories should remain solid at room temperature and melt at body temperature. Ointments and gels must also have a uniform appearance and physical consistency without grittiness, discoloration, or inappropriate odors. Gels should not show any signs of separation of liquid from the gel.

29. C: Recall that solutions are homogeneous mixtures; the drug is completely dissolved in the liquid vehicle. Suspensions are heterogeneous mixtures in that the drug is not dissolved but rather dispersed (aka suspended) in the liquid vehicle and can float (or sink) freely. Signs of drug instability in compounded solutions can result in precipitation, discoloration, haziness, and gas formation resulting from microbial growth. Signs of drug instability in compounded suspensions can result in caking, difficulty resuspending, and crystallization.

30. A: Several factors can affect the stability of a drug. Although the primary container does affect the product stability, a tightly closed container is preferred for compounded preparations to prevent effects from environmental factors such as exposure to carbon dioxide, oxygen, and humidity. Furthermore, exposure to adverse temperatures and light can also affect preparation stability. Other factors that can influence stability include pH, molecular binding, particle size, specific chemical additives, etc.

31. C: Amoxicillin-clavulanate (Augmentin) reconstituted oral suspension must be stored under refrigeration and discarded after 10 days. The clavulanic acid in Augmentin is unstable to heat and can deteriorate quickly, making it less effective in killing bacteria. Clarithromycin (Biaxin) dry granules and reconstituted suspension should not be stored in the refrigerator. Cefdinir (Omnicef) and nitrofurantoin (Macrobid) do not require refrigeration and can be safely kept at room temperature.

32. D: Insulin detemir (Levemir) is a long-acting insulin used once or twice daily through subcutaneous injection for the treatment of diabetes. Both the pen (Levemir FlexTouch) and vials can be stored at room temperature (below 86 °F [30 °C]) for 42 days, regardless of whether the product has been opened or is unopened. Unopened pens and vials can be stored in the refrigerator until the expiration date assigned by the manufacturer.

33. C: All chemotherapy agents are sensitive to light exposure and should constantly be protected during processing, distribution, compounding, and administration. Exposure to light could lead to product degradation and result in either drug deactivation and/or creation of undesirable photodegradation and impurities. Daunorubicin, doxorubicin, and dacarbazine are all chemotherapy agents. Other common chemotherapy agents include epirubicin, paclitaxel, docetaxel, fluorouracil, cyclophosphamide, carboplatin, cisplatin, oxaliplatin, and topotecan, among others. Didanosine is a human immunodeficiency virus antiretroviral drug belonging to the class of nucleoside reverse transcriptase inhibitors.

34. B: The FDA recommends that used needles and other sharp waste be immediately placed in FDA-cleared sharps disposal containers. These containers must be rigid, leak resistant, impervious to moisture, puncture resistant, and safe to handle. Anything capable of cutting or penetrating skin or packaging material, such as needles, glass vials, microscope slides, and scalpels, should be disposed of in a sharps container. Autoclave bags are clear or orange polyethylene plastic bags used in an autoclave to decontaminate biological waste and sterilize medical instruments. Biohazard containers are used only for nonsharp biohazardous wastes (anything containing blood and other bodily fluids).

35. A: According to the Resource Conservation and Recovery Act (RCRA) of the U.S. Environmental Protection Agency, as long as the items contain less than 3% of the former volume left, such as only trace or residual amounts of chemotherapy waste, it is considered to be "RCRA empty" waste and must be placed in a yellow container or bag and labeled as nonhazardous chemotherapy waste. Examples of yellow-bin items include empty IV bags, empty syringes, empty vials, gloves, pads, gowns, etc. Bulk chemotherapy waste such as spills and broken vials that don't qualify as RCRA empty must be cleaned following strict protocols, and all items must then be placed in a black hazardous waste bin.

36. A: The outer chemotherapy gloves should be changed every 30 minutes or whenever they are torn, punctured, or contaminated. Hands must be washed with soap and water immediately after removing gloves. Hazardous drug-resistant gowns should be changed every 2 to 3 hours (unless otherwise indicated by the manufacturer) or immediately after a spill or splash.

37. A: Recall that Lortab (hydrocodone and acetaminophen) is a schedule II drug. Schedule II (C2) drugs are those that have an accepted medical use but possess a high potential for abuse with severe physical or psychological dependency. Unlike the other scheduled drugs, refills are not permitted for schedule II drugs and a new prescription must be obtained by the prescriber each time. Schedules III, IV, and V drugs can be refilled up to five times within six months of the date that the prescription was written.

38. B: Recall that zolpidem (Ambien) is a schedule IV drug that is used to treat insomnia. According to the Controlled Substances Act of 1970, the transfer of original prescription information for a controlled substance listed in schedules III, IV, or V for the purpose of refill dispensing is permissible between pharmacies on a one-time-only basis, as long as the pharmacies do not share a real-time online database. Pharmacies that share a real-time database, such as those within the same corporation or company, may transfer the prescription up to the maximum refills permitted by law and the prescriber's authorization.

39. D: Recall that the combination medication butalbital-aspirin-caffeine is a schedule III drug used in the treatment of tension (or muscle contraction) headaches. All prescriptions for controlled substances must include the following information: the date of issue; the prescriber's name, address, and DEA number; the patient's name and address; the drug name, strength, and dosage form; the quantity prescribed; the directions for use; the number of refills (if any) authorized; and a manual signature of the prescriber.

40. D: Tramadol (Qdolo) is a schedule IV controlled substance used to treat pain. Schedule IV drugs have a lower potential for abuse than schedule III drugs, but they can still lead to limited psychological or physical dependence. Other schedule IV drugs include benzodiazepines (lorazepam [Ativan], alprazolam [Xanax], clonazepam [Klonopin], and diazepam [Valium]) and Z-drugs (zolpidem [Ambien], zaleplon, and eszopiclone [Lunesta]).

(Note: Z-drugs are a group of drugs whose names usually begin with the letter Z and are used to treat insomnia.)

41. B: A Drug Enforcement Administration (DEA) number is a unique identifier assigned to healthcare providers that allows them to handle and write prescriptions for controlled substances. Pharmacy technicians should be able to manually verify the validity of a prescription's DEA number. A DEA number consists of nine characters. The first two characters are letters, whereas the last seven are numbers.

- The first letter identifies the type of prescriber:
  - A/B/F/G – Hospital/clinic/practitioner/teaching institution/pharmacy
  - M – Midlevel practitioner (NP/PA/OD/ET, etc.)
  - P/R – Manufacturer/distributor/researcher/analytical lab/importer/exporter/reverse distributor/narcotic treatment program.
- The second letter is the first initial of the registrant's last name.
- The next six numbers are unique digits randomly assigned by the DEA.
- The final digit is called the "check digit."

Manually verifying a DEA number requires the following:

1. Add the numbers in the first, third, and fifth positions together.
2. Add the numbers in the second, fourth, and sixth positions together and multiply by two.
3. Add both of the sums together.
4. The number in the right-hand position should match the check digit (the final number) in the DEA number.

BH8253285

B = The prescriber is a physician; therefore, the first letter should be A, B, F, or G.

H = The prescriber's last name is Howard; therefore, the second letter should be H.

1. 8 + 5 + 2 = 15.
2. 2 + 3 + 8 = 13 × 2 = 26.
3. 15 + 26 = 41.
4. The last number (check digit) in the registration number should be 1.

42. C: To order schedule II medications, pharmacies must neatly and thoroughly complete a DEA Form 222. These forms are specific to the pharmacy (meaning that they cannot be shared) and are valid only for 60 days. DEA Form 222 is a triplicate order form: copies 1 and 2 are sent to the supplier, whereas copy 3 is kept by the pharmacy in a secure location for a minimum of two years. These forms must be completed with a typewriter, pen, or indelible pencil and must be signed by the person whose name is listed on the DEA registration. Only one item can be listed per line, with a maximum of 10 different items per form. The DEA is transitioning to a new single-sheet format for DEA Form 222; during this two-year transition period, the carbon-copy forms may continue to be used. DEA Form 41 is used to request permission from the DEA to destroy controlled substances. DEA Form 106 is used to document and report thefts or significant losses of controlled substances. DEA Form 224 is used by pharmacies and facilities to register with the DEA in order to dispense controlled substances. This registration must be renewed every three years using DEA Form 224a.

43. B: Pursuant to Title 21 Code of Federal Regulations §1301.75 Physical Security Controls for Practitioners: "Controlled substances listed in schedules II, III, IV, and V shall be stored in a securely locked, substantially constructed cabinet. However, pharmacies and institutional practitioners may disperse such substances throughout the stock of noncontrolled substances in such a manner as to obstruct the theft or diversion of the controlled substances."

44. C: Morphine is a schedule II controlled substance; therefore, the accident must be reported to the DEA using DEA Form 41. Although this form is used to request permission from the DEA to destroy controlled substances, it can also be used to report accidental spillage or breakage of a controlled substance. Recall that DEA Form 106 is used to document and report thefts or significant losses of controlled substances.

45. A: Under the Food and Drug Administration Amendments Act of 2007 (FDAAA), the FDA implemented a program called the Risk Evaluation and Mitigation Strategy (REMS), which informs patients of the risks associated with certain prescription drugs. REMS has been established for drugs or groups of drugs with a high risk of addiction potential, high teratogenic risk, and/or those with the potential for very harmful adverse effects. Special requirements for dispensation are established by each drug's REMS in order to manage known or potential risks associated with the drug. The iPLEDGE Program is a REMS for isotretinoin (Amnesteem, Claravis, Myorisan, Absorica, and Zenatane). Clozapine is associated with severe neutropenia, which can lead to serious and fatal infections and therefore requires a REMS. The THALOMID REMS is for thalidomide, which is highly teratogenic. Naprosyn is the brand name for naproxen, which is an OTC and prescription nonsteroidal anti-inflammatory drug.

46. A: The Combat Methamphetamine Epidemic Act of 2005 (CMEA) regulates sales, storage requirements, and recordkeeping requirements of products containing ephedrine, pseudoephedrine (PSE), or phenylpropanolamine. Enforcement of this act falls under the purview of the DEA. CMEA requires that daily and monthly limits be placed on the sale of drug products containing ephedrine, PSE, and phenylpropanolamine. The maximum amount of PSE that can be purchased in a day, regardless of the number of transactions, is 3.6 grams. This affects single- and multi-ingredient sales. Per the CMEA, individuals are prohibited from purchasing more than 9 grams of PSE during a 30-day period. Mail order companies may not sell more than 7.5 grams of product per customer during a 30-day period.

47. D: First, we need to calculate the amount of pseudoephedrine (PSE) that the patient has already purchased:

Wal-Phed D = 120 mg PSE × 10 caplets per box × 2 boxes = 2,400 mg PSE.

Claritin-D 24 Hour = 240 mg PSE × 10 tablets per box = 2,400 mg PSE.

Sudafed 24-Hour = 240 mg PSE × 10 tablets per box = 2,400 mg PSE.

2,400 mg + 2,400 mg + 2,400 mg = 7,200 mg PSE.

The maximum amount of PSE allowed in a 30-day period is 9 grams (9,000 mg). Therefore, the patient can only purchase

9,000 mg PSE (the maximum allowed) – 7,200 mg PSE (the amount already purchased) = 1,800 mg PSE.

Now, calculate how much PSE the patient would be purchasing in this transaction and compare it to the amount left that they can purchase.

Sudafed Sinus Congestion = 30 mg PSE × 24 tablets per box × 2 boxes = 1,400 mg PSE.

Comparing the numbers above, it's apparent that the patient can, in fact, legally purchase the two boxes of Sudafed Sinus Congestion.

48. B: A class I recall is a situation in which there is a reasonable probability that the use of or exposure to the drug product will cause serious adverse health consequences or death. A class II recall is a situation in which the use of or exposure to the drug product may cause temporary or medically reversible adverse health consequences or when the probability of serious adverse health consequences is unlikely. A class III recall is a situation in which use of or exposure to the drug product is not likely to cause adverse health consequences. Under FDA regulations, class IV recalls do not exist.

49. C: Once a pharmacy is notified by the FDA, drug manufacturer, or wholesaler of a drug recall, the pharmacy technician must remove all of the recalled medication from the inventory and keep it separate from other medications. The recalled drug product(s) must be removed the same day that the recall notice is received in order to prevent patients from inadvertently receiving recalled medications.

50. C: Per the Dietary Supplement Health and Education Act of 1994 (DSHEA), the FDA regulates dietary supplements under a much looser set of regulations than those of drug products (both prescription and OTC) and medical devices. Dietary supplement manufacturers are not required to present any clinical studies or safety data prior to approval. In fact, dietary supplements do not require FDA approval prior to marketing. However, under the DSHEA, manufacturers are prohibited from marketing dietary supplements that are adulterated or misbranded. The FDA is responsible for taking action against any adulterated or misbranded dietary supplement product after it reaches the market.

51. D: High-alert medications are drugs that carry a higher than normal risk of causing significant patient harm when they are used or administered in error. Mistakes with these drugs may or may not be more common, but the consequences of such mistakes are more devastating to patients than other drugs. All anticoagulants, insulin, and opioid products are considered high-alert medications in all settings (acute care, community/ambulatory, and long-term care). Anticoagulants (blood thinners) are associated with a high incidence of bleeding events, especially if used improperly. If administered improperly (too much or too soon), insulin can cause a precipitous drop in blood glucose levels resulting in altered mental status, seizure, coma, or death. Antidepressants are not considered a high-alert medication, regardless of the setting.

52. A: The Institute for Safe Medication Practices (ISMP) provides guidelines and resources on black box warnings, error-prone abbreviations, confused drug name lists, "do not crush" lists, and high-alert medication lists, just to name a few. Their list of confused drug names is updated regularly and contains common look-alike/sound-alike (LASA) drug name pairs. LASA drug name pairs are drugs with similar-looking and similar-sounding names. However, even though the names are similar, their mechanisms of action are very different and could have potentially harmful effects if inadvertently interchanged. The only similarity between Zyrtec and Zovirax is the first letter and, although this creates a similarity, it is not enough to create confusion, unlike the other pairs listed.

53. D: The Institute for Safe Medication Practices (ISMP) is an organization dedicated to preventing medication errors and is considered the gold standard for medication safety information. Although the FDA provides some guidelines on medication safety, it usually entails labeling and packaging requirements. The DEA only provides enforcement and oversight on controlled substances. The Joint Commission (TJC) provides accreditation regulations and standards for healthcare organizations.

54. B: Tall man lettering is an error prevention strategy originally created by the FDA in 2001 but later expanded upon by the ISMP. The ISMP List of Look-Alike Drug Names with Recommended Tall Man Letters contains drug name pairs with recommended, bolded uppercase letters that help highlight the differences between look-alike drug names.

55. A: The ISMP has established a list of oral medications that should not be crushed, commonly known as the "do not crush" list. Medications belonging to the list should not be crushed primarily because of their special formulations and characteristics, such as dosage forms that are slow release, extended release, and enteric coated.

56. D: The Joint Commission (TJC) is an organization responsible for accrediting and certifying more than 22,000 healthcare organizations and programs, including hospitals, ambulatory care clinics, office-based surgery suites, behavioral health facilities, laboratories, and long-term-care centers. Any healthcare facility or program accredited by TJC must include a copy of TJC's "do not use" list in their formulary. The purpose of this list is to reduce the risk of medication errors, especially with high-alert medications. Some items on the "do not use" list include U (unit), IU (international unit), QD or QOD, trailing or leading zeros, MS, MSO_4, and $MgSO_4$.

57. D: Pharmacy technicians are not allowed to make suggestions. They can provide the location of where a specific medication can be found, but all suggestions and questions outside their scope of practice should be referred to the pharmacist. Some of the more common OTC allergy medications include cetirizine (Zyrtec), loratadine (Claritin), fexofenadine (Allegra), and diphenhydramine (Benadryl). Although all OTC drugs fall into the "antihistamine" drug class, they vary in their onset of action, duration of action, and potential for drowsiness. Desloratadine (Clarinex) is only available by prescription.

58. C: One of the main goals of Omnibus Budget Reconciliation Act of 1990 was to ensure the protection and safety of patients by requiring that pharmacists conduct a prospective drug utilization review (ProDUR) of each prescription and offer counseling at the point of sale. During the ProDUR process, a new prescription is checked against the patient's profile and active medication list to determine if any potential problems may arise. Potential issues commonly addressed by a ProDUR include drug interactions, contraindications, drug-allergy interactions, therapeutic duplication, incorrect dosage, inappropriate duration of therapy, etc. Pharmacy technicians must defer all clinical decisions to the pharmacist.

59. C: Although still an adverse event reporting system, the Vaccines Adverse Event Reporting System (VAERS) is used to report adverse events associated with vaccines, not medications. VAERS is a collaboration between the FDA and CDC. Similar to the FDA Adverse Event Reporting System (FAERS), VAERS collects and analyzes postmarketing safety information from reports of adverse events following the administration of vaccines. MedWatch is the FDA's medical product safety reporting program for health professionals, patients, and consumers. MedWatch collects, analyzes, and publishes safety reports for FDA-regulated products such as prescription and OTC medicines, biologics, medical devices, combination products, nutritional products (supplements, medical food, and infant formula), cosmetics, and foods. The ISMP established a voluntary error-reporting program called Medication Error Reporting and Prevention (MERP) in which information is collected anonymously to learn about and analyze medication errors.

60. A: A near-miss event is a medication error that took place but was discovered before reaching the patient. These types of events or situations are considered "close calls" because they are still a medication error, but one that did not reach the patient. A sentinel event is a medication error that results in death or serious injury to a patient.

61. C: Like most error reporting systems, MEDMARX is anonymous. The purpose of all of these medical product and vaccine safety reporting programs is to determine the causes of the errors in hopes of not repeating them again. Healthcare professionals and consumers are encouraged to report any concerns or errors without fear of punishment. MEDMARX is overseen by the USP and is designed for use by hospitals and health systems to collect, analyze, and report adverse drug reactions and medication errors.

Recall: MedWatch and FAERS are both overseen by the FDA. VAERS is cosponsored by the FDA and CDC. MERP, the Vaccine Errors Reporting Program, and C-MERP (consumer) are overseen by the ISMP. All of these systems collect information anonymously with the goal of preventing future errors.

62. B: The FDA defines a medication error as any preventable event that may cause or lead to inappropriate medication use or patient harm while the medication is in the control of a healthcare provider, patient, or consumer. A compliance error is defined as inappropriate patient behavior regarding adherence to a prescribed medication regimen. Lisinopril is an ACE inhibitor commonly used to treat hypertension. This medication is typically prescribed as a once-daily medication, meaning that if the patient were taking the medication appropriately, then they would require monthly refills.

63. A: A medication error is a preventable mistake that can occur at various steps in the patient care process, from the point of prescribing the medication to the time when the patient is administered the drug. A prescribing error is one that occurs at the ordering or prescribing stage. These types of errors typically involve the prescribing provider writing the wrong medication, the wrong route or dose, or the wrong frequency. Amoxicillin is an antibiotic belonging to the penicillin family and is considered inappropriate for use in patients with penicillin allergies. A dispensing error occurs at the pharmacy level. It can involve errors in prescription interpretation, transcription, calculations, and filling. Administration errors occur once the medication has left the pharmacy.

64. B: A dispensing error occurs at the pharmacy level and can involve errors in prescription interpretation, transcription, calculations, and filling. A prescribing error occurs at the prescriber level and can include not specifying the route of administration, quantity to be filled, or instructions for use on the prescription. Writing a prescription for a drug that a patient is known to be allergic to also falls under the "prescribing error" category. Administration errors occur once the drug leaves the pharmacy and involve incorrectly administering the medication to the patient (wrong route of administration). A deteriorated drug error is administration of an expired drug or one in which the physical or chemical dosage-form integrity has been compromised.

65. B: Nothing should be permitted to come in contact with the HEPA filter, including disinfecting solutions. Great care must be exercised to avoid getting HEPA filters wet to avoid contamination. Ampules should be broken away from the HEPA filter to avoid accidental contamination. Furthermore, laminar workflow benches must be inspected and certified every six months to ensure their proper working condition. If the HEPA filter becomes contaminated or wet at any point of use, the filter must be replaced immediately and the workbench requires recertification.

66. A: Before entering the anteroom, the compounding technician must remove any outwear (coat, hat, etc.), makeup (if applicable), and all hand and wrist jewelry. The technician will then enter the anteroom and begin the garbing process. Although the garbing and hand-washing order is determined by each facility and documented in the standard operating procedures manual, shoe covers are always put on first to minimize the risk of contamination. Logically, someone about to enter a sterile area would want to touch their shoes before moving onto hand washing; donning the face mask, gown, etc.; and ending with putting on sterile, powder-free gloves.

67. B: Finasteride (Proscar) is 5-alpha-reductase inhibitor used to treat androgenetic alopecia and benign prostatic hyperplasia. It is also available under the brand name Propecia. This medication is considered highly teratogenic (FDA pregnancy category X), and the residue powder from the tablets can be absorbed through the skin. Therefore, women who are pregnant or may be pregnant should not handle finasteride because of the possibility of absorption and the potential risk of fetal abnormalities to a male fetus. For this reason, any counting tray that may contain drug powder residue must be immediately and thoroughly wiped clean to prevent cross contamination. This is also true for drugs with high allergic rates such as penicillin and sulfa-drug groups, as well as antineoplastic agents with high teratogenicity such as tamoxifen (Soltamox) and methotrexate (Trexall, Otrexup, Rasuvo, and Xatmep).

68. B: Ophthalmic (from the root *ophthalm/o*, meaning "eye") preparations are administered to the eyes. The eye is a sensitive organ, and ophthalmic formulations must be prepared using the same standards as parenteral products with regard to sterility, buffers, and isotonicity. These products must be prepared using aseptic techniques to prevent microbial contamination, and they must also include preservatives to prevent microbial growth. In addition to sterility, these products should have the same tonicity as lacrimal fluid (0.9% sodium chloride). Excessive deviations outside of the range of 0.5–1.8% of sodium chloride can cause eye injury. (Hint: the root *ot/o* means "ear.")

69. D: A suspension is a dispersion of insoluble drug particles that is evenly distributed (suspended) in a liquid medium. If left undisturbed for an extended period of time, the drug particulates will settle out of the mixture and cause improper dosing. All suspensions should be marked with a "shake well" label. Recall that PO (Latin: *per os*) means "by mouth"; therefore, this product will not be used for external use or otic (ear) purposes. This type of medication does not affect the nervous system and will not cause dizziness.

70. C: Parenteral products must be sterile, isosmotic, isotonic with blood (0.9% sodium chloride), and made with USP-grade ingredients. Any products used to compound these products (all injectables) must be sterile in order to prevent infection and vascular injury. Sterile water for irrigation is indicated for use as an irrigant and not for IV injection. Unlike sterile water for injection, sterile water for irrigation is hypotonic with blood and can cause hemolysis.

71. C: It is important to be able to complete pharmacy calculations with speed, efficiency, and accuracy. One of the most common calculations that a technician will need to solve is quantity dispensed. The quantity dispensed is exactly as it sounds: the amount (or quantity) of medication that will need to be dispensed in order to fill the prescription. Incorrectly calculating the quantity dispensed can lead to a variety of problems, such as the patient receiving the wrong amount of medication (too little or too much), denied insurance claims, and insurance audit flags. In order to calculate the quantity dispensed, it is imperative that technicians have a strong grasp on sig codes and conversions. The simplest way to calculate the quantity dispensed is using the following formula: dose × frequency × duration = quantity dispensed. The dose is how much of the medication is to be taken. In this problem, the dose is one capsule. The frequency is how often this dose is going to be taken. In this problem, the frequency is TID, which is three times a day (or every eight hours). The duration is how long the patient will need to take the medication. In this problem, the duration is seven days. For this question, it is not necessary to know the weight or demographics of the patient. On the certification exam, this information is known as a distractor and is just extra information meant to confuse test takers.

Formula: Dose × frequency × duration

Answer: 1 capsule × 3 times a day × 7 days = 21 capsules to be dispensed to fulfill this prescription.

(Note: QS means quantity sufficient, which represents a large enough amount to fill the prescription or order.)

72. B: Test-takers can instantly eliminate both cefdinir 250 mg/5 mL because the prescription is written for 125 mg/5 mL.

1. First, to convert pounds to kilograms: 46.5 lb ÷ 2.2 kg = 21.

    (Remember that in pediatrics, doses are rounded down to err on the side of caution.)

2. Calculate the dose needed: 7 mg/kg × 21 kg = 147 mg.
3. Use the ratio-proportion method to calculate how many milliliters are needed for one dose (147 mg):

$$\frac{125 \text{ mg}}{5 \text{ mL}} = \frac{147 \text{ mg}}{x \text{ mL}} \rightarrow x = 5.8 \text{ mL}.$$

4. Now, calculate how many milliliters are needed for the duration of treatment:

$$5.8 \text{ mL} \times 2 \text{ doses per day (BID)} \times 7 \text{ days} = 81.2 \text{ mL}.$$

At least 81.2 mL will be needed to correctly fill this prescription.

73. C: In order to solve this type of problem, the pharmacy technician will need to use the alligation method, also commonly called the tic-tac-toe method. A prescriber may write a prescription for a medication in a strength that is not commercially available. This typically occurs in compounding pharmacy settings. The compounding technician may be required to mix two different strengths (or concentrations) of the same active ingredient of a drug to fulfill the prescription order. The alligation method is when a lower percent concentration of a drug is mixed with a higher percent concentration of a drug to make the desired concentration at a strength between the two.

(Note: A higher concentration of a drug cannot be made with two concentrations of lower value. For instance, a 10% solution cannot be compounded from a 2% solution and a 7% solution. The desired strength must fall in between the two concentrations in stock.)

In order to solve this problem, the pharmacist must correctly set it up using a tic-tac-toe board:

Have	Want	Need
A (higher percentage)		D = C – B (parts of higher percentage)
	B (desired percentage)	
C (lower percentage)		E = A – B (parts of lower percentage)

In the "Have" column, place the concentrations of the items the pharmacy has in stock or on hand with the higher percentage at the top (A) and the lower percentage at the bottom (C).

In the "Want" column, place the desired concentration (the prescription order) in the middle.

The "Need" column is calculated by cross subtracting the first two columns. This will provide the parts of each corresponding concentration needed to correctly compound the order.

1. Convert ounces to grams (30 g are in an ounce): 4.5 oz × 30 g/oz = 135 g of final product needed.
2. Set up the alligation grid:

Have	Want	Need
10%		3 = 4 – 1 (parts of higher percentage)
	4%	
1%		6 = 10 – 4 (parts of lower percentage)

As is evident from the grid, the pharmacist needs three parts 10% hydrocortisone and six parts 1% hydrocortisone in order to compound this order.

3. Calculate the total number of parts: 3 + 6 = 9 total parts.
4. Divide each individual part by the total number of parts: 3/9 = 0.3333 and 6/9 = 0.6666.
5. Multiply each portion by the total volume required. In this case, it's 135 g:

0.3333 × 135 g = 44.999 = 45 g.

0.6666 × 135 g = 89.991 = 90 g.

Therefore, the technician will need 45 g of 10% hydrocortisone and 90 g of 1% hydrocortisone to compound 135 g of 4% hydrocortisone cream.

10%		3 parts of 10%	3/9 × 135 g = 45 g (rounded) of 10% hydrocortisone cream
	4%		
1%		6 parts of 1%	6/9 x 135 g = 90 g (rounded) of 1% hydrocortisone cream

The answer can be verified by adding both quantities together to see if the sum corresponds with the quantity desired (the amount on the prescription):

$$45 \text{ g} + 90 \text{ g} = 135 \text{ g}.$$

74. D: This question tests a lot of the necessary concepts for pharmacy technicians to master in order to be successful not only on the certification exam, but also in their careers. To solve this problem, the percent strength must first be converted into a ratio. In this question, it is a w/v percent strength, meaning the top value of the ratio (aka fraction) will be a weight (g) and the bottom will be the volume (mL).

$$w/v = \frac{1 \text{ g}}{100 \text{ mL}} = 1\%.$$

Other percent strengths can be written as follows:

$$w/w = \frac{1 \text{ g}}{100 \text{ g}} = 1\% \quad \text{and} \quad v/v = \frac{1 \text{ mL}}{100 \text{ mL}} = 1\%.$$

If a drug is 3% in w/v strength, then it would be written as

$$w/v = \frac{3 \text{ g}}{100 \text{ mL}} = 3\%.$$

Moving back to solving this question—move onto the ratio-proportion method in order to finish solving this question. The ratio-proportion method involves comparing two ratios (aka fractions) separated by an equal sign (=) with one missing variable (x). It is essential that pharmacy technicians master the ratio-proportion method because it accounts for more than 60% of pharmacy calculations commonly done in a hospital setting.

It is established that 1% means 1 g/100 mL and that the medication order is for furosemide 150 mg. The question is asking "how many milliliters?" So the variable x will be in milliliters (mL). It is crucial that, when completing the ratio-proportion method, the units on each side of the equal sign match. In this example, either convert 1 g to mg or convert 150 mg to grams. This will show both ways.

1. $\dfrac{1\text{ g}}{100\text{ mL}} = \dfrac{0.15\text{ g}}{x\text{ mL}}.$

2. $\dfrac{1{,}000\text{ mg}}{100\text{ mL}} = \dfrac{150\text{ mg}}{x\text{ mL}}.$

Regardless of which setup is used, now solve for x by cross multiplying and getting x alone on one side.

1. $\dfrac{1\text{ g}}{100\text{ mL}} = \dfrac{0.15\text{ g}}{x\text{ mL}}$ → $1\text{ g}\,(x\text{ mL}) = 0.15\text{ g}\,(100\text{ mL})$ → $x = 15\text{ mL}.$

2. $\dfrac{1{,}000\text{ mg}}{100\text{ mL}} = \dfrac{150\text{ mg}}{x\text{ mL}}$ → $1{,}000\text{ mg}\,(x\text{ mL}) = 150\text{ mg}\,(100\text{ mL})$ → $x = 15\text{ mL}.$

75. D: One of the most common calculations performed in retail or community pharmacy is finding the day's supply of a medication. Correctly calculating the day's supply is crucial in ensuring that insurance claims are correctly processed to prevent claim rejections or audit red flags.

The first step is to examine the dosing instructions. In this case, the medication is being dosed every 8 to 12 hours. Now find out how many tablets a day that represents and which is the maximum:

$\dfrac{24\text{ hours}}{\text{day}} \times \dfrac{1\text{ tab}}{8\text{ hours}} = 3$ tablets per day (Q8).

$\dfrac{24\text{ hours}}{\text{day}} \times \dfrac{1\text{ tab}}{12\text{ hours}} = 2$ tablets per day (Q12).

Therefore, the maximum number of tablets that a patient can take during one day is three.

Now, divide the amount to be dispensed by the maximum number of tablets in a single day:

$24 \div 3 = 8$ days.

76. A: By definition, the percent concentration of a solution (w/v) is the number of grams in 100 mL.

$$\dfrac{x\text{ g}}{100\text{ mL}} = x\%$$

First, convert 250 mg → g: $\dfrac{250\text{ mg}}{1} \times \dfrac{1\text{ g}}{1{,}000\text{ mg}} = 0.25$ g.

Next, set up the ratio proportion to calculate the percentage (g): $\dfrac{x\%}{100\text{ mL}} = \dfrac{0.25\text{ g}}{50\text{ mL}}.$

Solve for x: $x\% = \dfrac{0.25\text{ g}\,(100\text{ mL})}{50\text{ mL}} = 0.5\%.$

77. D: Proventil HFA (albuterol sulfate) is a short-acting beta-agonist bronchodilator that is used to treat or prevent bronchospasm in people with reversible obstructive airway disease, typically asthma. Proper administration of metered-dose inhalers is difficult in most patients and even more so in pediatric patients. Therefore, a spacer is typically recommended to be attached to the metered-dose inhaler in order to hold the medication in place so that it is easier to move deep into the lungs. A spacer is a cylindrical tube that creates a space between the output of the inhaler and the patient's mouth.

78. A: In order to test blood glucose levels, diabetic patients require a host of medical devices, starting with an isopropyl alcohol swab, glucometer and glucometer strips, as well as a lancet. Although considered a medical device, oral syringes provided little value to patients with diabetes. On the other hand, hypodermic or insulin syringes used for subcutaneous drug administration are another medical device commonly used in diabetic patients.

79. A: A syringe needle has four major parts: the hub, the shaft, the bevel, and the lumen. The hub is the part that attaches to the syringe. The shaft is the long, thin, stainless-steel stem of the needle. The bevel is the angled tip (point) of the needle. The lumen (opening) is the hollow bore of the needle shaft. The diameter of the lumen is inversely proportional to the needle gauge size. This means that the higher the gauge, the smaller the diameter of the lumen. The lower the gauge, the larger the diameter of the lumen.

80. B: FDA-approved drug products are identified and reported using a unique 10- or 11-digit, three-segment number called the National Drug Code (NDC) number, which serves as a product identifier for drugs. The NDC number identifies the labeler, product, and trade package size. The first set of numbers (segment) is assigned by the FDA and is called the labeler code. This identifies the drug manufacturer or distributor. The second set of numbers is called the product code. This identifies the drug's specific strength, dosage form, and formulation. The third set of numbers is the package code and identifies package sizes and types (e.g., 100 tablets, 50 tablets, 125 mL, 100 mL, 80 mL, etc.). Both the product and package codes are assigned by the manufacturer. Drugs produced by the same manufacturer will always share the same first segment. In the example above, both Drug Bottle A and Drug Bottle B have a labeler code of 0093, meaning they are produced by the same manufacturer. Some drugs may share the same labeler and product code but come in different package sizes. The NDC number should be used when filling prescriptions, and all digits should be matched to the label generated by the computer. Some drugs may share the same middle segment (the product code), which is commonly bolded and/or enlarged on most labels, but they may still be completely different drugs. It is important that all pharmacy personnel check and match the entire NDC number when filling and verifying prescriptions.

81. C: For unit-dose repackaged products, USP General Chapter <1178> Good Repackaging Practices recommends that the expiration date NOT exceed (1) six months from the date of repackaging, (2) the manufacturer's expiration date, or (3) 25% of the time between the date of repackaging and the expiration date shown on the manufacturer's bulk article container of the drug being repackaged, whichever is earlier.

82. B: The dispense-as-written (DAW) code is a product selection code that is transmitted to third-party payers (e.g., insurance) with the claim that indicates special circumstances. DAW code 1 is used when the brand-name drug is deemed medically necessary by the prescriber and no generic substitution is allowed. Some prescribers are of the opinion that a brand-name drug, especially for that of a narrow-therapeutic-index (NTI) drug, has consistently received better results than the generic version; therefore, the brand-name drug is deemed necessary for treatment purposes. Other DAW codes include the following:

DAW 0 = No product selection indicated
DAW 2 = Substitution allowed – patient-requested product dispensed
DAW 3 = Substitution allowed – pharmacist-selected product dispensed
DAW 4 = Substitution allowed – generic drug not in stock
DAW 5 = Substitution allowed – brand-name drug dispensed as generic
DAW 6 = Override
DAW 7 = Substitution NOT allowed – brand-name drug mandated by law

DAW 8 = Substitution allowed – generic drug not available in the marketplace

DAW 9 = Other

83. C: Although the number of maximum days varies among the different chain and independent pharmacies, the procedure is similar. Once the pickup window has closed for a prescription, the technician will edit the prescription in the system as "not picked up" and the prescription will be stored on the patient's electronic profile for future filling. Pharmacies must immediately reverse any charges adjudicated to third-party providers (i.e., insurance) in order to avoid triggering an audit. The medication is then returned to stock. Pharmacies are prohibited from returning drug products back to their stock once they leave the pharmacy's possession. As long as the dispensed medication does not leave the pharmacy area, the medication can be returned to stock.

84. D: Medications damaged in transit to the pharmacy must be promptly reported to the drug wholesaler or manufacturer to ensure that the medication is promptly reordered and credit is provided to the pharmacy. The damaged medication is then returned to the distributor. Medications under FDA recall must be pulled from inventory and returned to the wholesaler or manufacturer. Medications close to expiration (open or not) can be sent back to the wholesaler or manufacturer for a full refund or partial credit, depending on how many months of good dating are left.

85. B: Vilazodone (Viibryd), trazodone, nefazodone, and vortioxetine (Trintellix) are all atypical antidepressants indicated for the treatment of major depressive disorder. They are considered atypical in that they do not belong to one of the four major classes of antidepressants: SSRIs, serotonin-norepinephrine reuptake inhibitors, tricyclic antidepressants, and monoamine oxidase inhibitors. Atypical antidepressants are each unique in different ways from one another. Other atypical antidepressants include bupropion (Wellbutrin) and mirtazapine (Remeron).

86. A: Atorvastatin (Lipitor), lovastatin (Mevacor), rosuvastatin (Crestor), and simvastatin (Zocor) belong to the "statin" drug class. Statins (also called HMG-CoA reductase inhibitors) are a class of lipid-lowering drugs commonly used in the treatment of hyperlipidemia. Other statins include pravastatin (Pravachol) and fluvastatin (Lescol). They are called "statins" because all of the generic drug names in this class end in the suffix *-statin*.

87. C: Fluticasone (Flovent HFA), albuterol (ProAir Digihaler, Proventil HFA, Ventolin HFA), and montelukast (Singulair) are all commonly used drugs in the treatment of asthma.

Fluticasone (Flovent HFA) is an inhaled corticosteroid (ICS) with potent anti-inflammatory activity. It is used as a maintenance treatment of asthma for prophylactic therapy. Inflammation is an important component in the pathogenesis (pathological process) of asthma. Corticosteroids have been shown to inhibit various inflammatory cell types and mediator production or secretion involved in the asthmatic response. These anti-inflammatory actions of corticosteroids contribute to their effectiveness in the treatment of asthma. These medications must be taken continuously, and levels need to build up in the body in order to have an effect. Other ICS drugs include beclomethasone dipropionate (Qvar), budesonide (Pulmicort), flunisolide (Aerobid), mometasone (Asmanex), and ciclesonide (Alvesco). Albuterol is a short-acting beta$_2$ agonist that works by relaxing bronchial smooth muscle (bronchial dilation). This drug is considered a "rescue" medication because it can be taken during a flare-up and provide relief. Montelukast (Singulair) is a leukotriene receptor antagonist indicated for prophylaxis and chronic treatment of asthma in patients 12 months and older. This class of asthma drug can help prevent symptoms for up to 24 hours. Other leukotriene synthesis inhibitors include zafirlukast (Accolate) and zileuton (Zyflo). Nadolol (Corgard) is a nonselective beta-blocker used in the treatment of hypertension and in the long-term management of angina. The generic names for beta-blockers typically end in -*olol*, except for carvedilol and labetalol. Beta-blockers are commonly used in the treatment of cardiovascular disorders such as angina, hypertension, and heart failure. Some are more selective than others and produce different results. Beta-blockers work by binding and blocking the action of beta-receptors. Beta-receptors can be found in the heart (beta$_1$) and lungs (beta$_2$). Blocking beta-receptors in the heart is useful for the treatment of cardiovascular disease, but blocking beta-receptors in the lungs can produce deleterious effects in patients with asthma. Beta-blockers, especially nonselective beta-blockers, not only reduce the benefits of beta$_2$ adrenergic bronchodilators (e.g., albuterol), but also cause life-threatening bronchospasms in patients with asthma and other obstructive airway diseases. Due to these opposing effects on beta$_2$ receptors, propranolol has been used in the treatment of albuterol overdose.

88. A: Understanding conversions is necessary to be successful on both the certification and in the field. For example, some common conversions include the following:

Weight			
	2.2 lb	1 kg	
Volume			
	5 mL	1 teaspoon (tsp)	
	15 mL	1 tablespoon (tbsp)	3 tsp
	30 mL	1 oz	2 tbsp
	8 oz	1 cup	
Apothecary			
	1 lb	454 g	
	1 oz	30 g	

(This is not an all-inclusive list.)

In this question, 1 oz must first be converted into 30 g. Then take 476/30 g = 15.866. Because the question asks how many jars can be filled, it is necessary to round down to 15 jars.

89. D: In order to solve this question, first convert 1/8 oz to g. Knowing that 1 oz = 30 g means that 1/8 oz = 0.125 oz (to convert fractions to decimals, divide the numerator by the denominator).

$$\frac{1 \text{ oz}}{30 \text{ g}} = \frac{0.125 \text{ oz}}{x \text{ g}}$$

$$x \text{ g} = 0.125 \times 30 = 3.75 \text{ g.}$$

Now the grams must be converted into micrograms. Converting between the different metric units is crucial for all technicians to master. There are two ways of learning this conversion. The first way is by either dividing or multiplying by 1,000, depending on the direction of conversion. The second way is by moving the decimal space either left or right, depending again on the direction of conversion.

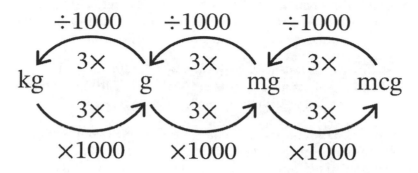

To convert from left (kg) to right (mcg), either multiply by 1,000 three times (once for each unit) or move the decimal space to the left nine times (three times for each unit).

Example: 1 kg = 1,000 g = 1,000,000 mg = 1,000,0000,000 mcg.

(Hint: If converting from a large unit of measurement [kg] to a smaller unit of measurement [mcg], the number should get bigger.)

To convert from right (mcg) to left (kg), either divide by 1,000 three times (once for each unit) or move the decimal space to the right nine times (three times for each unit).

Example: 1 mcg = 0.001 mg = 0.000001 g = 0.000000001 kg.

(Hint: If converting from a small unit of measurement [mcg] to a larger unit of measurement [kg], the number should get smaller.)

For this question, the objective is to convert 3.75 g → mcg. Using the image above, this can be done in one of two ways:

- Multiply by 1,000 twice: 3.75g x 1,000 = 3,750mg x 1,000 = 3,750,000 mcg.
- Move the decimal space to the right six times (adding zeros in place of each empty space):

$$3.75g \rightarrow mcg$$

$$3.750. = 3,750 \ mg$$

$$3.750000. = 3,750,000 \ mcg$$

90. A: USP General Chapter <795> Pharmaceutical Compounding—Nonsterile Preparations focuses on applying good compounding practices to the process of preparing nonsterile compounded medications. This includes, but is not limited to, the compounding process, facility requirements, personnel training, documentation, and quality controls.

USP General Chapter <797> Pharmaceutical Compounding—Sterile Preparations provides the procedures and requirements for compounding sterile medications. This includes, but is not limited to, training and responsibilities of compounding personnel, environmental monitoring and controls, storage and testing of finished preparations, and infection control methods. USP <797> covers compounding standards for nonhazardous and hazardous sterile products.

USP General Chapter <800> Hazardous Drugs—Handling in Healthcare Settings focuses on standards for the safe handling of hazardous drugs in healthcare settings to minimize the risk of exposure to personnel, patients, and the environment.

USP General Chapter <825> Radiopharmaceuticals—Preparations, Compounding, Dispensing, and Repackaging provides standards for the preparation, compounding, dispensing, and repackaging of sterile and nonsterile radiopharmaceuticals for use in humans and animals.

Four Additional PTCB Practice Tests

To take these additional PTCB practice tests, visit our bonus page:
mometrix.com/bonus948/ptcb

PTCB Image Credits

Licensed Under CC BY 4.0 (creativecommons.org/licenses/by/4.0/)

Diltiazem Generics: "Diltiazem 3" by Mark Oniffrey
(https://commons.wikimedia.org/wiki/File:Diltiazem_3_(cropped).jpg)

Syringe: "Insulin Syringe" by rebcenter-moscow.ru
(https://commons.wikimedia.org/wiki/File:Insulin_syringe_foto.jpg)

Syringe Disassembled: "Insulin Syringe in Disassembled Form" by rebcenter-moscow.ru
(https://commons.wikimedia.org/wiki/File:Insulin_syringe_in_disassembled_form.jpg)

Pen Needle Pen: "Insulin Analog 100 IU-1ml Novomix Pen" by Wikimedia user Wesalius
(https://commons.wikimedia.org/wiki/File:Insulin_analog_100_IU-1ml_novomix_pen_white_background.jpg)

Unit Dose Packaging: "Pharmaceutical Blister Pack B" by Wikimedia user Michiel4
(https://commons.wikimedia.org/wiki/File:Pharmaceutical_Blister_Pack_b.png)

Licensed Under CC BY-SA 3.0 (creativecommons.org/licenses/by-sa/3.0/deed.en)

Asthma Spacer: "Asthma spacer" by Wikimedia user Tradimus
(https://commons.wikimedia.org/wiki/File:Asthma_spacer.JPG)

Planes of Movement: "Human anatomy planes" by YassineMrabet
(https://commons.wikimedia.org/wiki/File:Human_anatomy_planes.svg)

Automated Dispenser: " File:Kirby Lester KL60 fully-automated dispensing system" by Kirby Lester, LLC (https://commons.wikimedia.org/wiki/File:Kirby_Lester_KL60_fully-automated_dispensing_system.jpg)

How to Overcome Test Anxiety

Just the thought of taking a test is enough to make most people a little nervous. A test is an important event that can have a long-term impact on your future, so it's important to take it seriously and it's natural to feel anxious about performing well. But just because anxiety is normal, that doesn't mean that it's helpful in test taking, or that you should simply accept it as part of your life. Anxiety can have a variety of effects. These effects can be mild, like making you feel slightly nervous, or severe, like blocking your ability to focus or remember even a simple detail.

If you experience test anxiety—whether severe or mild—it's important to know how to beat it. To discover this, first you need to understand what causes test anxiety.

Causes of Test Anxiety

While we often think of anxiety as an uncontrollable emotional state, it can actually be caused by simple, practical things. One of the most common causes of test anxiety is that a person does not feel adequately prepared for their test. This feeling can be the result of many different issues such as poor study habits or lack of organization, but the most common culprit is time management. Starting to study too late, failing to organize your study time to cover all of the material, or being distracted while you study will mean that you're not well prepared for the test. This may lead to cramming the night before, which will cause you to be physically and mentally exhausted for the test. Poor time management also contributes to feelings of stress, fear, and hopelessness as you realize you are not well prepared but don't know what to do about it.

Other times, test anxiety is not related to your preparation for the test but comes from unresolved fear. This may be a past failure on a test, or poor performance on tests in general. It may come from comparing yourself to others who seem to be performing better or from the stress of living up to expectations. Anxiety may be driven by fears of the future—how failure on this test would affect your educational and career goals. These fears are often completely irrational, but they can still negatively impact your test performance.

Elements of Test Anxiety

As mentioned earlier, test anxiety is considered to be an emotional state, but it has physical and mental components as well. Sometimes you may not even realize that you are suffering from test anxiety until you notice the physical symptoms. These can include trembling hands, rapid heartbeat, sweating, nausea, and tense muscles. Extreme anxiety may lead to fainting or vomiting. Obviously, any of these symptoms can have a negative impact on testing. It is important to recognize them as soon as they begin to occur so that you can address the problem before it damages your performance.

The mental components of test anxiety include trouble focusing and inability to remember learned information. During a test, your mind is on high alert, which can help you recall information and stay focused for an extended period of time. However, anxiety interferes with your mind's natural processes, causing you to blank out, even on the questions you know well. The strain of testing during anxiety makes it difficult to stay focused, especially on a test that may take several hours. Extreme anxiety can take a huge mental toll, making it difficult not only to recall test information but even to understand the test questions or pull your thoughts together.

Effects of Test Anxiety

Test anxiety is like a disease—if left untreated, it will get progressively worse. Anxiety leads to poor performance, and this reinforces the feelings of fear and failure, which in turn lead to poor performances on subsequent tests. It can grow from a mild nervousness to a crippling condition. If allowed to progress, test anxiety can have a big impact on your schooling, and consequently on your future.

Test anxiety can spread to other parts of your life. Anxiety on tests can become anxiety in any stressful situation, and blanking on a test can turn into panicking in a job situation. But fortunately, you don't have to let anxiety rule your testing and determine your grades. There are a number of relatively simple steps you can take to move past anxiety and function normally on a test and in the rest of life.

Physical Steps for Beating Test Anxiety

While test anxiety is a serious problem, the good news is that it can be overcome. It doesn't have to control your ability to think and remember information. While it may take time, you can begin taking steps today to beat anxiety.

Just as your first hint that you may be struggling with anxiety comes from the physical symptoms, the first step to treating it is also physical. Rest is crucial for having a clear, strong mind. If you are tired, it is much easier to give in to anxiety. But if you establish good sleep habits, your body and mind will be ready to perform optimally, without the strain of exhaustion. Additionally, sleeping well helps you to retain information better, so you're more likely to recall the answers when you see the test questions.

Getting good sleep means more than going to bed on time. It's important to allow your brain time to relax. Take study breaks from time to time so it doesn't get overworked, and don't study right before bed. Take time to rest your mind before trying to rest your body, or you may find it difficult to fall asleep.

Along with sleep, other aspects of physical health are important in preparing for a test. Good nutrition is vital for good brain function. Sugary foods and drinks may give a burst of energy but this burst is followed by a crash, both physically and emotionally. Instead, fuel your body with protein and vitamin-rich foods.

Also, drink plenty of water. Dehydration can lead to headaches and exhaustion, especially if your brain is already under stress from the rigors of the test. Particularly if your test is a long one, drink water during the breaks. And if possible, take an energy-boosting snack to eat between sections.

Along with sleep and diet, a third important part of physical health is exercise. Maintaining a steady workout schedule is helpful, but even taking 5-minute study breaks to walk can help get your blood pumping faster and clear your head. Exercise also releases endorphins, which contribute to a positive feeling and can help combat test anxiety.

When you nurture your physical health, you are also contributing to your mental health. If your body is healthy, your mind is much more likely to be healthy as well. So take time to rest, nourish your body with healthy food and water, and get moving as much as possible. Taking these physical steps will make you stronger and more able to take the mental steps necessary to overcome test anxiety.

Mental Steps for Beating Test Anxiety

Working on the mental side of test anxiety can be more challenging, but as with the physical side, there are clear steps you can take to overcome it. As mentioned earlier, test anxiety often stems from lack of preparation, so the obvious solution is to prepare for the test. Effective studying may be the most important weapon you have for beating test anxiety, but you can and should employ several other mental tools to combat fear.

First, boost your confidence by reminding yourself of past success—tests or projects that you aced. If you're putting as much effort into preparing for this test as you did for those, there's no reason you should expect to fail here. Work hard to prepare; then trust your preparation.

Second, surround yourself with encouraging people. It can be helpful to find a study group, but be sure that the people you're around will encourage a positive attitude. If you spend time with others who are anxious or cynical, this will only contribute to your own anxiety. Look for others who are motivated to study hard from a desire to succeed, not from a fear of failure.

Third, reward yourself. A test is physically and mentally tiring, even without anxiety, and it can be helpful to have something to look forward to. Plan an activity following the test, regardless of the outcome, such as going to a movie or getting ice cream.

When you are taking the test, if you find yourself beginning to feel anxious, remind yourself that you know the material. Visualize successfully completing the test. Then take a few deep, relaxing breaths and return to it. Work through the questions carefully but with confidence, knowing that you are capable of succeeding.

Developing a healthy mental approach to test taking will also aid in other areas of life. Test anxiety affects more than just the actual test—it can be damaging to your mental health and even contribute to depression. It's important to beat test anxiety before it becomes a problem for more than testing.

Study Strategy

Being prepared for the test is necessary to combat anxiety, but what does being prepared look like? You may study for hours on end and still not feel prepared. What you need is a strategy for test prep. The next few pages outline our recommended steps to help you plan out and conquer the challenge of preparation.

STEP 1: SCOPE OUT THE TEST

Learn everything you can about the format (multiple choice, essay, etc.) and what will be on the test. Gather any study materials, course outlines, or sample exams that may be available. Not only will this help you to prepare, but knowing what to expect can help to alleviate test anxiety.

STEP 2: MAP OUT THE MATERIAL

Look through the textbook or study guide and make note of how many chapters or sections it has. Then divide these over the time you have. For example, if a book has 15 chapters and you have five days to study, you need to cover three chapters each day. Even better, if you have the time, leave an extra day at the end for overall review after you have gone through the material in depth.

If time is limited, you may need to prioritize the material. Look through it and make note of which sections you think you already have a good grasp on, and which need review. While you are studying, skim quickly through the familiar sections and take more time on the challenging parts.

Write out your plan so you don't get lost as you go. Having a written plan also helps you feel more in control of the study, so anxiety is less likely to arise from feeling overwhelmed at the amount to cover.

STEP 3: GATHER YOUR TOOLS

Decide what study method works best for you. Do you prefer to highlight in the book as you study and then go back over the highlighted portions? Or do you type out notes of the important information? Or is it helpful to make flashcards that you can carry with you? Assemble the pens, index cards, highlighters, post-it notes, and any other materials you may need so you won't be distracted by getting up to find things while you study.

If you're having a hard time retaining the information or organizing your notes, experiment with different methods. For example, try color-coding by subject with colored pens, highlighters, or post-it notes. If you learn better by hearing, try recording yourself reading your notes so you can listen while in the car, working out, or simply sitting at your desk. Ask a friend to quiz you from your flashcards, or try teaching someone the material to solidify it in your mind.

STEP 4: CREATE YOUR ENVIRONMENT

It's important to avoid distractions while you study. This includes both the obvious distractions like visitors and the subtle distractions like an uncomfortable chair (or a too-comfortable couch that makes you want to fall asleep). Set up the best study environment possible: good lighting and a comfortable work area. If background music helps you focus, you may want to turn it on, but otherwise keep the room quiet. If you are using a computer to take notes, be sure you don't have any other windows open, especially applications like social media, games, or anything else that could distract you. Silence your phone and turn off notifications. Be sure to keep water close by so you stay hydrated while you study (but avoid unhealthy drinks and snacks).

Also, take into account the best time of day to study. Are you freshest first thing in the morning? Try to set aside some time then to work through the material. Is your mind clearer in the afternoon or evening? Schedule your study session then. Another method is to study at the same time of day that you will take the test, so that your brain gets used to working on the material at that time and will be ready to focus at test time.

STEP 5: STUDY!

Once you have done all the study preparation, it's time to settle into the actual studying. Sit down, take a few moments to settle your mind so you can focus, and begin to follow your study plan. Don't give in to distractions or let yourself procrastinate. This is your time to prepare so you'll be ready to fearlessly approach the test. Make the most of the time and stay focused.

Of course, you don't want to burn out. If you study too long you may find that you're not retaining the information very well. Take regular study breaks. For example, taking five minutes out of every hour to walk briskly, breathing deeply and swinging your arms, can help your mind stay fresh.

As you get to the end of each chapter or section, it's a good idea to do a quick review. Remind yourself of what you learned and work on any difficult parts. When you feel that you've mastered the material, move on to the next part. At the end of your study session, briefly skim through your notes again.

But while review is helpful, cramming last minute is NOT. If at all possible, work ahead so that you won't need to fit all your study into the last day. Cramming overloads your brain with more information than it can process and retain, and your tired mind may struggle to recall even previously learned information when it is overwhelmed with last-minute study. Also, the urgent nature of cramming and the stress placed on your brain contribute to anxiety. You'll be more likely to go to the test feeling unprepared and having trouble thinking clearly.

So don't cram, and don't stay up late before the test, even just to review your notes at a leisurely pace. Your brain needs rest more than it needs to go over the information again. In fact, plan to finish your studies by noon or early afternoon the day before the test. Give your brain the rest of the day to relax or focus on other things, and get a good night's sleep. Then you will be fresh for the test and better able to recall what you've studied.

STEP 6: TAKE A PRACTICE TEST

Many courses offer sample tests, either online or in the study materials. This is an excellent resource to check whether you have mastered the material, as well as to prepare for the test format and environment.

Check the test format ahead of time: the number of questions, the type (multiple choice, free response, etc.), and the time limit. Then create a plan for working through them. For example, if you have 30 minutes to take a 60-question test, your limit is 30 seconds per question. Spend less time on the questions you know well so that you can take more time on the difficult ones.

If you have time to take several practice tests, take the first one open book, with no time limit. Work through the questions at your own pace and make sure you fully understand them. Gradually work up to taking a test under test conditions: sit at a desk with all study materials put away and set a timer. Pace yourself to make sure you finish the test with time to spare and go back to check your answers if you have time.

After each test, check your answers. On the questions you missed, be sure you understand why you missed them. Did you misread the question (tests can use tricky wording)? Did you forget the information? Or was it something you hadn't learned? Go back and study any shaky areas that the practice tests reveal.

Taking these tests not only helps with your grade, but also aids in combating test anxiety. If you're already used to the test conditions, you're less likely to worry about it, and working through tests until you're scoring well gives you a confidence boost. Go through the practice tests until you feel comfortable, and then you can go into the test knowing that you're ready for it.

Test Tips

On test day, you should be confident, knowing that you've prepared well and are ready to answer the questions. But aside from preparation, there are several test day strategies you can employ to maximize your performance.

First, as stated before, get a good night's sleep the night before the test (and for several nights before that, if possible). Go into the test with a fresh, alert mind rather than staying up late to study.

Try not to change too much about your normal routine on the day of the test. It's important to eat a nutritious breakfast, but if you normally don't eat breakfast at all, consider eating just a protein bar. If you're a coffee drinker, go ahead and have your normal coffee. Just make sure you time it so that the caffeine doesn't wear off right in the middle of your test. Avoid sugary beverages, and drink enough water to stay hydrated but not so much that you need a restroom break 10 minutes into the test. If your test isn't first thing in the morning, consider going for a walk or doing a light workout before the test to get your blood flowing.

Allow yourself enough time to get ready, and leave for the test with plenty of time to spare so you won't have the anxiety of scrambling to arrive in time. Another reason to be early is to select a good seat. It's helpful to sit away from doors and windows, which can be distracting. Find a good seat, get out your supplies, and settle your mind before the test begins.

When the test begins, start by going over the instructions carefully, even if you already know what to expect. Make sure you avoid any careless mistakes by following the directions.

Then begin working through the questions, pacing yourself as you've practiced. If you're not sure on an answer, don't spend too much time on it, and don't let it shake your confidence. Either skip it and come back later, or eliminate as many wrong answers as possible and guess among the remaining ones. Don't dwell on these questions as you continue—put them out of your mind and focus on what lies ahead.

Be sure to read all of the answer choices, even if you're sure the first one is the right answer. Sometimes you'll find a better one if you keep reading. But don't second-guess yourself if you do immediately know the answer. Your gut instinct is usually right. Don't let test anxiety rob you of the information you know.

If you have time at the end of the test (and if the test format allows), go back and review your answers. Be cautious about changing any, since your first instinct tends to be correct, but make sure you didn't misread any of the questions or accidentally mark the wrong answer choice. Look over any you skipped and make an educated guess.

At the end, leave the test feeling confident. You've done your best, so don't waste time worrying about your performance or wishing you could change anything. Instead, celebrate the successful completion of this test. And finally, use this test to learn how to deal with anxiety even better next time.

> **Review Video: Test Anxiety**
> Visit mometrix.com/academy and enter code: 100340

Important Qualification

Not all anxiety is created equal. If your test anxiety is causing major issues in your life beyond the classroom or testing center, or if you are experiencing troubling physical symptoms related to your anxiety, it may be a sign of a serious physiological or psychological condition. If this sounds like your situation, we strongly encourage you to seek professional help.

Additional Bonus Material

Due to our efforts to try to keep this book to a manageable length, we've created a link that will give you access to all of your additional bonus material:

mometrix.com/bonus948/ptcb